Return to:
Berthaud Living

The Source for Dysphagia

Updated & Expanded

Nancy B. Swigert

| Skill Area: | Dysphagia |
| Age Level: | Adults |

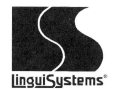

LinguiSystems, Inc.
3100 4th Avenue
East Moline, IL 61244-9700

800-776-4332

Fax: 800-577-4555
E-mail: service@linguisystems.com
Web: linguisystems.com

Printed in the U.S.A.
ISBN 0-7606-0363-4

About the Author

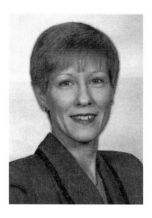

Nancy B. Swigert, M.A., CCC-SLP, is director of Swigert & Associates, Inc., a private practice which has been providing services in the Lexington, Kentucky area for over 20 years. The practice is contracted by Central Baptist Hospital in Lexington to administer and staff the inpatient and outpatient departments where Nancy spends the majority of her time. Nancy developed the multi-disciplinary Dysphagia Team at the hospital. She has also served as a consultant to a variety of other health care facilities in Kentucky concerning their dysphagia programs.

Nancy has lectured extensively on dysphagia at state, regional, national, and international conferences. She is the author of two other books for LinguiSystems, *The Source for Dysarthria* and *The Source for Pediatric Dysphagia*. Nancy has also published information on functional outcomes for dysphagia in other resources. She is very active in the American Speech-Language-Hearing Association, including serving as its president in 1998.

Dedication

To Jeri Logemann, whose teaching and writing initially sparked my interest in dysphagia, and whose continued mentorship is invaluable.

To the colleagues in my private practice who take on extra work to allow me time for projects such as this. Thanks especially to Verity, Michelle, Janice, Hope, Kim, and Holley. Interacting with them on a daily basis keeps it fun!

Most of all, to my husband, Keith, whose patience and support never cease to amaze me.

Acknowledgment

I am fortunate to provide services at Central Baptist Hospital and to work with talented and dedicated professionals there. Special thanks to Larry Gray, M.Div., Vice-President for Mission Effectiveness, for his guidance concerning medical ethics; to Sharon Wallace, RD/LD, DSc., for teaching me about nutrition; to Ronald G. Mobley, B.S., R.R.T., for sharing his expertise on respiratory care; and to Lonnie Wright, M.S.L.S. and Jeff Kurz, medical librarians who manage to find the most obscure references just when I need them.

Illustrated by Margaret Warner and Cindy Maxwell
Edited by Lauri Whiskeyman
Page Layout by Lisa Parker

Table of Contents ———————————————————————————

Table of Contents, *continued*

Introduction

Working with adults with dysphagia is a challenging and rewarding part of the practice of speech-language pathology. I am fortunate to have the opportunity to evaluate and treat patients in a variety of settings and find that I continually learn from them how to be a better dysphagia clinician. This book is a compilation of what I have learned and how I have applied that information to different practice settings. It is meant to be a practical resource for you to use on a day-to-day basis, but also has reference information which will help you when you encounter a challenging patient. It should be just one of many you use to build your knowledge and skills in dysphagia management.

The Source for Dysphagia was first printed in 1996. Since that time, advances in research have resulted in new treatment techniques and enhancements in the evaluation of patients with dysphagia. This edition provides up-to-date information in these areas. In addition, we have continued to develop more teaching materials, handouts, etc. that have made our work easier. I wanted to share those materials with you.

Most chapters contain significant revisions, such as:

- updated information on billing and coding issues

- numerous patient and staff education materials on issues from gag reflex to why instrumental exams are needed

- more in-depth information on videofluoroscopic studies and how to perform and interpret them, as well as information on FEES®

- an entirely new framework for short-term goals and treatment objectives based on symptoms observed and the physiological cause of each symptom which should make it much easier to plan treatment

In addition, the book contains two new chapters:

- special considerations in the ICU, including information on tracheostomies, ventilators, the blue dye test, and suctioning

- outcomes and efficacy data, including information you can use to document effectiveness of your treatment

In these challenging times in health care, patients with dysphagia are fortunate that speech-language pathologists remain dedicated to providing quality services. I hope *The Source for Dysphagia* helps you evaluate and treat patients more effectively and more efficiently, and helps in your quest to become the best dysphagia clinician you can be.

Nancy

Chapter 1

Preparing for a
Patient Assessment

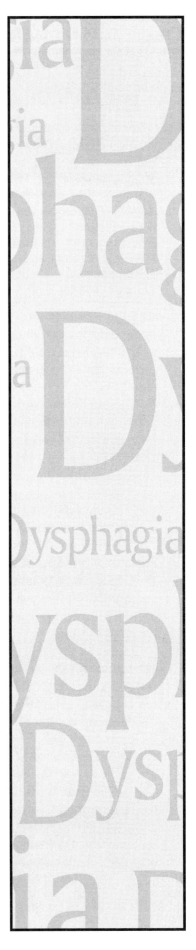

Have you ever been rushed for time and thought to yourself, "I'll go into my patient's room and take a quick look at her swallowing abilities. I can always review the chart later"? If so, here are a few extreme examples of why you shouldn't wait to review the chart:

- The patient goes limp after taking a drink and appears to have no pulse. Do you call a code? How would you know whether to call a code if you haven't checked the patient's resuscitation status on his chart?

- You take some foods from the department refrigerator and begin to assess the patient. A nurse walks in at the end of the session and is angry because you've just given a diabetic patient foods loaded with sugar.

- You begin feeding your patient from the test tray, and halfway through your assessment, the physician walks in, informs you that the patient is NPO for a procedure, and asks why you didn't notice it in the chart.

Of course, there are many more reasons a thorough review of a patient's medical history is essential before completing an evaluation.

1. You'll know what to expect from the patient.

2. You may be able to determine which food consistencies to present in the bedside evaluation.

3. You may also learn whether the patient's physical condition will preclude full participation in the evaluation.

The information on the following pages is important to obtain BEFORE you evaluate a patient's swallowing abilities.

Interviewing the Patient

You may find critical information by asking the patient for a description of the problem. It may be necessary to reword your question in order to get the information. For example, you might ask a patient if he ever chokes when eating and he answers, "No." If you reword your question and ask if food or liquid ever goes down the wrong way, the patient may reply, "Yes."

The questionnaire on pages 15-17 provides several different ways to ask questions. Information on pages 18-19 will help you interpret what the patient tells you during your interview.

The Patient's Chart

The following information can usually be found on the patient's chart.

1. Medical History

Admit diagnosis — Determine if the patient has a diagnosis which might account for the dysphagia. For instance, the patient might have had a recent stroke or may have a progressive disorder like Parkinson's disease or Multiple Sclerosis.

If the patient is in an acute care setting, the admit diagnosis might not seem to be related to the dysphagia. He may have been admitted for pneumonia or cardiac problems. In this case, it would be necessary to delve more deeply into the patient's medical record to see what might have happened to the patient after he was admitted to cause the dysphagia.

Medicare cannot deny intervention services based on a diagnosis, but it will deny intervention if there's a decreased expectation and/or a lack of skilled treatment being provided.

Functional problems observed — This information can often be obtained from nursing notes. Look for terminology such as *coughing or choking when drinking*, *refusing to take certain foods*, or *drooling*.

Level of alertness — The more alert a patient is, the better the candidate he is for therapeutic intervention. If a patient isn't alert, it may be best to delay the intervention until a later time.

Previous diagnoses and treatment — Note any other diagnosis the patient may have had. The patient may have had several strokes that resulted in oral-motor problems affecting swallowing. Also note whether the patient has had any previous treatment for dysphagia or related disorders.

Advance directive — Check to see whether the patient has filled out an advance directive indicating his wishes for resuscitation.

Premorbid status — Find out what the patient's status was before the most recent event that caused the dysphagia. It may be that the patient has eaten pureed foods for some time and therefore it may not be reasonable to expect the patient to return to a regular diet at this time.

2. Referral

Reason for referral — Your evaluation should state the reason the patient was referred to you. If you don't have the information, look through the patient's records to find out why he was referred. The patient may have been referred to you because of functional problems like those described previously, to rule out silent aspiration as a possible cause for pneumonia, or to determine if dysphagia is related to a recent weight loss.

Signed physician's order — Be sure you have a signed physician's order or have obtained a verbal order before you assess the patient.

3. Signs and Symptoms of Dysphagia

Temperature — Review the chart for any spiking of temperatures. An elevated temperature can indicate that the patient has an infection in the lungs from aspirated foods. There is no defined amount of time at which the temperature spike will occur after an aspiration event. It could happen within an hour of the event. Other patients may run a low grade fever without a significant spike in temperature. If the patient is already on antibiotics for treatment of an infection, his temperature may not increase at all.

Drooling/increased secretions — A patient showing drooling or complaining of "excess saliva" (usually means he isn't swallowing his secretions as well as he did previously) may indicate dysphagia.

Weight loss — If a patient has experienced an unintentional weight loss, dysphagia is a possible cause. A patient may have trouble swallowing certain food consistencies and avoids eating them. He then experiences weight loss.

Coughing/choking — Coughing and choking are very obvious symptoms of dysphagia.

Pocketing — If the patient has poor oral skills, you may find information indicating that the nurses have to clean food out of the patient's mouth long after a meal.

Pneumonia — If a patient has aspirated, he may develop pneumonia within several hours, or it may be several weeks or months before any pneumonia develops. It's very difficult for a physician to determine if pneumonia is due to aspiration unless the pneumonia developed soon after an observable episode of aspiration. It's just as difficult for a radiologist to look at a chest x-ray and determine aspiration pneumonia vs. other lung disorders like atelectasis. Therefore, question any mention of pneumonia on a patient's chart.

Changes in diet — If the patient has recently begun to eat or drink different textures or types of food, it may be an unconscious reaction to difficulty in handling certain foods.

Patient complaint — Often a patient's complaint about difficulty swallowing will spur the referral even though problems may have been previously noted by the nursing staff. All it may take for a referral is for the patient or a family member to mention to the doctor that the patient is having trouble eating eggs at breakfast. The doctor will then write an order for the evaluation.

Dehydration — Patients who have become dysphagic may begin to avoid liquids and become dehydrated. The dehydration may not be mentioned specifically in the chart. If not, some signs that the patient may be dehydrated include confusion, constipation, poor skin turgor/skin breakdown, and renal insufficiency. Dehydration can contribute to patient falls, to stroke, and to renal failure.

Dehydration may also result from conditions that cause water loss (e.g., fever/infection, high environmental temperature or low environmental humidity, dry oxygen therapy, use of air fluidized beds, diuretic therapies) as well as from conditions that cause both water and electrolyte loss (e.g., vomiting, diarrhea, food/fluid malabsorption or losses through a fistula or an ostomy).

Older adult patients (over age 55) are at risk for dehydration if they take less than 30 ml of fluid per kg body weight per day (35 ml per kg body weight for younger adults) or less than 1 ml per calorie in the daily diet.

You can perform a simple screening by pinching the skin on the back of the patient's hand. If the patient is well hydrated, the skin should immediately fall back into place. If the patient is dehydrated, the skin may remain "tented" for a second or two.

Reflux — Look for any mention of the patient's complaints of heartburn, reflux, or tightness in the chest. For more information on reflux and other esophageal disorders, see pages 21-23.

4. Nutrition/Hydration

Current diet — Find out what the patient's current diet is. If a patient is in an acute care setting and recently had surgery, he may initially be placed on a clear liquid or full liquid diet. This is done to reduce the risk of upsetting the patient's stomach and causing vomiting.

However, the clear liquid diet may be the most difficult for the dysphagic patient to handle. The patient may have been on a modified diet for some time. For instance, if the patient has had all his teeth removed, he may have already altered the kinds of food he is eating. Patients with dementia may have been placed on a pureed diet for ease of feeding. It's important to know what the baseline is before going in to evaluate the patient.

Dietary restrictions — There may be restrictions other than the texture of a patient's diet that need to be considered. For instance, many patients will be on the American Heart Association diet or a diabetic, carbohydrate-controlled diet.

Alternate method of feeding — Determine if the patient is on an NG/NJ or PEG tube or is receiving parenteral nutrition. (See chart on pages 24-25 for information about different kinds of feeding tubes.)

5. Medication

Mental Status Change, Confusion, Sedation — Elderly patients are at risk for confusion caused by drugs, especially if they already have some cognitive impairments. Drugs that may cause confusion include anticholinergics, analgesics, psychotropics, and anti-epileptics. Many of these drugs can also cause drowsiness. If a patient is on sedatives, it's important to time your evaluation so the patient is alert. You must consider that even if you evaluate the patient when alert and make recommendations, he may be sedated a large part of the day and not able to do as well at mealtimes as during your evaluation.

Antibiotics — If the patient is on an antibiotic, it may suppress any possible lung infection secondary to aspiration. Therefore, he may not show signs of early pneumonia simply because he is on antibiotics for something else.

Medications specific to disorders — If the patient is taking a medication for treatment of a specific neurological disorder, it is important to find out if that medicine has any effect on enhancing or interfering with the swallow function. Two specific examples come to mind. Many patients with Parkinson's disease are treated with levodopa (L-dopa), commonly called Sinemet. One case study (Fonda, Schwarz, & Clinnick, 1995) reports an improvement in swallowing with adjustment of timing of medication. Sinemet seems to have peak effect one hour after administration. We have observed that some patients with Parkinson's do show an improvement if given their medication one hour prior to meals (we usually document this via instrumental examination). Patients with Myasthenia Gravis are typically treated with Mestinon which has its peak effect at two hours post administration. Therefore, changing the timing of medication may significantly improve the patient's ability to swallow.

Medications can also cause dysphagia. For example, nitrates are used to treat coronary artery disease but they can cause reflux disease to worsen. This is because the nitrates contribute to reduced tension in the lower esophageal sphincter. Side effects of certain medications can also worsen dysphagia. For example, antipsychotic drugs can cause tardive dyskinesia, which usually involves the muscles in the face and tongue. If it is severe, the patient may not be able to chew or swallow.

Many medications can cause dry mouth, or xerostomia (e.g., decongestants, beta blockers and benzodiazepines).

Gastroesophageal Reflux Disease (GERD) is often treated with medications so it is important to note if the patient is currently taking any of the following: antacids to neutralize stomach acid and help increase the pressure in the lower esophageal sphincter; a group of drugs called Histamine-2 receptor antagonists (e.g., Zantac, Pepcid, Tagamet); or proton pump inhibitors (e.g., omeprazole, Prilosec) to block the formation of acid. If the patient is also experiencing esophageal dismotility, a prokinetic drug (e.g., Propulsid) may have been prescribed.

How presented to patient — Determine how medications are being given to the patient. If he is NPO with an NG tube, is he still getting his medications by mouth?

6. Respiratory Status

Lung sounds — Respiratory therapists, nurses, and physicians may make comments about the patient's lung sounds. Look for terms such as:

rhonchi	coarse, dry rale in the bronchial tubes
rale	abnormal respiratory sound
wheeze	whistling respiratory sound

Chest x-rays — Look at recent chest x-rays to determine if any infiltrates have been observed.

Remember that something may not be reported as aspiration-related when it actually is. In addition, if the patient has actually aspirated, the area of infiltrate in the lung will be the area of the lung which was dependent at the time of the aspiration event, not necessarily the right lower lobe. What this means is that if the patient lies down a lot, then both lower lobes may be affected or even the mid-lobes. If the patient aspirated and was then lying on his left side, the aspiration may be in the left lobe.

Oxygen therapy and mode of delivery — If the patient is on oxygen therapy, it will give you some indication of his lung status. Determine whether he is receiving oxygen through a nasal cannula or face mask. (See illustrations below.) If the patient is using a face mask, find out if it can be changed to a nasal cannula so you can present food during your assessment.

Recent intubations — If the patient has recently been orally intubated, he may have some edema of the vocal cords. This alone may be enough to cause some decreased laryngeal closure and possible aspiration during swallowing.

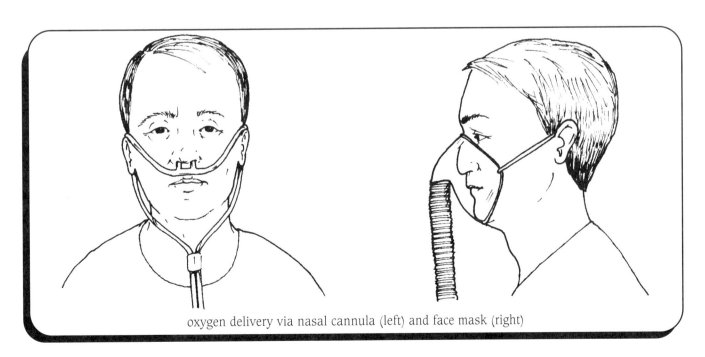

oxygen delivery via nasal cannula (left) and face mask (right)

Ventilator, Tracheostomy/type of tube, and Tracheostomy speaking valve — For information on these and their effects on swallowing, see Chapter 9, pages 241-246.

7. Nursing Assessment

Cognitive assessment — Nursing notes usually make some statement about the patient's cognitive skills. This is important information when you're going to assess a patient.

Observations of patient — Nursing notes may also provide some information about signs or symptoms of dysphagia.

Previous living situation — You may want to find out what kind of previous living situation the patient has had to help determine whether he was cooking for himself and to determine the type of meals he ate.

Family support/involvement — Find out if there are family members or others who can be taught safe techniques for feeding the patient. If the patient is discharged from your facility, what kind of support will the patient have for following the techniques at home?

Sensory impairments — It's also important to consider whether the patient can see the food in front of him, listen to your directions, and smell and taste the food.

8. Other Evaluations

GI series — The patient may have had an upper or lower GI because of initial complaints of dysphagia. Helpful information can be found in these reports.

Barium swallow — Some physicians don't carefully delineate between a barium swallow and a modified barium swallow. Therefore, a patient who complains of dysphagia or

"choking" may have had a barium swallow performed. Read the report carefully for any information about aspiration.

There are several important differences between a modified barium swallow study and a barium swallow study. A modified barium swallow study is designed to assess the oral and pharyngeal phases of the swallow. A barium swallow study assesses the esophageal phase and the function of the stomach. The modified barium swallow study is performed while the patient sits up and is presented with small amounts of various consistencies. The barium swallow study is done with the patient lying down, drinking a whole bottle of liquid barium.

The reason for the modified barium swallow is only partially to diagnose the problem. In large part, the modified barium swallow is to identify the physiological causes of the symptoms and to select appropriate treatment techniques based on the physiology. Modifications to texture, different postures, and compensatory techniques may be tried to determine their effect on swallowing. The barium swallow is strictly a diagnostic procedure, designed to determine if there is a problem and what the possible cause is. No trial treatment techniques are used.

Neurological consult — If a patient has had a recent neurological consult, read carefully for any information about etiology that may be the cause of the dysphagia.

Dietary consult — The dietary consult may have important information about nutritional status. A dietitian's note may include target levels for calorie and protein intake, diet modifications that are required based on the patient's diagnosis. The note may also include laboratory values indicative of both nutritional status and treatment progress. The dietitian should clearly state when lab values can and cannot be used as nutrition indicators. For

12

example, a serum albumin is seldom a valid indicator of nutritional status during an illness as the value is affected by most disease conditions, including simple stress.

A patient may present with protein calorie malnutrition such that their physical condition is significantly weakened. Malnutrition can be the sole cause of a patient's dysphagia.

Surgery — If the patient has had recent surgery, there may be several ways the surgery can impact swallowing. Patients may be debilitated and weak as a result of the surgery and have a short term swallowing problem as a result. If the surgery was to the chest or neck, there may have been some compromise of the laryngeal nerve or one of its branches which contributes to swallowing. If the surgery was to the oral or pharyngeal region (e.g., cancer), the structures for swallowing may have changed along with the physiology. If the surgery was to the brain, control of swallowing may be affected.

Radiation treatment — Radiation treatment to the head or neck will almost certainly have an effect on swallowing. Patients may experience these problems immediately, or may not present their first symptoms for three to ten years after the completion of radiation due to the cumulative effects of radiation which stays in the body.

A list is provided on the next page to remind you of the information you need to gather about a patient before beginning a swallowing evaluation.

Information to Obtain from Chart Review _____

Patient _____

Medical History
❏ Admit diagnosis
❏ Functional problems observed
❏ Level of alertness
❏ Previous diagnoses and treatment
❏ Advance directive
❏ Premorbid status

Referral
❏ Reason for referral
❏ Signed physician's order

Signs and Symptoms of Dysphagia
❏ Temperature
❏ Drooling/increased secretions
❏ Weight loss
❏ Coughing/choking
❏ Pocketing
❏ Pneumonia
❏ Changes in diet
❏ Patient complaint
❏ Dehydration
❏ Reflux

Nutrition/Hydration
❏ Current diet
❏ Dietary restrictions
❏ Alternate method of feeding

Medications
❏ Cause mental status change/sedation
❏ Antibiotics
❏ GERD meds
❏ How presented to patient
❏ Other meds:

_____

Respiratory Status
❏ Lung sounds
❏ Chest x-rays
❏ Oxygen therapy and mode of delivery
❏ Recent intubations
❏ Ventilator
❏ Tracheostomy
    ❏ status of cuff
    ❏ tracheostomy speaking valve

Nursing Assessment
❏ Cognitive assessment
❏ Observations of patient
❏ Previous living situation
❏ Family support/involvement
❏ Sensory impairments

Other Evaluations/Procedures
❏ GI series
❏ Barium swallow
❏ Neurological consult
❏ Dietary consult
❏ Surgery
❏ Radiation therapy

Swallowing Questionnaire to Provide Additional History

Patient _____   SLP _____

Date _____

1. Do you have any problems with swallowing?   ❐ yes   ❐ no

   If so, when did the problem start? _____

   _____

   Briefly describe the difficulty. _____

   _____

2. Did the start of your swallowing problem relate to other medical
   problems you have?   ❐ yes   ❐ no

   If so, please describe: _____

   _____

3. When you eat or drink, do you have episodes of coughing?   ❐ yes   ❐ no

   When you eat or drink, do you have episodes of choking?   ❐ yes   ❐ no

4. Do you wear dentures when you eat?   ❐ yes   ❐ no

5. Does food or drink ever "go down the wrong way"?   ❐ yes   ❐ no

6. Does your food generally require special preparation before
   you can eat it?   ❐ yes   ❐ no

   If so, please describe: _____

   _____

7. Do you avoid certain foods because they are difficult to swallow?   ❐ yes   ❐ no

   If so, please list examples: _____

8. Do you find food in your mouth after you swallow? ❑ yes ❑ no

9. Do you have difficulty keeping food or drink in your mouth? ❑ yes ❑ no

10. Do liquids ever come back through your nose when you swallow them? ❑ yes ❑ no

11. Do you ever feel that food gets "stuck" in your throat? ❑ yes ❑ no

    If so, describe where it feels stuck. _____

12. Do you regularly wake up at night coughing? ❑ yes ❑ no

13. Do you often wake up with a bad/sour taste in your mouth? ❑ yes ❑ no

14. Is your swallowing problem intermittent / constant? (Circle one.)

15. Has your swallowing problem changed over time? ❑ yes ❑ no

    If so, please describe: _____

    _____

16. Are there any factors that make your swallowing problem worse? ❑ yes ❑ no

    If so, please describe: _____

    _____

17. Do you have more difficulty swallowing when in any certain position? ❑ yes ❑ no

    If so, please describe: _____

    _____

18. Have you had pneumonia recently?   ❒ yes   ❒ no

    If so, when? _____

    _____

19. Has your voice changed in the past year?   ❒ yes   ❒ no
    If so, check all that apply:

    ❒ hoarse   ❒ quieter

    ❒ whispery/breathy   ❒ other _____

20. Did the changes in your voice start gradually / suddenly? (Circle one.)

21. What was the date of onset of your voice change? _____

22. Has your speech changed in the past year?   ❒ yes   ❒ no
    If so, check all that apply:

    ❒ slurring

    ❒ need to clear your throat more

    ❒ talking through your nose

    ❒ other _____

23. Did the changes in your speech start gradually / suddenly? (Circle one.)

24. What was the date of onset of your speech change? _____

25. Have you had any previous swallowing or throat problems?   ❒ yes   ❒ no

    If so, please describe: _____

    _____

Interpreting Patient Information _____

Obstruction or Pain	The medical term for this is *odynophagia*. Ask the patient to point to the area where this occurs. If it's a sharp pain, it could indicate an ulcerative lesion of the pharynx or esophagus. If the patient describes a dull or squeezing pain, it could likely be an esophageal spasm.
Globus	This is a descriptive term for a lump or fullness in the throat, sometimes caused by a mass or gastroesophageal reflux (GER). Some patients may just be more sensitive to esophageal distention and describe the sensation. Globus may be a better symptom of GER than heartburn. Eighty percent of patients complaining of globus have a functional cause, and it's often related to GER.
	Patients are usually fairly accurate when identifying where the problem is in the pharynx, but if a patient is having problems with the esophagus, he'll often tell you that he feels the sensation much higher in his throat. This is called *referral of the symptoms* and is often caused by food remaining in the esophagus which is then jetted up against a closed upper esophageal sphincter. Globus is often momentarily relieved by a swallow.
Heartburn	This is a very common symptom of esophageal reflux disease. However, the severity does not correlate with the severity of the reflux-induced damage to the esophagus. Ask if the patient's heartburn is more common after meals or at night.
Terrible Taste in Mouth	Ask if the patient often has a bad taste in his mouth upon awakening. Also determine whether the patient has excessive burping. These symptoms are frequently caused by esophageal reflux.
Nasal Burning and Dripping	A patient who reports burning in his nose, sniffs frequently, or wipes his nose excessively during a meal may be experiencing reflux of food/liquid into the nasal cavity.
Burning or Tickling at Back of Throat	Patients with good sensation may report this when they have food pocketing in the valleculae.
Choking/Coughing	A patient often answers negatively when asked if he feels like he's choking when he swallows. You may want to reword your question. You might ask if the patient ever feels like the food goes down the wrong way or if he's unable to breathe when food gets caught.
Late Regurgitation	If the patient is vomiting hours after a meal, it probably indicates an esophageal disorder such as GER or achalasia, an esophageal disorder in which food backs up in the esophagus.

Appetite	Ask if the patient has noticed a decrease in his appetite. Poor appetite might be because the patient is afraid of choking or could also be caused by early muscle fatigue while eating. The patient may be so fatigued by eating that he stops eating and doesn't finish his meal.
Taste	Taste deficits, especially if accompanied by olfactory disturbances, may interfere with the sensory component of swallowing and the desire to eat. Pathological damage to cranial nerves VII and IX may reduce or eliminate the ability to taste.
Changes in Speech or Voice	Ask the patient to be specific when describing any changes to his speech or voice. You may need to give examples such as "Is your speech slurred?" "Does your voice sound breathier?" "Are you talking through your nose?" or "Do you need to clear your throat more?" Any problems related to the voice may warrant a referral to otolaryngology/ENT.

Problems Related to Phases of Swallowing

The symptoms being described or those which are found in the medical chart may relate to a particular phase of swallow. There are many possible causes for these symptoms.

Oral Dysphagia

Having only an oral dysphagia (referring to the oral preparatory and oral voluntary phases) is fairly uncommon. It could be caused by a neurogenic disorder, decreased salivary flow, painful lesions in the mouth, or as a result of oral surgery for cancer. Diminished salivary flow makes it very difficult to prepare the bolus to swallow. Be aware that over 400 commonly-used drugs can affect salivary flow including anticholinergics, antihistamines, antidepressants, antihypertensives, and diuretics.

Also, patients with dementia may show an oral dysphagia only. They often don't recognize food (an agnosia). When food is placed in their mouths, it's as if they have forgotten what to do with the bolus of food (swallowing apraxia). The staff or family may report that patients won't swallow even when persuaded to take some food into their mouths.

You may occasionally find patients with isolated neurogenic oral dysphagia showing up prior to the onset of other neurological findings. Watch this very carefully so you can make a referral to neurology if difficulty swallowing is the first symptom to appear. Some oral dysphagia may be psychogenic in nature. Patients may describe a fear of choking or state that the food just won't go down. They may eat only certain types of foods, and this selection may not always make sense if textures are analyzed (e.g., a patient stating that he can swallow coffee, but not water).

19

Pharyngeal Dysphagia

Pharyngeal dysphagia can have many causes. Some of these include neurological disorders of acute, chronic, or progressive nature; status post-surgery or radiation to head and neck; overall weakness; history of intubation; placement of tracheostomy tube; and/or surgery to neck/chest with damage to nerves important for swallowing. It is important to determine the etiology as improvement is expected in some cases, but not in others.

Neurological Causes

Stroke — Patients who have had a stroke comprise the largest group of patients with neurological diseases who have dysphagia. There is no specific site of lesion that results in dysphagia. Dysphagia may be observed in patients who have had cortical strokes (either hemisphere), subcortical strokes, or unilateral or bilateral brainstem lesions. Logemann (1998) provides an excellent summary of the literature describing the kinds of problems that may be observed as a result of lesions in different areas of the brain.

Closed Head Injury — Patients who have suffered closed head injuries often have severe dysphagia. The kinds of problems they present may be complicated because of the type of neurological insult (e.g., coup and contra-coup damages result in the areas of damage being more diffuse) and possible structural injuries to the head and neck (e.g., fractures). The management of the patient has to be guided by the level of his recovery. For instance, if a patient is in the combative stage, it is not likely he will allow for physical help to achieve a compensatory posture.

Spinal Cord Injury — Patients with closed head injury may also have spinal cord injuries which will compound their swallowing problems. Patients with spinal cord injuries alone can also present with dysphagia, including problems such as a delay in triggering the pharyngeal swallow and impaired movement of the larynx.

Myasthenia Gravis — This causes an impairment at the juncture of the muscle and the nerve which diminishes the input to the muscle. The hallmark feature is that performance worsens on repetitive trials with fatigue. Therefore, swallowing is usually worse at the end of the meal and at the end of the day.

Guillain-Barré — This is a viral-based disease with rapid onset of paresis. It may progress to the point that the patient requires ventilatory support. One of the first signs of this disease may be swallowing difficulty. As the disease progresses, it is not unusual for the patient to require tube feeding.

Alzheimer's Dementia — In addition to the oral phase difficulties described above, patients with dementia may also have problems in the pharyngeal phase, such as delayed initiation of pharyngeal swallow and impaired laryngeal movement. Coupled with the food-holding behavior, these problems may make it impossible to safely feed the patient orally in a reasonable amount of time.

Amyotrophic Lateral Sclerosis (ALS) — This progressive disease affects swallowing in both the oral and pharyngeal phases. Impaired swallowing may be one of the first symptoms reported by the patient.

Parkinson's Disease — This disease may also affect oral and pharyngeal phases. These swallowing problems may be one of the first signs of the disease. Logemann (1998) indicates that the progression of the dysphagia often begins with reduced tongue base retraction and repetitive tongue rolling, followed by delayed initiation of the pharyngeal swallow, and then impaired elevation and closure of the larynx.

Multiple Sclerosis — This results in plaque-like deposits throughout the neurological system. Patients may present with any type of swallowing disorder depending on where the lesions are.

Head and Neck Cancer

Pharyngeal dysphagia may be caused by surgery to the oral or pharyngeal regions. In addition, radiation therapy can have a significant impact on pharyngeal swallowing, sometimes years after the radiation therapy. For a comprehensive source on dysphagia related to cancer, you might read *Swallowing Guidelines in Oncology* by Sullivan & Guilford (1999).

Intubation and Tracheostomy

Information about intubation and tracheostomy tubes can be found in Chapter 9, pages 241-246.

Esophageal Dysphagia

It's important to understand esophageal dysphagia because symptoms in the esophageal phase are often referred to the area of the throat. That means the patient may be describing symptoms that sound as if they are occurring in the pharynx when really they are esophageal.

In addition, patients with pharyngeal dysphagia may also have esophageal dysphagia. It's important to understand the relationship between these two. Esophageal dysphagia begins with problems at the level of the cricopharyngeus and below as the food travels through the esophagus to the stomach. Remember the patient will probably not be accurate at indicating where the problem is when it is in the esophagus.

There are two main causes of problems with swallowing in the esophageal phase:

1. There can be a narrowing of the opening to the stomach. Often the first symptoms noted will be with solid foods, particularly chewy meats. The patient may change his diet to pureed food and liquids. If the progression has been very rapid (1-3 months) and the patient has had a large weight loss, then it's more likely that the obstruction or narrowing is caused by a malignancy.

2. There can be interference in some part of the swallowing sequence with relaxation of the muscle followed by squeezing or peristalsis. These motility abnormalities can occur with liquids and solid boluses and typically the onset is intermittent. The patient may report that episodes occur when he's distracted and not paying close attention to swallowing. Oftentimes these episodes may occur when eating out and may be mistakenly attributed to emotional tension.

Gastroesophageal Reflux Disease (GERD)

If the dysphagia is associated with chest pain which goes away after the bolus passes into the stomach or after it's regurgitated, then the patient may be showing esophageal spasm.

One of the most common esophageal disorders is gastroesophageal reflux disease (GERD). GERD occurs when gastric contents pass through the lower esophageal sphincter into the esophagus. This is different from intraesophageal reflux in which material never empties from the esophagus and moves upwards in a retrograde fashion, or to-and-fro movement. When screening the esophageal phase during a modified barium swallow, it is important to note whether gastroesophageal reflux or intraesophageal reflux has been observed.

Many individuals have some degree of reflux and may never know it because they do not present with any symptoms. Such symptoms include the burning sensation called "heartburn," feeling of tightness or fullness in the chest area (i.e., globus), bad taste in the mouth, a feeling of being unable to breathe when lying flat, nasal burning or dripping, and/or frequent burping. There is some indication that prevalence of GERD may be increased in the elderly. Mold et al. (1990) report a prevalence as high as 20% in older primary care patients.

Damage to the mucosa of the esophagus can result from reflux. GERD has also been implicated as a cause, or at least as an exacerbation, of other diseases of the larynx and lungs. Koufman (1991) reported varying degrees of association between GERD and carcinoma of the larynx; laryngeal and tracheal stenosis; reflux laryngitis; globus pharyngeus (i.e., sensation of a lump in the throat); dysphagia; and chronic cough. Hamilos (1995) reported on reflux and sinusitis in asthma and indicates that it has long been argued that GERD may be a causative factor in asthma, but that clinical studies have yielded conflicting results. He concludes that GERD should be considered as a potential contributing factor in any patient with poorly controlled asthma. There is also, of course, the risk that gastric contents/acid may be aspirated. This is more likely in patients with impaired laryngeal sensation/reflex and impaired pharyngeal peristalsis (DePaso, 1991).

Certain factors may cause, or aggravate the symptoms of reflux in individuals prone to the disorder. These include cigarette smoking, obesity, some medications (e.g., anticholinergics), alcohol, clothing that is tight around the waist, lifting heavy objects (especially if leaning over to do so), and eating very large meals. Certain foods can also worsen the symptoms of reflux. These include caffeine, chocolate, mint, spicy foods, foods with high acid content, pepper, pickled items and processed meats (e.g., hot dogs, sausage), and foods with high fat content.

Treatment depends on how severe the problem is. GERD can be managed through one or a combination of approaches: lifestyle modifications, drugs, or surgery. Lifestyle modifications include avoiding foods and activities that aggravate the reflux. (For a patient handout, see Chapter 4, page 92.) Drug treatment may be as simple as over-the-counter antacids. If the problem is more severe, other types of medications may be prescribed. Surgery is usually considered if the GERD does not respond to medication and lifestyle changes, and especially if it is contributing to pulmonary disease. Surgery, called Nissen fundoplication, involves surgically reducing the size of the opening into the stomach by wrapping the stomach around the distal esophagus, although several variations are performed (Little, 1996).

Other Esophageal Disorders

Esophageal dismotility is a decrease in the primary contraction wave of the esophagus. This results in slower movement of the bolus into the stomach, and in the case of severe dismotility, may result in subsequent boluses "piling up" in the esophagus. The patient may report feeling full or may state he is unable to swallow the next bite. Esophageal dismotility is typically treated with motility drugs such as Reglan or Propulsid. *Esophageal spasm* is just what the names implies: a tightening of the esophagus which causes a sharp pain. Patients may also experience *medication-induced esophageal injury*. This occurs if the pill gets stuck and dissolves in the esophagus, or stays in the esophagus too long secondary to esophageal dismotility. It may also occur if the medication returns to the esophagus through reflux action. The symptoms are acute substernal pain, odynophagia, and dysphagia. A *Zenker's diverticulum* is a small pouch that develops on the posterior esophageal wall like a hernia. It occurs near the upper esophageal sphincter. The pouch can be very small or as large as a golf ball. Food and liquid collect in the pouch. Sometimes the food flows out of the pouch and is swallowed, but there is the risk of aspirating the material. Because of this retention of food, patients may report a very bad taste in their mouth, bad breath, and may even state that they cough up pieces of food they haven't eaten in days. The diverticulum can be surgically repaired.

Esophageal Dysphagia and Cricopharyngeal Dysfunction

The cricopharyngeus, which is the primary muscle in the upper esophageal sphincter, must relax in order for opening into the esophagus to take place. If the problem is failure of the cricopharyngeus to relax, a cricopharyngeal myotomy may be indicated (Buchholz, 1995). However, the problem is often not one of the cricopharyngeus failing to relax, but is due to limited laryngeal elevation and limited anterior movement of the hyolaryngeal complex. If this lifting and forward movement is inadequate, then there is insufficient mechanical action to pull open the cricopharyngeus. Before a myotomy is considered, careful assessment of the neuromuscular aspects of the swallow should be assessed to determine if swallowing therapy rather than surgery is indicated.

How Feeding Tubes Compare

Types of Tubes	Description	Indications	Advantages	Disadvantages
Nasogastric (NG tube)	• available in a variety of sizes • placed into the nares through the naso-pharynx, down the esophagus, into the stomach • radiopaque (shows up on an x-ray to verify placement)	• usually used short term (less than 6 weeks) • patient's GI tract has to be functioning • often used for patients with swallowing disorders secondary to neurological impairment, tumors of the head and neck or esophagus	• putting tube into the stomach is more natural than directly into the intestine • stomach acid helps destroy microorganisms and may reduce the risk of infection • intermittent feedings may be better tolerated in the stomach	• some patients find the tube uncomfortable • sometimes difficult for the patient to self-feed around a feeding tube • sometimes patients pull at the tubes and have to have their hands restrained • may be contraindi-cated for patients at high-risk for aspiration as it keeps the lower esophageal sphincter slightly open and may permit reflux • easily dislodged by the patient or can be placed incorrectly into the trachea
Nasoduodenal or Nasojejunal	• very similar to NG tube, but the tip goes through the stomach into the duodenum or jejunum • may be used post-operatively if the patient has had gastric surgery	• same as NG tube	• may be less risk for aspiration	• same as NG tube

How Feeding Tubes Compare, *continued*

Types of Tubes	Description	Indications	Advantages	Disadvantages
Gastrostomy (G-tube)	• surgically placed directly into the stomach (very few tubes are surgically placed unless the patient is already undergoing abdominal surgery)	• used for long-term feedings • patient's GI tract has to be functioning • often used for patients with swallowing disorders secondary to neurological impairment, tumors of the head and neck or esophagus	• same as NG tube but more comfortable and aesthetic	• requires surgery to place
Percutaneous Endoscopic Gastrostomy (PEG tube)*	• same as G-tube but placed under local anesthesia or conscious sedation at bedside	• same as G-tube	• same as G-tube	• contraindicated for patients with peritonitis, esophageal obstruction, morbid obesity, or severe gastroesophageal reflux
Jejunostomy (J-tube)	• tube surgically placed directly into the jejunum	• for long-term feeding • also used for short-term feeding after GI tract surgery	• may be lower aspiration risk since the tube is in the jejunum and not in the stomach • tube can't be misplaced in the trachea • more comfortable and aesthetic	• same as PEG tube

* Percutaneous Endoscopic Jejustomy (PEJ tube) — similar to PEG tube; tube inserted in jejunostomy

Chapter 2

Medicare Expectations and Other Billing Issues

The *Medicare Intermediary Manual* provides specific instructions for medical review of dysphagia claims. It provides guidance to claims reviewers regarding the type of documentation that indicates reasonable and necessary care. Sections 3910, "Special Instructions for Medical Review of Dysphagia Claims," and 3589 give all the specific information. The instructions are almost identical to section 504 in the *Medicare Outpatient Physical Therapy and Comprehensive Outpatient Rehabilitation Facility Manual*. The information provided here is a summary from these documents.[1] In addition, the Health Care Finance Administration (HCFA) periodically releases Program Memoranda which contain interpretations of the regulations and answers to specific questions. To obtain these program memoranda, visit HCFA's website at *www.hcfa.gov*.

Covered Services

The following services are allowed by Medicare for patients with dysphagia:

- patient/caregiver training in feeding and swallowing techniques
- analysis of proper head positioning
- analysis of amount of intake per swallow
- appropriate diet analysis
- treatment for facilitating the swallow
- analyzing the need for self-help eating or feeding devices
- facilitation of more normal tone or oral facilitation techniques
- food consistencies (texture & size)
- oral-motor and neuromuscular training and instruction to improve oral-motor control
- training in laryngeal and vocal cord adduction exercises
- compensatory swallow techniques
- oral sensitivity training

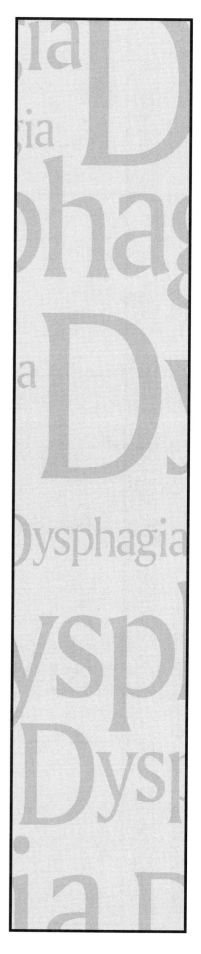

---

[1] Similar guidelines appear in the *Medicare Hospital Manual* (section 450) and *Medicare Skilled Nursing Facility Manual* (section 544.3).

Dysphagia Patient Criteria

In addition, the patient should present at least one of the following:

• presence of oral-motor disorders such as drooling, oral food retention, or leakage of food or liquids placed in mouth

• history of aspiration problems or a definite risk of aspiration, aspiration pneumonia, or signs and symptoms of aspiration

• significant weight loss directly related to non-oral nutritional intake (non-oral feedings) and reaction to textures and consistencies

• poor coordination, sensation loss, or abnormalities affecting oropharyngeal abilities necessary to close the lips; squeeze the cheeks; or to bite, chew, suck, shape, and squeeze the food bolus into the upper esophagus while protecting the airway

• post-surgical reaction affecting the ability to adequately use oropharyngeal structures used in swallowing

• existence of other conditions such as presence of tracheotomy tube; reduced or inadequate laryngeal elevation, labial closure, velopharyngeal closure, or pharyngeal peristalsis; and cricopharyngeal dysfunction

• impaired salivary gland performance and/or presence of local structural lesions in the pharynx resulting in threatening oropharyngeal swallowing difficulties like head and neck cancer

Medical Workup

Medical diagnostic evaluation by the physician must precede treatment for medical coverage. You must indicate that you consulted with the physician and that there is a dysphagia that needs to be addressed. You must also document which stage of swallowing is involved.

There are currently several Medicare intermediaries who require a hands-on examination by the physician prior to treatment authorization. This is a strict interpretation of the Medicare policy manual's dysphagia medical review guidelines and is of particular concern to SLPs in nursing facilities who must frequently delay initiation of treatment while waiting for the physician's visit. The intermediaries who require the physician exam expect the SLP to provide the physician with information as needed, such as on the sample form on page 35. However, the underlying reason for the physician's exam is to "force" physicians to become more knowledgeable about dysphagia.

Assessment

The medical workup and your assessment needs to document the patient's history, current eating status, and specific clinical observations. These clinical observations must include:

• presence/absence of a feeding tube
• presence/absence of paralysis
• presence/absence of coughing or choking
• oral-motor structure and function
• oral sensitivity
• muscle tone
• cognition
• positioning
• laryngeal function
• oropharyngeal reflexes
• swallowing function

Your assessment must then list a very specific diagnosis, describing the phase or phases of swallowing which are affected and a recommended treatment plan.

Duration and Intensity

Medicare will allow for services to continue at a duration and intensity appropriate to the severity of the impairment and the patient's response to the treatment.

The Source for Dysphagia　　　　　27

Reasonable Expectation When Planning Care

As with any rehabilitation service, Medicare expects you to recognize that the patient will make "material improvement within a reasonable period of time." In addition, our Code of Ethics (ASHA) holds us responsible for providing patient treatment only when benefit can reasonably be expected.

When More Than One Profession Is Involved

Medicare guidelines don't distinguish between SLPs, OTs, and PTs regarding dysphagia services. Occupational therapy and physical therapy often provide service with SLPs but it's important that these services don't duplicate one another. If you're involved in a team approach in which two or more of these professions are providing intervention for a feeding disorder, the notes documented by each must reflect the different areas addressed.

Example Notes

Speech
"Patient able to close lips around spoon with tactile assistance on 8 of 10 trials during therapeutic feeding at lunch. Analysis of patient's ability to actively close lips around spoon revealed patient unable to do so without the tactile stimulation. If support is not provided to the right lower corner of the lip, patient has anterior loss with thin liquids. Patient able to manipulate bolus of pureed consistency from front to back of mouth with minimal oral residue on 10 of 10 trials. Patient used chin-down posture for thin liquids without cues 100% of the time when small sips were presented from a straw."

Occupational Therapy
An occupational therapist feeding the patient, who would certainly follow all the precautions described above, might document such as:

"Patient positioned at upright at the beginning of meal with extra pillow placed behind her head. Patient able to maintain head at midline for approximately 3 minutes at a time. Patient could reposition head at midline with tactile cues on 6/7 trials. Patient showed adequate sensation to wipe residue from right side of face without cues. Patient using weighted handle spoon for presentation of pureed foods."

Relationship to Safety Issues

Medicare is very specific in stating that the treatment should be designed to make it safe for the patient to swallow during oral feedings. The guidelines even state that the primary emphasis and goal of treatment should be to improve the patient's safety and quality of life by reducing or eliminating alternative nutritional support systems and moving the patient to a higher dietary level with improved nutritional intake. You must have a reasonable expectation that you can achieve this goal and that skilled intervention is needed to do so.

If you don't believe you can improve the patient's safety or quality of life or move the patient to a higher level of dietary input, then there's no justification to begin service. If the patient can achieve her goals, but doesn't require intervention by a licensed and certified SLP to do so, the services will probably not be reimbursed. Medicare reimburses for *skilled* rehabilitation services.

Skilled Level of Care

Remember that if all you're doing is routine, repetitive observation, or standby cueing, it's probably not going to be viewed as skilled rehabilitation. Services of a certified and licensed SLP are needed because you're able to observe and analyze what the patient is doing and make changes based on your observations. These changes may be in treatment techniques, positioning techniques, diet, etc.

However, a note such as the one below would probably indicate that the services being provided are not skilled in nature. There's nothing in the note which indicates that a nursing assistant or family member couldn't do the same thing.

> "Watched patient at lunchtime. Fed patient pureed diet by spoon and thin liquids from cut-out cup. Patient consumed 80% of pureed foods and 100% of liquids."

Tube Feeding and Oral Feeding

There continues to be confusion as to whether a patient receiving tube feeding can also receive intervention to improve oral feeding and have Medicare reimburse both. The answer is *yes*.

The presence of an NG tube or G-tube does *not* preclude the need for dysphagia treatment. (This is stated specifically in section 3910 of the *Medicare Intermediary Manual*.) Remember that Medicare states the importance of improving the patient's safety and quality of life by *reducing* or eliminating alternative nutritional support systems. If a physician has ordered tube feeding to maintain the patient's nutrition and hydration, then Medicare will pay for the tube feeding. If, in addition, the physician orders dysphagia services, then Medicare will also reimburse those services if all the other requirements are met (reasonable expectation for improvement, need for skilled service, etc.).

Reimbursement Changes as a Result of the Balanced Budget Act of 1997

The Balanced Budget Act of 1997 (BBA) resulted in tremendous changes in the way all Medicare services are reimbursed. It is beyond the scope of this book to explain all of the changes and how they have impacted each type of facility. In addition, legislative and regulatory changes and interpretation of the regulations are occurring frequently, and therefore, the information provided may soon be out of date. However, it is important that this book address some of the basics of the BBA so you

understand how the reimbursement changes have had an impact on the provision of dysphagia services. Three of the major changes will be described here: Prospective Payment System, $1500 cap, and the Medicare Fee Schedule.

Prospective Payment System (PPS)

In the past, services were rendered and a bill was submitted and paid. This was a retrospective payment system, in which none of the risk was placed on the provider. Prospective payment systems are structured differently. The payer agrees to pay a certain amount of money "up front" to the provider and the provider has to figure out a way to provide the services for that amount of money. The amount paid might be per diagnosis (as in the Diagnosis Related Groups [DRG] system used in acute IP hospital settings), per month (as when managed care plans pay a certain amount for every member of their plan per month to the physician who then has to provide all the care needed by those members), or per diem (as in the amount paid per day to the skilled nursing facility). This shifts the risk to the provider. Acute inpatient settings have been under a PPS for a long time with DRG reimbursement. (DRGs provide pre-established payment amounts to the hospital based on the patient's medical diagnosis, regardless of how long the patient stays or how many services she receives.)

Skilled nursing facilities were placed under the per diem PPS beginning in 1998 and are phasing in according to their cost-reporting period. The facility receives a certain amount per day for each resident in a Part A stay, depending on the category in which they are placed. These categories are called Resource Utilization Groups III (RUGS) and reflect the level of care needed by the patient. The skilled nursing facility has to use this per diem to pay for all the services the patient needs, including nursing care and ancillary services such as speech-language pathology. Each RUG category requiring rehabilitation services specifies how many minutes per week of therapy the patient must receive in order to stay in that reimbursement category. It is up to the three rehab disciplines to determine how to share those minutes so the patient receives the maximal benefit. Home health settings and IP rehabilitation hospitals are scheduled to transition to prospective payment systems, but as of this writing, details were not available.

Consolidated Billing

Consolidated billing requires that the skilled nursing facility be the only one who can bill Medicare for any services the patient receives during her stay (at the present time, consolidated billing has been instituted for Part A stays, but implementation for Part B stays has been delayed). Consolidation billing means that if the skilled nursing facility sends a patient out for an instrumental assessment of swallowing, the facility (usually a hospital) performing the procedure will send the bill to the nursing facility (not to Medicare), and the nursing facility will have to pay the hospital out of the per diem amount. This has resulted in some nursing facilities pressuring SLPs not to request instrumental assessments. (See Chapter 3, pages 36-37, for information on the dangers of planning treatment without appropriate instrumental assessment.)

$1500 Cap

The BBA also included an arbitrary $1500 cap on rehabilitation services reimbursed under Part B. OT has its own $1500 cap, while PT and SLP share a cap. This is not what Congress thought would happen when it passed the legislation, but was a later interpretation by the Health Care Finance

Administration (HCFA). HCFA based its interpretation on wording in the Medicare statute which was added when speech-language pathology services were added. When that happened, speech-language pathology services were listed under the physical therapy section with words similar to "physical therapy services, to include speech-language pathology services." HCFA interpreted that to mean that the cap was meant to be a shared cap.

At this writing, HCFA is unable to keep track of when a beneficiary has reached her $1500 limit and has determined it will interpret the cap per provider. Therefore, if an outpatient is able to go to one facility for outpatient physical therapy services and to another facility to receive outpatient speech-language pathology services, the patient could receive $1500 of PT and $1500 of SLP services. The patient could then go to another facility to receive more services (up to $1500). Of course, patients in nursing homes are usually unable to go to different providers and thus receive only the combined $1500 for PT and SLP. Hospital outpatient departments are exempt from the cap so a patient may receive as much service as needed, as long as the guidelines described earlier in this chapter are followed.

Note: In November 1999, Congress passed a bill placing a two-year moratorium on the caps. During this time, HCFA will study alternative reimbursement systems.

Medicare Fee Schedule

Part B services used to be billed by a facility at a cost determined by the facility. Medicare determined if that cost was within the reasonable and customary allowance and reimbursed the facility for 80%. The patient had to pay 20% (co-pay). Patients are still responsible for the co-pay, but now all of Part B outpatient services are covered under a fee schedule. This fee schedule sets specific amounts which the facility can bill for each Current Procedural Terminology (CPT) code.

Since 1992, the Resource-Based Relative Value Scale (RBRVS) payment system has been in effect for Part B physician services rendered to Medicare recipients. However, because SLPs cannot bill directly for their services, the RBRVS did not apply to us until now. The fee schedule on which our services are paid is based on an RBRVS. That means that HCFA used a formula to assign a relative value to each CPT. This value is then used to determine the actual fee.

Coding Issues

Coding systems were designed to collect data for research and health statistics and to aid in the payment of claims. There are three coding systems of which SLPs should be aware: ICD-9-CM, Current Procedural Terminology (CPT), and HCFA Common Procedure Coding System (HCPCS). The HCPCS is simply the descriptive term used by HCFA to indicate the CPT codes.

The ICD-9-CM stands for the International Classification of Diseases, 9th Revision, Clinical Modification. It is published by the U.S. Department of Health and Human Services, Public Health Service, and is intended to standardize disease and pro-cedure classification throughout the United States. According to the ICD-9-CM Manual, "medical codes today are utilized to facilitate payment of health services, to evaluate utilization patterns, and to study the appro-priateness of health care costs. Coding provides the basis for epidemiological studies and research into the quality of health care" (ASHA).

The diagnostic code reported must match the services rendered. For instance, if a patient is coded with a broken hip, services for dysphagia might be called into question. Sometimes patients have apparent diagnoses which have not been documented. For example, the patient may have been admitted to your facility with a broken hip, but also demonstrated mental status change which might indicate a stroke. If the mental status change is not identified and coded, then it might appear you are rendering services inappropriately. Dysphagia can be the medical diagnosis listed without a medical cause of the dysphagia. The ICD-9 code for Dysphagia (difficulty in swallowing) is 787.2. Asking that this medical diagnosis code be added will easily demonstrate to a reviewer that dysphagia services are warranted.

Current Procedural Terminology (CPT) Codes
These codes are approved by the American Medical Association (AMA) and are used for billing. You need to know these codes when billing your dysphagia services. CPT manuals are available from the AMA. In addition, for an extra charge, you can receive the CPT Code Companion and the CPT Code Assistant. These provide periodic updates and answers to frequently asked questions.

Use of CPT codes simplifies the reporting of services. This became increasingly important as of January 1, 1999, when sweeping Medicare changes took place. Medicare requires that a CPT code be listed for each procedure billed. Therefore, it is crucial that you know and understand all of the CPT codes available for use, and that you communicate the information about these codes to the billing office at the facility. Inaccurate or inappropriate use of codes may result in Medicare charging the facility with fraud or abuse.

Fraud is defined as knowingly and willfully executing, or attempting to execute, a scheme to defraud any health care benefit program. Abuse is any action which directly or indirectly results in unnecessary cost to the Medicare or Medicaid program, improper payment, or payment for services which fail to meet professionally recognized standards of care or are medically unnecessary. Therefore, if you choose codes which do not accurately reflect the service rendered but might bring a higher reimbursement rate to the facility, it could be viewed as fraudulent.

On pages 33 and 34 is a list of CPT codes which may apply to dysphagia evaluation and treatment. It is important that you read the descriptions of each code and choose one which accurately describes what you have done with the patient. Some examples of how these codes are used have been provided, but this information must be interpreted by you. HCFA does not provide any concrete examples (called scenarios) of how each code can be used. Such scenarios are provided as exemplary for OT and PT, but not for SLP. HCFA indicates that any of the codes may be used by any discipline, as long as the code accurately reflects the service provided. The facility then attaches a discipline specific modifier, which indicates which rehabilitation professional rendered the service. These modifiers are very important, as more than one discipline may be billing the same CPT code on the same day. The revenue code for speech-language pathology is 440. Some of these CPT codes do not have a time unit attached, whereas some of the physical medicine codes (those in the 97000 series) do. If you are billing

under a code without timed units (e.g., 92525 - evaluation of swallowing/oral-function for feeding or 92526 - treatment of swallowing dysfunction/oral function for feeding), it is important to communicate to your billing office that they may bill for only one of those codes, whether you were with the patient for 15 minutes or an hour.

Impact on the Care of Patients with Dysphagia

As a result of the reimbursement changes, patients with dysphagia are at risk of not receiving all the services they require. As mentioned above, some patients may not be receiving the instrumental assessments they need in order for the SLP to accurately plan treatment. Patients in skilled nursing facilities may be receiving less than the optimal amount of therapy and may receive very short bedside evaluations, as evaluation minutes do not count towards the number of minutes of service that must be rendered during the week. Hospitals and other facilities that offer outpatient services may provide only short visits to Medicare outpatients for those procedures which do not have time units attached. For example, the hospital will receive only $XX for 92526 (treatment of swallowing dysfunction and/or oral function for feeding), whether the patient is seen for 15 minutes or an hour. The facility may pressure the SLP to schedule Medicare outpatients for short visits only. All of these pressures for productivity place extreme demands on the SLP trying to provide quality services.

CPT Codes for Dysphagia Evaluation & Treatment _____

CPT Code	Description from manual	Time units?	Example of use
92525	Evaluation of swallowing and oral function for feeding (includes both clinical bedside evaluation and instrumental assessment [i.e., videofluoroscopy])	No	Used for bedside dysphagia evaluation and/or instrumental assessment (i.e., MBS or FEES® if you did not pass the scope)*
92526	Treatment of swallowing dysfunction and/or oral function for feeding	No	Treatment provided during therapeutic trials with food/ liquid; training patient in use of any compensatory strategies
92511	Nasopharyngoscopy with endoscope	No	With FEES® if you actually inserted the endoscope; could be billed as separate procedure which occurred along with 92525 (bedside evaluation)
97530	Therapeutic activities, direct (one-on-one) patient contact by the provider—use of dynamic activities to improve performance	Yes, per each minute unit	During therapeutic feeding at a meal, you may be instructing the patient to carry over use of the super-supraglottic swallow maneuver to increase safety of swallow. This may include some caregiver training.
97112	Neuromuscular re-education of movement, balance, coordination, kinesthetic sense, posture, and proprioception	Yes, each 15-minute unit	Performing thermal/tactile stimulation to reestablish quick initiation of pharyngeal swallow; performing oral neuromuscular facilitation exercises

* It is not appropriate for the SLP to bill her part of the modified barium swallow under 74230. That code is for the Radiologist.

CPT Code	Description from manual	Time units?	Example of use
97110	Therapeutic procedures, one or more areas; therapeutic exercises to develop strength and endurance, range of motion, and flexibility	Yes, each 15-minute unit	Performing the effort swallow to strengthen base of tongue and posterior pharyngeal wall movement; performing range of motion exercises
97535	Self care/home management training (e.g., activities of daily living [ADL] and compensatory training, meal preparation, safety procedures, and instructions in use of adaptive equipment); direct one-on-one contact by provider	Yes, each 15-minute unit	Teaching patient and caregiver about the kinds of textures the patient can take safely, and making sure the caregiver can help the patient follow compensatory techniques

For those codes which are associated with 15-minute units, HCFA has provided the following guide to help you determine how many units to list:

1 unit	=		1 minute to <	23 minutes
2 units	= >	23 minutes to <	38 minutes
3 units	= >	38 minutes to <	53 minutes
4 units	= >	53 minutes to <	68 minutes
5 units	= >	68 minutes to <	83 minutes
6 units	= >	83 minutes to <	98 minutes
7 units	= >	98 minutes to <	113 minutes
8 units	= >	113 minutes to <	128 minutes

Physician Referral Form _____

Patient _____ Date _____

The patient appears to present:

- ❒ oral dysphagia
- ❒ pharyngeal dysphagia
- ❒ esophageal dysphagia

Patient exhibits the following symptoms of oral dysphagia:

- ❒ drooling
- ❒ holding food in mouth
- ❒ decreased ability to chew
- ❒ impaired salivary gland performance
- ❒ oral lesions
- ❒ increased time to complete meal

Patient exhibits these conditions which may indicate an oral and/or pharyngeal dysphagia:

- ❒ tracheostomy tube
- ❒ weight loss
- ❒ surgery to head/neck

Patient exhibits the following clinical signs of aspiration or possible pharyngeal dysphagia:

- ❒ coughing
- ❒ choking
- ❒ history of pneumonia
- ❒ temperature spikes
- ❒ wet vocal quality
- ❒ breathy vocal quality
- ❒ decreased lung sounds

Speech-Language Pathologist: Please complete the following:

- ❒ Bedside/Clinical Evaluation Needed
- ❒ Referral for instrumental exam (e.g., modified barium swallow, FEES®)

Physician's Signature _____

Chapter 3

Clinical Bedside Screening

A clinical or bedside evaluation is usually the first step in a complete assessment of a patient with dysphagia. The bedside evaluation should be considered a screening, rather than a diagnostic procedure. Very often an instrumental procedure (a modified barium swallow study [MBS] or fiberoptic endoscopic evaluation of swallowing [FEES®]) is recommended for more complete assessment of the pharyngeal phase. Unfortunately, there are situations in which only a clinical evaluation can be completed because there is no access to a facility at which an instrumental exam of swallowing can be completed.

Clinicians who are treating patients with suspected pharyngeal disorders based solely on results obtained at bedside place themselves and the patient at risk, as a bedside evaluation has definite limitations. Aspiration cannot be confirmed nor ruled out during a bedside evaluation. The bedside evaluation simply allows you to observe for any clinical signs of aspiration. However, up to 60% of patients may be silent aspirators as they don't show clinical signs such as coughing or throat clearing. The bedside evaluation can reveal very important information that will help decide which types and textures of food the patient can eat and which positions are appropriate for the patient.

How Accurate are Bedside Screenings?

Research continues to determine if the bedside evaluation can become more sensitive (i.e., to accurately identify patients who are aspirating). In 1999, HCFA instructed the Agency for Health Care Policy Research (AHCPR) to conduct a review of the literature to determine what efficacy literature exists to support dysphagia management. AHCPR contracted with an agency called ECRI, an evidence-based practice center, to conduct the study. The press release about their report, which was based on studies related to stroke patients, concluded that "The use of full bedside examinations in dysphagia management programs are capable of identifying up to 80% of cases of aspiration, which is often difficult to detect because about half of patients with dysphagia who aspirate do so silently (without a cough)" (AHCPR, 1999). Of course, what this conclusion fails to state is that it is not enough to know who is or is not aspirating. In order for SLPs to plan treatment for pharyngeal dysphagia appropriately, an instrumental exam is necessary to identify the physiological cause of the symptom observed. A symptom observed on a bedside screening may be the result of different physiological problems. For example, if you observe a patient coughing during the bedside evaluation, this might mean that the patient has inadequate laryngeal closure and is aspirating during the swallow; has poor back of tongue control and has let the bolus slip over the back of the tongue and has aspirated before the swallow; or has limited laryngeal elevation with pyriform sinus residue which was aspirated after the swallow. Without the instrumental exam to identify which of those physiological problems the patient is presenting, you are just guessing when choosing short-term goals and treatment objectives. (See Chapter 7, pages 180-181.)

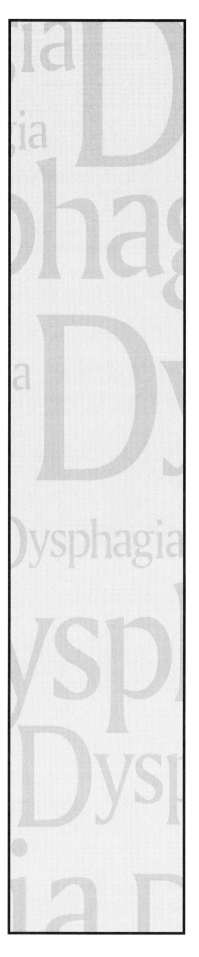

ECRI reached its conclusions based on a meta-analysis of several studies. ASHA challenged the conclusions in a report entitled "AHCPR Report: Diagnosis and Treatment of Dysphagia/Swallowing Disorders in the Elderly - Questions and Answers for ASHA Members" (June 1999). ASHA raised questions about the methodology (meta-analysis) used in the report, indicating that the five studies used in the meta-analysis reflected a very heterogenous group according to age range and percent with stroke. It also challenged the fact the report focused primarily on prevention of aspiration as the outcome of dysphagia treatment even though it acknowledged that prevention of malnutrition and dehydration and improving quality of life were important outcomes.

SLPs who assess patients with dysphagia at bedside should carefully follow current research results. Work is being done to determine which characteristics a patient exhibits at bedside are more likely to indicate that the patient is aspirating or is at risk of aspirating. This will help us to more accurately determine which patients need the instrumental assessment. For example, Logemann et al. (1999) studied the sensitivity and specificity of a 28-item screening test in identifying patients who aspirate or who have an oral stage disorder, a pharyngeal delay, or a pharyngeal stage disorder. Their results identified variables that could classify whether or not patients aspirated (71%), have an oral stage disorder (69%), have a pharyngeal delay (72%), or a pharyngeal stage swallowing problem (70%).

Medicare Guidelines Related to Evaluation

Medicare provides guidelines for the evaluation and treatment of dysphagia which will be helpful as you conduct your assessment. (See pages 26-29.)

The patient should have had a previous medical workup before you do a clinical evaluation. That is, a physician should have seen this patient and referred the patient for a specific problem. The problem may not always be stated clearly on the patient's chart, but you may find statements such as *decreased appetite*, *refusing food*, or *patient had trouble with pills this morning*. More complete information about the patient's problems can usually be found by talking with the nurse.

Your assessment needs to address whether the patient is alert and able to participate in the evaluation and whether the patient is motivated to work for improvement. The patient's cognitive skills need to be briefly assessed and mentioned.

Medicare indicates that patients with dementia (and other types of progressive disorders) don't usually show improvement in swallowing function, but Medicare will allow for short-term assistance or instruction in things such as positioning, diet, or feeding modifications, or even in the use of self-help devices. Therefore, decreased cognition should **not** rule out the possibility of a patient benefitting from short-term intervention.

The assessment must reveal any problems the patient is having with swallowing. The patient has to present one of several conditions in order for Medicare to cover the service. (See Chapter 2, page 27.) Your report should also include statements about the patient's current ability to eat.

At the conclusion of the screening, document your clinical observations with a definitive diagnosis that identifies which phase of swallowing is affected. You also need to establish a treatment plan and indicate why intervention is needed. A helpful way to do this is to indicate what would happen to the patient if you did not treat him.

Test Tray

Work with the Dietary Department at your facility to design a test tray which includes samples of a variety of types and textures of foods and liquids. You'll also need to include a thickening agent. A test tray might include the following:

    1/4 c. pureed fruit
    1/4 c. ground meat
    1/4 c. regular meat

1/4 c. mixed vegetables
1/4 c. rice or noodles
1 slice of white bread
1 pineapple ring
1 sugar cookie
1 c. Cheerios
1 c. 2% milk
1 c. grape juice
1/4 c. food thickener
margarine

Team vs. Solo Approach

You may work in a facility where speech-language pathology performs the bedside dysphagia screening alone. If that's the case, you'll want to consult with the occupational therapist and physical therapist as needed for help on positioning the patient, adaptive equipment, etc. On the other hand, you may work in a facility where speech-language pathology and occupational therapy or speech-language pathology and physical therapy work together to assess the patient. Each discipline should be looking at different aspects of the patient's ability to eat.

Benefits to the solo approach are:

1. It's efficient and convenient for you to complete the evaluation at a time suitable for you without having to coordinate schedules for two therapists.

2. You get the whole picture, from chart review to the evaluation to the recommendations.

3. The patient and his family work with one professional and become familiar with that individual.

Disadvantages:

1. If the patient could benefit from an assessment for positioning or adaptive equipment, you need to make a referral and have this done at a later time.

2. You may overlook an area needing evaluation due to lack of expertise in that area.

If designed carefully, the team approach has several benefits:

1. Two professionals assessing the patient and discussing the case may come up with a more comprehensive assessment and better treatment plan.

2. The specific team players look at their own areas of expertise during the evaluation.

3. Any problem areas, like positioning, can be assessed during the evaluation rather than having to wait until later.

4. Team evaluations promote the development of rapport with other professionals.

5. In a facility where maintaining adequate staffing is a problem, the patient may receive more intensive treatment if two disciplines are sharing the feeding therapy.

Disadvantages you may encounter with a team approach are:

1. There may be some controversy over who will assess each area. For example, some occupational therapists may assess oral-motor skills. For guidance about what is appropriate for each discipline to do, consult the scope of practice in your state licensure law and in the occupational therapy law.

2. You may encounter some difficulty scheduling the evaluations so all professionals can be available at the same time.

3. You may disagree on the findings or the treatment focus.

4. If the evaluation and progress notes aren't written appropriately, there may be funding and reimbursement issues for what appears to be two professionals performing the same task.

If you decide to use a team approach, remember that it may not be necessary for all members of the team to be at every evaluation. For example, an ambulatory patient who's quite obviously able to self-feed may need to be seen only by speech-language pathology for assessment of oral and pharyngeal stages. On the other hand, a patient whose PO intake has declined because arthritis in the hands prevents self-feeding may need to see occupational therapy only.

Procedures Sometimes Used During Bedside Swallowing Screenings

Sometimes you can supplement the information you obtain during a bedside screening. You may use cervical auscultation, the Blue Dye Test, or Pulse Oximetry. The latter two procedures will be discussed in more detail in Chapter 9, pages 246-248. You should also be aware of the *3-oz. Water Swallow Test*, which is described as a screening protocol, and is sometimes used by physicians instead of referring for a more complete screening by the SLP. Another procedure, called the *Timed Test of Swallowing*, is sometimes used by physicians. Both the *3-oz. Water Swallow Test* and the *Timed Test of Swallowing* have the potential to result in the patient aspirating a large amount of water.

Cervical Auscultation

Cervical auscultation is a general term that describes several techniques for listening to a patient's breath sounds. In research, a laryngeal microphone is used for auscultation. In clinical settings, the flat diaphragm of a stethoscope is placed laterally on the thyroid cartilage on the side of the neck. Placement is adjusted until cervical breath sounds can be heard. Cervical breath sounds are generally hollow or "tubular" in nature compared with breath sounds heard over the lungs. Some clinicians now routinely use cervical auscultation to assess swallowing, although great caution must be taken in making summary statements based on what is heard.

A normal swallow is thought to "sound" like this:

- breath sounds are heard
- breathing stops (usually in the middle of an exhalation)
- a sound often described as a "clunk" or "swish" is heard
- breath sounds are heard again, similar to how the breath sounded before the swallow

Some clinicians who use cervical auscultation say they can "hear" aspiration. Zenner et al. (1995) state that aspiration is suspected if a flushing sound of material is heard prior to initiation of the swallow, or when wet breath sounds, coughing, or a distorted voice is heard after the swallow. However, there is no scientific evidence to indicate that this technique can accurately predict aspiration. Zenner et al. performed cervical auscultation on 50 patients at bedside who then underwent an MBS study (mean of 14.5 days later). That means that the ratings for cervical auscultation were not made on the same swallows that were viewed during the MBS, and in fact, some of the patients weren't evaluated until weeks after their assessment via cervical auscultation. The authors report the following levels of agreement between what they "heard" at bedside and then saw on videofluoroscopy weeks later: pharyngeal delay 66%, pharyngeal residue 42%, and tracheal aspiration 76%.

These results must be viewed with skepticism given the design flaws in the study. Even the authors conclude: "At this time, cervical auscultation is an imprecise clinical method for evaluating risks of tracheal aspiration." In addition, clinicians using cervical auscultation don't always use the same terms to describe what they are hearing. This is a highly technical skill, and many clinicians are using it without any training. The technique holds some promise, and perhaps in the future will be refined enough to yield useful information, but at this time, cervical auscultation is considered an imprecise clinical method for evaluating risks of tracheal aspiration.

3-oz. Water Swallow Test

DePippo et al. (1992) described a procedure called the *3-oz. Water Swallow Test for Aspiration Following Stroke*. The patients in their study were given 3 oz. of water in a cup and asked to drink without interruption. The authors considered an abnormal response to be coughing during or for one minute after completion of the swallow, or a wet-hoarse vocal quality after the swallow. The patients then underwent an MBS (it is not clear if there was a lapse in time between the timed swallow test and the MBS). On the MBS, 16 of 20 patients who had had an abnormal response on the water swallow test showed evidence of aspiration (reported as 76% sensitivity) and 11 patients had an abnormal response on the water swallow test, but did not aspirate on the modified (reported as 59% specificity). The authors concluded that their test is sensitive enough to be useful as a screening tool for MBS referral. However, the authors recommend that the 3-oz. Water Swallow Test be used in conjunction with a clinical symptom checklist when determining which patients should be referred for further study. This test is not meant to take the place of instrumental examinations, but to help determine which patients should have such examinations.

Garon et al. (1995) tested the reliability of the 3-oz. Water Swallow Test with 100 consecutive patients with a variety of diagnoses. After evaluating the patients at bedside with the 3-oz. Water Swallow Test using cough reflex as the sole indicator, they performed MBS studies on the patients. They found 54 who aspirated and of those, only 19 (35%) had coughed at bedside. This leaves an alarming 65% as silent aspirators.

Timed Test of Swallowing

Nathadwarawala et al. (1992) described a timed test of swallowing capacity to be used with patients with neurogenic dysphagia. The authors state that swallowing speed could be used as an index of abnormal swallowing. They defined abnormal swallowing as the patient's perception of a problem. Therefore, they used the *Timed Test of Swallowing* to confirm the complaint of the patient. However, even these authors conclude that the swallowing test itself "will be potentially hazardous where the patient has overt aspiration or is strongly suspected of silent aspiration."

Blue Dye Test

This test is described in detail in Chapter 9, pages 247-248. It involves suctioning the patient at the trach to determine if there is evidence of aspirated material.

Pulse Oximetry

This procedure is described in detail in Chapter 9, pages 240 and 246. It involves monitoring the patient's oxygen saturation and watching for changes during a swallow.

Drawing Conclusions and Making Recommendations

After your assessment is complete, you'll have to draw conclusions and make recommendations. Your first decision is whether you have obtained enough information to make an informed decision about this patient's management.

If You Don't Have Enough Information

What other assessments do you need to obtain?

An instrumental exam (MBS or FEES®) is indicated if the patient showed clinical signs of aspiration which couldn't be eliminated with compensatory techniques. Even if you did eliminate the symptom (e.g., chin-down eliminated the coughing), you can't be sure there still isn't some silent aspiration. An instrumental exam is also indicated if the patient is thought to be at high risk for aspiration.

What are some risks for pharyngeal dysphagia that you should consider when deciding whether to refer for an instrumental exam?

- coughing or throat clearing during bedside screening

- multiple swallows

- wet vocal quality/breath sounds

- breathy vocal quality

- reduced laryngeal elevation on trial swallows

- not managing own secretions

- history of pneumonia

- recent temperature spikes

- decreased lung/breath sounds

- significant fatigability

- history of long-term intubation

- presence of tracheostomy

There may be times when the patient is *not* ready for an MBS:

- if the patient isn't alert enough to eat anyway

- if all the problems appear to be in the oral phase and you don't suspect aspiration or pharyngeal problems

- if the patient refuses to eat

- if the patient won't open his mouth for food or liquid (In this case, the patient may need some work to get ready for an MBS study as he may be orally defensive, his dementia may be so advanced he doesn't understand what to do, or he may be very apraxic.)

Is there a need to consult with other physicians?

An ENT consult may be indicated if the patient presents a change in vocal quality and you think reduced laryngeal closure may be a factor in aspiration. Be sure to specify what you want the ENT to assess, such as "ENT eval to check movement of vocal folds for closure, especially at posterior chink" or "ENT fiberoptic exam of laryngeal function during swallow, suspect possible aspiration after swallow."

A referral to a gastroenterologist may be needed if the patient presents symptoms which seem more esophageal in nature.

A neurologist may need to see the patient if the change in swallowing seems related to a change in overall cognitive/neurological status.

Be sure to discuss any findings with the patient's primary care physician before making a referral.

If You Have Enough Information

Is it safe for the patient to eat by mouth?

If so, determine the type of diet the patient can safely tolerate and identify any compensatory techniques that help the patient eat.

- food texture

- liquid consistency

- feeding position for the patient

- presentation of the food or liquid

- compensatory techniques

Can the patient maintain adequate nutrition and hydration when eating by mouth?

Some patients may be able to eat safely by mouth but may fatigue easily or may be on such a restrictive diet (e.g., pureed with no sticky foods, no eggs, pudding-thick liquids) that they cannot get adequate nutrition or hydration by mouth. Consult with the dietitian and physician to help make this determination. It certainly isn't appropriate to recommend that a patient eat by mouth and to select a diet, yet not mention the concern that the patient may not be able to eat enough by mouth. You may find that within a week the patient is dehydrated and in the early stages of malnutrition.

If you have concerns about the patient not being able to eat or drink enough, request a three-day calorie count. Then the dietitian can determine if the patient is getting adequate intake. Some patients may just need oral supplements like Ensure or Sustacal to reach adequate levels.

Can a patient receive some PO feedings AND be tube fed?

Keep in mind that the most important factor is to maintain the health of the patient. The physician and the dietitian will determine the specifics such as type of tube feeding, type of tube, and rate of tube feeding.

As the patient gains strength and seems ready to eat more, you may want to speak to the dietitian about turning off the tube feeding an hour before meals or running it only at night. Even if the patient is never able to take enough food or liquid by mouth to maintain nutrition, he may be able to have pleasure feedings. Pleasure feedings often enhance the quality of a patient's life.

If Medicare is the payment source, keep in mind the payment guidelines. Medicare will pay for tube feeding if ordered by the physician and if it's necessary to maintain adequate nutrition and hydration. Medicare will also pay for swallowing therapy if the patient meets the guidelines (e.g., there is a reason-

able expectation that the patient will improve, that the patient's safety is an issue if treatment is not initiated, and the patient is alert enough to participate). It's *not* true that Medicare will stop paying for tube feeding when feeding therapy is initiated.

When should a patient be NPO only?

There are no hard and fast rules about who should and shouldn't be NPO. General guidelines are that if you can't find any consistency the patient can eat without aspiration, then the patient should be NPO.

Keep in mind the situation in which the patient will normally be fed. Perhaps during a modified barium swallow, it's determined that the patient can safely take pudding-thick liquids with chin-down and head rotation to the right, swallowing twice to clear the pooling. If these techniques are for a patient who has dementia and will be fed most meals by staff who may not follow your recommendations, the patient might be safer NPO except for therapeutic feeds when you are present.

What should I consider when recommending that a patient be NPO?

Be careful with your wording when recommending NPO. Depending on the physician with whom you're working, you may need to state your findings and suggest consideration of an alternative means for nutrition and hydration. Some physicians feel boxed into a corner when you make a strong recommendation that the patient shouldn't be fed by mouth. Then if the physician or physician in conjunction with the patient's wishes makes a determination to feed the patient, it looks like it's contraindicated. You may need to give your findings and offer options such as:

> "Clinical evaluation of the patient reveals significantly impaired oral skills. The patient isn't able to masticate and form a bolus with any materials. Of more concern is the fact that aspiration is strongly suspected. The patient showed the following clinical signs of aspiration:

- coughed with thin liquids despite a variety of compensatory techniques

- showed intermittent throat clearing with foods of mixed textures

- showed occasional throat clearing with pureed textures

Consideration should be given to making the patient NPO until an instrumental exam can be completed to rule out the possibility of aspiration. However, if the patient is to continue eating, a diet of pureed texture and pudding-thick liquids may reduce, but not entirely eliminate, the risk for aspiration."

Or you may want to leave it even more open-ended by simply stating:

"Patient has significantly impaired oral skills and the pharyngeal stage is also suspected to be impaired. Patient has many clinical signs of aspiration. An instrumental exam is needed to confirm or rule out aspiration. Safer textures for the patient appear to be pudding-thick liquids and purees, although aspiration of these materials can't be entirely ruled out."

If you're making a recommendation of NPO, have a prognosis in mind. If you think the patient is likely to regain enough skills to be able to take the majority of nutrition and hydration by mouth within six to eight weeks, consider placement of an NG tube.

"This patient shows clinical signs of aspiration of all materials. These signs could not be eliminated with a variety of compensatory techniques. This needs to be confirmed via an instrumental exam, but it appears that the patient is not safe for any PO at this time.

Because the prognosis is good for a return to safe intake of some PO within four to five weeks, consideration might be given to placement of an NG tube while intensive

indirect therapy (therapy without presentation of foods) proceeds."

If the patient is not expected to improve, or the improvement will take months, then a PEG tube or PEJ tube is probably indicated.

"This patient shows clinical signs of aspiration on all consistencies which could not be eliminated with postural or diet texture changes. The aspiration can be confirmed or ruled out via an instrumental exam. Patient's decreased cognitive skills preclude using other compensatory techniques. Therefore, pending the results of an instrumental exam, it's recommended that the patient be NPO and consideration be given to an alternative form of nutrition. Since this dysphagia is not likely to resolve quickly, a PEG tube is suggested."

What can I do to help a patient regain PO status?

We often forget that there's more to therapy with a patient with dysphagia than therapeutic feedings. If the patient is NPO, has a PEG tube, and is deteriorating, then there's no indication that therapy should be provided. If, however, the patient is NPO but expected to return to PO feeding, there may be deficits you can address without presenting food to the patient. For example:

- oral-motor exercises for bolus control to improve the patient's ability to form and manipulate a bolus

- strengthening of the back of the tongue to prevent premature movement of the bolus over the base of the tongue

- laryngeal closure exercises

- laryngeal elevation exercises

Besides feeding, what other things might I recommend for a patient?

- determining who can safely feed the patient

- family training

- where the patient should eat

- how medications should be given

- how patients with NG tubes should be positioned

- how oral care should be performed

- the status of the tracheostomy cuff during feeding

What about patients who enter my facility with a tube?

Example 1

Step 1 Patient enters facility with tube feedings and radiographic data to support NPO status.

Step 2 Initiate indirect therapy.

Step 3 Patient appears able to initiate swallow on command; demonstrates adequate oral-motor control; exhibits adequate laryngeal closure on phonation.

Step 4 Request an instrumental exam to determine if it's safe to resume intake by mouth. Once the instrumental exam is done, there are three possible outcomes:

    A. The study reveals that the patient can eat safely by mouth. Therapy can be continued, if warranted, and you can consult with the physician and dietitian to determine if the tube can be removed.

    B. The study reveals that the patient can have some food by mouth in therapy only. Therapy is continued and the tube remains in place until the patient shows significant improvement. Repeat Step 4.

    C. The study reveals that it is still unsafe for the patient to take any food by

mouth. Indirect therapy is continued and the tube remains in place until there is significant improvement. Repeat Step 4.

Example 2

Step 1 Patient enters facility with tube feedings and radiographic data to indicate direct therapy.

Step 2 Therapy includes trying recommended types, amounts, and consistencies of foods.

Step 3 Patient appears able to handle larger amounts of food.

Step 4 Consult with the physician and dietitian regarding calorie count and the possibility of removing the tube.

Example 3

Step 1 Patient enters facility with tube feeding, but no radiographic data to indicate whether intake by mouth is safe.

Step 2 Patient status is such that he can tolerate an instrumental exam, so you request the procedure before introducing food. Indirect therapy may begin before the instrumental exam is completed.

Do I use direct or indirect therapy with a patient with a feeding tube?

A patient may have a feeding tube (NG Tube, G-tube, or J-tube) placed for one of two reasons.

    1. The patient may be able to tolerate some PO intake, but not able to get enough nutrition by mouth.

    2. The patient may not safely have any intake by mouth and must receive all nutrition by tube.

Direct therapy may be used in the first situation. Direct therapy involves the presentation of food and liquid in controlled amounts to attempt to reinforce appropriate behaviors during swallowing.

In the latter situation, you may work with the patient to improve his swallowing so intake by mouth can be resumed. This treatment will be *indirect*. Indirect therapy may involve:

- exercises to improve oral-motor control of the bolus and the voluntary stage of the swallow

- stimulation of the swallowing reflex to heighten the sensitivity when a swallow is attempted

- exercises to increase adduction of tissues at the top of the airway to improve airway protection during the swallow

Medicare Guidelines

These guidelines are found in the *Medicare Intermediary Manual*. The case examples on pages 60 and 67 reference these specific guidelines to give you an example of how they might be addressed in a patient summary report.

1. Medical Workup

2. Dysphagia Criteria

   A. Level of alertness
   B. Motivation
   C. Cognitive
   D. Deglutition
   E. One of these conditions:
   - history of aspiration
   - oral-motor disorders
   - structural lesion
   - neuromotor disturbances
   - post-surgical reaction
   - significant weight loss
   - other conditions

3. Assessment
   A. History
   B. Current eating status
   C. Clinical observations
   D. Definitive diagnosis
   E. Identification of swallowing phase affected
   F. Recommended treatment plan

4. Care Planning
   A. Goals
   B. Type of care planned
   C. Reasonable expectation for improvement
   D. Safety issues

5. Need for Skilled Rehabilitation
   (What would happen if you didn't treat the patient?)

Bedside Dysphagia Evaluations

The forms in this chapter can be used when assessing a patient's swallowing abilities. Form C (pages 56-57) is used in all settings.

Form A (page 47) and Form B (page 48) are cover sheets that are designed to go with Form C. Once you have completed the evaluation using Form C, summarize the information on either Form A or Form B, depending on whether you did the assessment alone or with an OT. Form D (pages 63-64) is used in skilled nursing facilities where more specific documentation for Medicare is required.

Directions are provided on how to complete the forms. Completed sample forms are also included in this chapter, except for Form B. This form is virtually the same as Form A, except that it includes long-term goals and recommendations as identified by the OT.

You may work in a setting that requires a narrative format. Examples of narrative patient summary reports for each setting are also included on pages 60 and 67. Please note, however, that the influence of managed care and Medicare changes has precipitated more efficient methods of documentation. Reference to the Medicare Guidelines is made throughout the written summaries with superscript numbers and letters.

Directions for Bedside Dysphagia Evaluation – Summary Sheets for Form A or B

The top part of the summary sheets on pages 47 and 48 contain the history you should obtain from the patient's chart. (See Chapter 1 for more detailed information.) The bottom of the forms are completed at the conclusion of the evaluation.

Identifying Information

- *Admit Date* — When was the patient admitted to your facility?

- *Physician* — Who ordered the dysphagia consult?

- *Admit Diagnosis* — What caused the patient to be admitted to the facility?

- *Medical History* — Include information pertinent to the assessment you are about to perform, including the diagnosis related to the swallowing problem.

- *Medications* — Note if the patient is currently on, or has been on in the past, any medications which might reduce the level of alertness, cause confusion, or cause dry mouth.

- *Current Method of Nutrition* —Check if the patient is receiving a PO diet, and then indicate what that diet is. If the patient is NPO, check that box and then indicate if the patient is receiving nutrition via NG, PEG/PEJ, or total parenteral nutrition (TPN).

- *History/Duration of Swallowing Problems* — If the patient is in an acute care facility, this may simply state "since admit." If the patient is in another type of facility, note the date and related cause of the swallowing disorder. For example, "Patient has been unable to swallow w/o choking since CVA on 2/12/99."

- *Respiratory Status* — If the patient is receiving oxygen, check the box and then circle how the oxygen is being delivered. This might be via nasal cannula or a face mask. If the patient has a tracheostomy, the oxygen will be at the trach via trach collar. Determine if the patient has had a recent intubation and how long the intubation lasted. Write a note if it was a traumatic emergency intubation. If the patient has a tracheostomy, note when the surgery was done and the type of trach placed. If the patient is on a ventilator, list number of hours/day patient is mechanically ventilated and whether your evaluation was completed while the patient was on or off the vent. You will also want to note if the cuff on the trach tube was inflated or deflated during the evaluation and if the patient wore a tracheostomy speaking valve.

Dysphagia Diagnosis

List your diagnosis and the swallowing phases affected. For example, you might write, "moderate oral dysphagia with anterior loss and pocketing. Suspected pharyngeal dysphagia with clinical signs of aspiration including coughing and wet vocal quality." If you're using a team approach, have all therapists list their diagnoses here. For example, OT might write "impaired ability to self feed related to decreased visual perception."

Long-Term/Functional Goals

Circle all goals appropriate for the patient. More than one goal may be appropriate. For example, goals 1 and 3 might be addressed at the same time. Also indicate the period of time for which the goals are being set.

Recommendations

You may want to make some of your recommendations pending the results of an instrumental exam. If you aren't certain the patient is safe to eat by mouth, defer those recommendations until the instrumental exam confirms that it is safe to proceed. Mark any pending recommendations with an asterisk (*). For example, you may have decided that the patient can only handle a pureed diet because of significant problems in the oral phase of swallowing. You suspect that the patient is aspirating that texture, so an * is placed next to that recommendation until you have more information.

Bedside Dysphagia Evaluation – Summary Sheet for Speech-Language Pathology – Form A

Date _____ Patient _____

Admit Date _____ Physician _____

Admit Diagnosis _____

Medical History _____
_____

Medications _____

Current Method of Nutrition: ❐ PO _____ diet ❐ NPO NG/PEG/TPN

History/Duration of Swallowing Problems _____
_____

Respiratory Status: ❐ O$_2$ nasal/face mask/trach collar ❐ Intubated from _____ to _____
❐ Trach placed on _____ Trach type _____ ❐ Ventilatory support: _____ hours
❐ Eval done with patient on/off vent ❐ Cuff inflated/deflated ❐ Passy-Muir valve on/off

Dysphagia Diagnosis _____
_____

Long-Term/Functional Goals (Circle goals to be addressed.)

These goals are set for a _____ time period.
1. Patient will safely consume _____ diet with _____ liquids without complications such as aspiration pneumonia.
2. Patient will be able to eat foods and liquids with more normal consistency.
3. Patient will be able to complete a meal in less than _____ minutes.
4. Patient will maintain nutrition/hydration via alternative methods.
5. Patient's quality of life will be enhanced through eating and drinking small amounts of food and liquid.

Recommendations

_____ NPO — consider alternative feeding: _____
_____ NPO until instrumental exam
_____ trial therapeutic feeding only (no meal trays)
_____ tube feedings will be held a minimum of two hours before each meal
_____ PO: _____
      liquids: _____ spoon / cup / straw
      meds: _____
_____ supplemental tube feedings
_____ SLP to treat _____ meals/day
_____ no therapeutic feeding by SLP indicated
_____ instrumental exam ❐ MBS ❐ FEES®
_____ Speech/language eval
_____ OT eval
_____ ENT consult re: _____
_____ re-eval pending: _____
_____ positioning/feeding precautions as posted
      _____ chin-down   _____ upright 90°   _____ liquid wash
      _____ head rotation R/L   _____ multiple swallows
_____ reflux precautions
_____ Dietitian to interview patient/family to determine food preferences
_____ calorie count
_____ review chart for spiked temps
_____ feed with trach cuff   up / down
       Passy-Muir   off / on
_____ suction per trach after each meal
_____ other: _____
_____ Treatment by SLP (See Treatment Plan)

> *Recommendations marked with * are pending results of an instrumental exam revealing if patient is safe to eat.

Patient/Family Teaching Goals

Was patient/family teaching completed? ❐ yes ❐ no
(See *Teaching Fact Sheet for PO Feeding*.)

_____
Speech-Language Pathologist

Bedside Dysphagia Evaluation – Summary Sheet for Speech-Language Pathology and Occupational Therapy – Form B

Date_____ Patient _____

Admit Date_____ Physician _____

Admit Diagnosis _____

Medical History _____

_____

Medications _____

Current Method of Nutrition: ❐ PO _____ diet ❐ NPO NG/PEG/TPN

History/Duration of Swallowing Problems _____

_____

Respiratory Status: ❐ O$_2$ nasal/face mask/trach collar   ❐ Intubated from _____ to _____

❐ Trach placed on _____ Trach type _____ ❐ Ventilatory support: _____ hours

❐ Eval done with patient on/off vent   ❐ Cuff inflated/deflated   ❐ Passy-Muir valve on/off

Dysphagia Diagnosis _____

_____

Long-Term/Functional Goals (Circle goals to be addressed.)

These goals are set for a _____ time period.

1. Patient will safely consume _____ diet with _____ liquids without complications such as aspiration pneumonia.
2. Patient will be able to eat foods and liquids with more normal consistency.
3. Patient will be able to complete a meal in less than _____ minutes.
4. Patient will maintain nutrition/hydration via alternative methods.
5. Patient's quality of life will be enhanced through eating and drinking small amounts of food and liquid.

Recommendations

_____ NPO — consider alternative feeding: _____

_____ NPO until instrumental exam

_____ trial therapeutic feeding only (no meal trays)

_____ tube feedings will be held a minimum of two hours before each meal

_____ PO: _____

     liquids: _____ spoon / cup / straw

     meds: _____

_____ supplemental tube feedings

_____ SLP to treat _____ meals/day   OT to treat _____ meals/day

_____ no therapeutic feeding by SLP indicated   _____ no treatment at meals by OT

_____ instrumental exam   ❐ MBS   ❐ FEES®

_____ Speech/language eval

_____ OT eval

_____ ENT consult re: _____

_____ re-eval pending: _____

_____ positioning/feeding precautions as posted

    _____ chin-down   _____ upright 90°   _____ liquid wash

    _____ head rotation R/L   _____ multiple swallows

_____ reflux precautions

_____ Dietitian to interview patient/family to determine food preferences

_____ calorie count

_____ review chart for spiked temps

_____ feed with trach cuff   up / down

    Passy-Muir   off / on

_____ suction per trach after each meal

_____ other: _____

_____ Treatment by SLP (See Treatment Plan)   _____ Treatment by OT (See Treatment Plan)

> *Recommendations marked with * are pending results of an instrumental exam revealing if patient is safe to eat.

Patient/Family Teaching Goals

Was patient/family teaching completed?   ❐ yes   ❐ no

(See *Teaching Fact Sheet for PO Feeding*.)

_____
Occupational Therapist

_____
Speech-Language Pathologist

Sample – Form A

Date _____ Patient Fred _____
Admit Date _____ Physician _____
Admit Diagnosis (L) CVA _____
Medical History ASCVD, HTN, IDDM _____
_____
Medications N/A _____
Current Method of Nutrition: ❑ PO _____ diet   ☑ NPO (NG) PEG/TPN given ice chips
History/Duration of Swallowing Problems since admit with CVA; referred by M.D. for "choking" _____
_____
Respiratory Status: ☑ O₂ (nasal) face mask/trach collar   ❑ Intubated from _____ to _____
       ❑ Trach placed on _____   Trach type _____   ❑ Ventilatory support: _____ hours
       ❑ Eval done with patient on/off vent   ❑ Cuff inflated/deflated   ❑ Passy-Muir valve on/off

Dysphagia Diagnosis oral dysphagia, suspected pharyngeal dysphagia _____
_____

Long-Term/Functional Goals (Circle goals to be addressed.)

These goals are set for a _____ one month _____ time period.
1. Patient will safely consume _____ pureed _____ diet with _____ honey thick _____ liquids without complications such as aspiration pneumonia.
2. Patient will be able to eat foods and liquids with more normal consistency.
3. Patient will be able to complete a meal in less than _____ minutes.
4. Patient will maintain nutrition/hydration via alternative methods.
5. Patient's quality of life will be enhanced through eating and drinking small amounts of food and liquid.

Recommendations

_____ NPO — consider alternative feeding: _____
✓ NPO until instrumental exam
_____ trial therapeutic feeding only (no meal trays)
✓ tube feedings will be held a minimum of two hours before each meal
*✓ PO: _____ pureed _____
    liquids: honey thick _____ (spoon) / cup / straw
    meds: crush and mix
_____ supplemental tube feedings
✓ SLP to treat _____ 2 _____ meals/day
_____ no therapeutic feeding by SLP indicated
✓ instrumental exam   ☑ MBS   ❑ FEES®
✓ Speech/language eval
_____ OT eval
_____ ENT consult re: _____
_____ re-eval pending: _____
✓ positioning/feeding precautions as posted
    ✓ chin-down   ✓ upright 90º   _____ liquid wash
    _____ head rotation R/L   ✓ multiple swallows
_____ reflux precautions
_____ Dietitian to interview patient/family to determine food preferences
_____ calorie count
_____ review chart for spiked temps
_____ feed with trach cuff   up / down
    Passy-Muir   off / on
_____ suction per trach after each meal
_____ other: _____
✓ Treatment by SLP (See Treatment Plan)

> *Recommendations marked with * are pending results of an instrumental exam revealing if patient is safe to eat.

Patient/Family Teaching Goals

Was patient/family teaching completed?   ☑ yes   ❑ no
(See *Teaching Fact Sheet for PO Feeding*.)

_____
Speech-Language Pathologist

Directions for Bedside Dysphagia Evaluation for All Care Settings – Form C

Oral-Motor Evaluation

Examining a patient's ability to use oral-motor skills in isolation does not necessarily tell how the patient will be able to use these same structures for swallowing. Therefore, this oral-motor examination is fairly brief, but is a good precursor to examining the use of the same structures when food is presented. Remember to wear gloves when performing any oral-motor evaluation.

1. **Structure**
   Carefully examine for any structural abnormalities of the lips, tongue, gums, and hard and soft palates.

   Find out if the patient has no teeth (edentulous) and if so, note if the patient has dentures and if he usually eats with his dentures. You may be surprised at the textures many individuals can eat if they've been without teeth for a long period of time.

   Note whether or not dentures are worn during your evaluation. If the patient wants to wear dentures, you may need to clean the dentures and help the patient put them in.

   If the patient has had a stroke with hemiparesis, he will probably try to put the dentures in the side of his mouth in which he still has feeling, catching the denture on the side of the mouth in which he has no feeling. You may need to assist him in getting the dentures into his mouth, starting on the weaker side.

   Sometimes the patient doesn't want to put the dentures in for an evaluation. If he hasn't worn them for a while, they may not fit or they may even cause some gagging.

2. **Awareness/Control of Secretions**
   Note if the patient is unable to control secretions with drooling or is retaining secretions in the mouth. Listen to the patient's quiet breathing before you begin your exam to determine if the patient has a gurgly, wet sound to his breathing, possibly indicating he is not swallowing his own secretions.

3. **Assessing Jaw, Lips, and Tongue**
   Circle + if the movements assessed appear within normal limits. Note decreased movement by circling — followed by ( ) indicating whether it is decreased in strength (S), speed (SP), amplitude (A), accuracy (AC), or if groping movements indicate apraxia (APR). Use a ✓ if an abnormal characteristic is noted like asymmetry. CNA indicates that you could not assess. Circle this if you could not assess that area (e.g., laryngeal function) at all.

   Jaw Control
   Assess the patient's ability to open his jaw adequately and to maintain good jaw closure.

   Labial Function
   Assess the patient's range of motion when asked to repeat /i/ and /u/. Note lip closure at rest, indicating if there is symmetry or droop on either side. Have the patient repeat /pʌpʌpʌ/. Note lip closure during this activity. Have the patient smack his lips. Observe for strength and symmetry. Also note lip closure during repetition of sentence or connected speech. Remember that the ability to use the articulators for speech does **not** have a direct correlation to the ability to use the articulators for swallowing.

Lingual Function

You may demonstrate any of the following tasks if the patient does not understand your instructions.

protrusion/retraction — Ask the patient to stick his tongue out as far as he can and then retract it entirely within his mouth.

lick lips — Ask the patient to lick his lips all the way around in a circular motion.

lateralization to corners — Ask the patient to touch the tip of his tongue to each corner of his lips.

lateralization to buccal cavity — Ask the patient to put his tongue in the lower buccal cavity on either side.

elevation of tip — Ask the patient to place his tongue tip on his alveolar ridge with his mouth open and jaw steady.

elevation of back — Have the patient produce /k/ with as much force as possible.

repetitive elevation of tip — Have the patient repeat /tʌ tʌ tʌ / as sharply as possible.

repetitive elevation of back — Ask the patient to repeat /kʌ kʌ kʌ /, making each sound as sharp as possible.

fine lingual shaping — Ask the patient to repeat a sentence such as "Say something nice to Susan on Sunday." Listen to how carefully articulated the phrase is. Remember that the ability to use the articulators for speech does not have a direct correlation to the ability to use the articulators for swallowing.

4. Velar Function

Using a tongue depressor to stabilize the tongue and a penlight to visualize the oral cavity, ask the patient to produce a prolonged /a/. Watch for symmetry on elevation of the velum. Listen to the patient's resonance in connected speech or have him repeat "my pie" several times.

5. Reflexes

Swallow Reflex

Place a small amount of iced water (a drop or two) near the anterior faucial arch through a pipette and ask the patient to swallow. This can also be accomplished without giving the patient anything and just asking him to swallow. If the oral cavity is very dry, you may need to stop and clean the patient's mouth (oral care) before the patient will be able to elicit a swallow.

Gag Reflex

Although there is no data to support a relationship between gag and swallowing ability (Leder, 1996, 1997; Davies et al., 1995), it should be tested to provide more information about the patient's sensation. The gag reflex is elicited by touching the back of the tongue or posterior pharyngeal wall with a tongue blade or laryngeal mirror. Watch for symmetrical contraction of the pharyngeal wall and soft palate. Any asymmetry may indicate a unilateral pharyngeal weakness (Logemann, 1998). If your patient is less than cooperative, you may want to forego testing the gag reflex.

Palatal Reflex
Test for the palatal reflex by touching a cold laryngeal mirror to the juncture of the hard and soft palate (DeJong, 1967). You should see the soft palate move up and back, but the pharyngeal walls should not move.

Laryngeal Examination

Tracheostomy Tube — If the patient has a tracheostomy, identify the type of tracheostomy tube and whether it is cuffed. Also indicate whether you used finger occlusion or the patient had a Passy-Muir valve or other tracheostomy speaking valve on for the assessment.

Vocal Quality — Note the patient's vocal quality during conversation before any food is given. A breathy vocal quality may indicate decreased vocal fold closure. Wet quality may be related to poor management of secretions.

Voluntary Cough — Note if the patient coughs spontaneously. If not, ask the patient to cough.

Throat Clearing — Note if the patient clears his throat spontaneously. If not, ask the patient to clear his throat.

Pitch Range — It's important to assess the patient's ability to control his pitch range as this indicates his ability to elevate his larynx. Ask the patient to sing /a/ up the scale. Indicate the number of notes the patient is able to produce.

Volume Control — Ask the patient to count from 1 to 5, starting quietly on 1 and getting louder on each number.

Phonation Time — Ask the patient to take in a breath and prolong /a/. Count how many seconds the patient is able to prolong phonation. Normal phonation time is 12 - 15 seconds.

Valving for Speech — Have the patient repeat sentences or listen to the patient's conversational speech and determine how many syllables per breath group the patient typically produces. The average production is 12 - 15 syllables per breath group.

Respiratory Status

Patients with respiratory disorders (e.g., chronic obstructive pulmonary disease, dyspnea) may have difficulty coordinating a swallow with their breathing. In addition, patients with compromised respiratory status may fatigue very easily. They may exhibit better skills at the beginning of the meal and compromised skills as they fatigue. Most people with normal swallowing skills hold their breath for a swallow during the exhalation phase. Observe if the patient is doing that or is stopping in the middle of an inhalation.

See if the patient can hold his breath at all, as this may be needed if the patient is to use the supraglottic or super-supraglottic swallow. Observe if the patient is breathing through his mouth or nose. If the patient is a mouth breather, it may be difficult for him to stop breathing while he chews and swallows.

Cognition/Communication

Orientation — Ask the patient to identify the day, date, year, and place.

One-Step Directions — Ask the patient to follow some basic one-step commands such as "Close your eyes," "Point to the door," and "Pick up the spoon." Note whether these commands are followed accurately or if cues are required.

Two-Step Directions — Ask the patient to follow several two-step commands such as "Open your mouth and touch your head" or "Point to the door and pick up the fork." Again note whether these commands are followed accurately or if cues are required

Expressive Language — Provide a judgment about the patient's basic expressive skills.

Intelligibility — Indicate whether intelligibility is impaired by the presence of dysarthria, apraxia, or confused speech.

Short-Term Memory — If the patient is going to have to use any techniques to assure safe swallowing, indicate whether the patient is able to restate them.

Hearing Acuity — Note if the patient's hearing has been informally or formally assessed. Add any observation about hearing acuity that may interfere with dysphagia treatment. For example, does the patient fail to follow a direction because he can't hear it accurately? Also note whether the patient wears hearing aids and if he is wearing them during the evaluation.

Swallowing

Indicate the variety of textures tried with the patient. If the patient shows adequate skill, indicate **+**. If there's a problem with the skill, indicate **—**. Use **N/A** if it's not applicable for that texture.

Note that some of the blocks are divided by diagonal lines. If you use a compensatory technique with a specific texture, note which compensatory technique you used with the appropriate two-letter code below the diagonal line. Indicate **+** if the technique was successful in eliminating the problem and **—** if it was not helpful.

If the compensatory technique was simply using a different texture, record this information in a blank column.

When presenting liquids, use a separate column each time you use a different method of presentation (e.g., spoon, cup, cut-out cup) and indicate with the appropriate abbreviation.

Ability to prepare bolus
To prepare a bolus, several specific skills are needed. The patient must be able to maintain adequate *labial closure* to prevent anterior loss of the bolus. In addition, adequate labial closure helps to keep the bolus from falling into the anterior lateral sulcus (between gums and teeth). *Lingual elevation* is necessary to scoop the bolus, particularly liquid boluses, from the floor of the mouth so they are on the tongue. *Lingual lateralization* is necessary to move the bolus from midline to the chewing surface and from the chewing surface back to midline. *Mastication* skills are required for many textures to prepare an adequate bolus.

Ability to manipulate bolus

To manipulate the bolus from front to back, adequate *lingual function* is necessary. In addition, the patient's *oral transit time* should be observed. The average time to move a bolus from the front of the oral cavity to the back is one second or less.

Ability to maintain bolus

While the patient is preparing the bolus and manipulating the bolus, he must keep the bolus on the tongue and avoid pocketing in the sulci. In addition, he must maintain the bolus to prevent either premature loss over the back of the tongue or anterior loss. However, our previous belief that no food passed over the back of the tongue during mastication was questioned by Hiiemae et al. (1999) who provided a description of how people with normal swallowing skills handle masticated foods. It seems that normal individuals move small parts of the bolus over the back of their tongues while they continue to chew the rest of the bolus. The accumulated bolus on the pharyngeal surface of the tongue is maintained there during that additional chewing without the help of the soft palate. From a screening perspective at bedside, we want to observe any behaviors that might lead us to believe that the food is not remaining on the pharyngeal surface of the tongue, but has prematurely fallen into the airway. Therefore, assess for *back of tongue control* and make a judgment as to whether any of the material may be falling over the back of the tongue in a premature fashion. This might be indicated by a cough before the swallow. You can only make a supposition about this. *Labial closure* is more easily assessed because you can observe for anterior loss. You can also observe for *decreased tone in the cheeks* as the patient will demonstrate pocketing in the sulci. *Lingual lateralization* skills will allow the patient to return the bolus to the midline of the tongue.

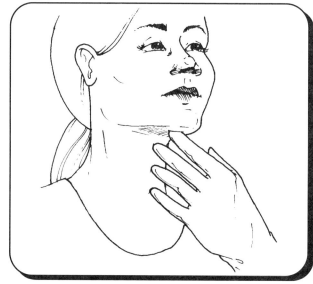

After the swallow, check to see if the oral cavity is empty to determine if the patient is able to *clear his oral cavity with one swallow*. If not, note the *number of swallows per bolus* necessary for the patient to clear his oral cavity. One good way to monitor this is to place the forefinger of one hand immediately under the patient's chin, the middle finger under the chin near the base of the tongue, and the ring finger and small finger on the larynx to monitor laryngeal elevation, indicating a probable swallow.

Pharyngeal Phase

When the head of the bolus passes over the back of the tongue, the swallowing reflex should occur within one second. Some patients exhibit a delay in the initiation of the reflex. When this occurs, the bolus falls to the valleculae and sometimes all the way to the pyriform sinuses before the reflex is initiated. A delayed reflex can only be accurately judged with videofluoroscopy. Once the head of the bolus passes the back of the tongue at the point of the mandible, you can start counting the time before the swallow is initiated. At bedside, you can make a rough guess about reflex initiation by counting the time from when the patient stops moving his tongue until you feel laryngeal elevation.

Laryngeal Characteristics

After the patient's swallow, assess his *vocal quality*. A gurgly vocal quality can indicate possible penetration or aspiration. Also note any *coughing or throat clearing* (+ indicates presence of coughing/throat clearing) and give an estimation of adequacy of *elevation of the larynx* (+ indicates adequate elevation). This is very difficult to judge at bedside.

Short-Term Goals/Treatment Objectives

Circle the appropriate oral phase short-term goal(s) and then write in the abbreviation codes for the treatment objectives you have chosen. (See Chapter 7, pages 182-197.) Indicate the period of time for which these goals apply. Pharyngeal phase goals are not included on this bedside screening since they cannot accurately be determined without an instrumental exam. You may write in some pharyngeal goals if you want to begin to work on them while you await the instrumental exam. For instance, if the patient presents with a very breathy vocal quality and weak cough, you might choose to begin work on laryngeal closure activities or teach the super-supraglottic swallow so that the patient will be able to perform the technique if needed during the instrumental exam.

Bedside Dysphagia Evaluation for All Settings – Form C

Patient _____ Date _____

Facility _____ SLP _____

Oral-Motor Evaluation   ❑ CNA

1. Structure
   Note any abnormalities _____

edentulous	yes	no	dentures	yes	no
wears dentures when eating	yes	no	dentures in during eval	yes	no

2. Awareness/Control of Secretions

   _____ drooling   _____ excess secretions in mouth   _____ wet breath sounds

3. Assessing Jaw, Lips, and Tongue

   Jaw Control   CNA   + / —

   Labial Function   CNA

lip spread /i/	+ / —		lip round /u/	+ / —
lip closure at rest			lip smacking	+ / —
symmetry	+ / —		lip closure on /pʌpʌpʌ/	+ / —
droop	R L			

   sentence (*Please put the paper by the back door.*) + / —

   Lingual Function   CNA

protrusion	+ / —		retraction	+ / —
lick lips	+ / —		lateralization to corners	R + / — L + / —
lateralization to buccal cavity	R + / — L + / —		elevation of tip	+ / —
elevation of back	+ / —		repetitive elevation of tip	+ / —
repetitive elevation of back	+ / —			

   fine lingual shaping (*Say something nice to Susan on Sunday.*)   + / —

4. Velar Function   CNA

   prolonged /a/: symmetry during elevation   + / —

   Resonance: _____ normal   _____ hypernasal   _____ hyponasal

5. Reflexes   CNA

   swallow reflex   + / —   gag reflex   + / —   palatal reflex   + / —

Laryngeal Examination   ❑ CNA

Tracheostomy Tube: _____   yes   no

   cuffed   yes   no

   finger occluded   PM valve   other _____

Vocal Quality: normal   hoarse   breathy   wet

Voluntary Cough: strong   weak   absent

Throat Clearing: strong   weak   absent

Pitch Range: # of notes _____

Volume Control: noticeable change in loudness   + / —   ability to control loudness   + / —

Phonation Time: # seconds prolonged /a/ _____

Valving for Speech: # syllables/breath group _____

Respiratory Status   ❑ CNA

Patient swallows during inhalation/exhalation.   Patient can hold breath for _____ seconds.

Patient breathes from nose/mouth.

Cognition/Communication   ❑ CNA

Orientation	day _____	date _____	year _____	place _____
Follows One-Step Directions	+ / —	with cues	without cues	
Follows Two-Step Directions	+ / —	with cues	without cues	
Expressive Language	gestures/points	uses single words	uses phrases	
Intelligibility	unintelligible	dysarthria	apraxia	confused speech

Short-Term Memory

   Can patient retell techniques?   yes   no

Hearing Acuity _____

wears hearing aid(s)	yes	no	right _____	left _____	
hearing aid(s) in for eval	yes	no			

Comments: _____

Patient _____ Patient # _____

Swallowing

	Key					Compensatory Techniques	
+	skill is adequate		S	straw		TS	thermal stimulation
—	skill is inadequate		SP	spoon		CD	chin down
N/A	not applicable for that texture		C	cup		HR	head rotation
			CO	cut-out cup		BS	bolus size
						EP	external pressure

Texture								
Ability to prepare bolus								
labial closure	+ / —							
lingual elevation	+ / —							
lingual lateralization	+ / —							
mastication	+ / —							
Ability to manipulate bolus								
lingual function	+ / —							
oral transit time	+ / —							
Ability to maintain bolus								
back of tongue control	+ / —							
labial closure	+ / —							
cheeks	+ / —							
lingual lateralization	+ / —							
clears oral cavity in one swallow	+ / —							
# swallows per bolus								
Pharyngeal Phase								
initiate reflex in _____ seconds	+ / —							
Laryngeal Characteristics								
vocal quality	+/describe							
cough/throat clearing	+ / —							
elevation of larynx	+ / —							

Comments _____

Oral Phase Short-Term Goals/Treatment Objectives

(Circle goals to be addressed.) These goals are for ____ days/weeks. For related treatment objectives, see SLP Treatment Plan.

1. (AL/jc)	Patient will improve jaw closure to reduce anterior loss to keep food and liquid in the mouth while eating.	
2. (AL/lc)	Patient will improve lip closure to reduce anterior loss to keep food and liquid in the mouth while eating.	
3. (AL/os)	Patient's oral sensation will improve to reduce anterior loss to keep food in the mouth while eating.	
4. (BF/os)	Patient's oral sensation will increase to improve the ability to put food/liquid into a cohesive bolus to reduce the risk of food residue falling into the airway.	
5. (BF/tm)	Patient will increase tongue movement to improve the ability to put food and liquid into a cohesive bolus to reduce the risk of food falling into the airway.	
6. (BF/tc)	The tone in patient's cheek(s) will increase to improve the ability to put food and liquid into a cohesive bolus to reduce the risk of food residue falling into the airway.	
7. (BP/tm)	Patient will increase tongue movement to improve the ability to move a bolus to the back of the mouth in a coordinated fashion to reduce the risk of it falling into the airway.	
8. (BP/oc)	Patient will increase oral coordination to improve the ability to move a bolus to the back of the mouth in a coordinated fashion to reduce the risk of it falling into the airway.	
9. (BP/os)	Patient's oral sensation will increase to improve the ability to move a bolus to the back of the mouth in a coordinated fashion to reduce the risk of it falling into the airway.	
10. (BP/ag)	Patient will increase awareness of food/liquid and utensils in the mouth to improve the ability to move a bolus to the back of the mouth in a coordinated fashion to reduce the risk of it falling into the airway.	

_____ _____ _____ _____
Speech-Language Pathologist   Date   Time   Procedure

Sample – Form C

Patient __Fred__   Date _____

Facility _____ SLP _____

Oral-Motor Evaluation   ☐ CNA

1. Structure

   Note any abnormalities _____

   edentulous   (yes) no   dentures   (yes) no

   wears dentures when eating   (yes) no   dentures in during eval   (yes) no

2. Awareness/Control of Secretions

   _____ drooling   _____ excess secretions in mouth   ✓ wet breath sounds

3. Assessing Jaw, Lips, and Tongue

   Jaw Control   CNA   (+) —

   Labial Function   CNA

   lip spread /i/   (+) —   lip round /u/   + /(—) (A)

   lip closure at rest   lip smacking *CNA - oral apraxia* + / —

     symmetry   + /(—)   lip closure on /pΛpΛpΛ/   CNA   + / —

     droop   (R) L

   sentence (*Please put the paper by the back door.*) + / —

   Lingual Function   CNA

   protrusion   (+) —   retraction   + / —

   lick lips   (+) —   lateralization to corners   R (+) —   L (+) —

   lateralization to buccal cavity R (+)/ —   L (+) — elevation of tip   + /(—) (SP)

   elevation of back   (+) —   repetitive elevation of tip   + /(—) (SP)

   repetitive elevation of back   + (—) (A)

   fine lingual shaping (*Say something nice to Susan on Sunday.*)   + /(—) (AC)

4. Velar Function   CNA

   prolonged /a/: symmetry during elevation (+) —

   Resonance: ✓ normal   _____ hypernasal   _____ hyponasal

5. Reflexes   CNA

   swallow reflex (+)/ —   gag reflex + (—)   palatal reflex (+)/ —

Laryngeal Examination   ☐ CNA

Tracheostomy Tube: _____   yes   (no)

  cuffed   yes   no

  finger occluded   PM valve   other _____

Vocal Quality: normal   hoarse   breathy   (wet)

Voluntary Cough: (strong)   weak   absent

Throat Clearing: (strong)   weak   absent

Pitch Range: # of notes ___3___

Volume Control: noticeable change in loudness (+) —   ability to control loudness + / —

Phonation Time: # seconds prolonged /a/ ___6___

Valving for Speech: # syllables/breath group ___DNA___

Respiratory Status   ☐ CNA

Patient swallows during inhalation/(exhalation)   Patient can hold breath for __4__ seconds.

Patient breathes from (nose)/mouth.

Cognition/Communication   ☐ CNA

Orientation   day ___✓___   date ___✓___   year ___✓___   place ___✓___

Follows One-Step Directions   (+) —   with cues   without cues

Follows Two-Step Directions   + /(—)   with cues   without cues

Expressive Language   (gestures/points)   (uses single words)   uses phrases

Intelligibility   (unintelligible)   (dysarthria)   apraxia   confused speech

Short-Term Memory

  Can patient retell techniques?   yes   (no) *but he's alert* _____

Hearing Acuity __appears adequate__

  wears hearing aid(s)   yes   (no)   right _____   left _____

  hearing aid(s) in for eval yes   no

Comments: _____

Patient __Fred__   Patient # _____

Swallowing

Key						Compensatory Techniques	
+	skill is adequate		S	straw		TS	thermal stimulation
—	skill is inadequate		SP	spoon		CD	chin down
N/A	not applicable for that texture		C	cup		HR	head rotation
			CO	cut-out cup		BS	bolus size
						EP	external pressure

Texture		liquids	pureed	eggs	honey		
Ability to prepare bolus							
labial closure	+ / —	—	—	—	—		
lingual elevation	+ / —	+	+	+	+		
lingual lateralization	+ / —	N/A	+	+	+		
mastication	+ / —	N/A	N/A	—	N/A		
Ability to manipulate bolus							
lingual function	+ / —	+	+	—	+		
oral transit time	+ / —	+	+	—	+		
Ability to maintain bolus							
back of tongue control	+ / —	— CO+	+	+	+		
labial closure	+ / —	—	—	—	—		
cheeks	+ / —	— EP+	EP+	EP+	EP+		
lingual lateralization	+ / —	N/A	+	+	+		
clears oral cavity in one swallow	+ / —	—	—	—	—		
# swallows per bolus		2	2	2-3	2		
Pharyngeal Phase							
initiate reflex in _____ seconds	+ / —						
Laryngeal Characteristics							
vocal quality	+/describe	wet	wet	wet	wet		
cough/throat clearing	+ / —	+	+	+	+		
elevation of larynx	+ / —	+	+	+	+		

Comments _____

Oral Phase Short-Term Goals/Treatment Objectives

(Circle goals to be addressed.) These goals are for __2__ days/weeks. For related treatment objectives, see SLP Treatment Plan.

1.	(AL/jc)	Patient will improve jaw closure to reduce anterior loss to keep food and liquid in the mouth while eating.	
2.	(AL/lc)	Patient will improve lip closure to reduce anterior loss to keep food and liquid in the mouth while eating.	Tx Obj 1, 2, 4, 6
3.	(AL/os)	Patient's oral sensation will improve to reduce anterior loss to keep food in the mouth while eating.	
4.	(BF/os)	Patient's oral sensation will increase to improve the ability to put food/liquid into a cohesive bolus to reduce the risk of food residue falling into the airway.	
5.	(BF/tm)	Patient will increase tongue movement to improve the ability to put food and liquid into a cohesive bolus to reduce the risk of food falling into the airway.	
6.	(BF/tc)	The tone in patient's cheek(s) will increase to improve the ability to put food and liquid into a cohesive bolus to reduce the risk of food residue falling into the airway.	Tx Obj 1, 2, 3, 6, 9
7.	(BP/tm)	Patient will increase tongue movement to improve the ability to move a bolus to the back of the mouth in a coordinated fashion to reduce the risk of it falling into the airway.	
8.	(BP/oc)	Patient will increase oral coordination to improve the ability to move a bolus to the back of the mouth in a coordinated fashion to reduce the risk of it falling into the airway.	Tx Obj 2, 3
9.	(BP/os)	Patient's oral sensation will increase to improve the ability to move a bolus to the back of the mouth in a coordinated fashion to reduce the risk of it falling into the airway.	
10.	(BP/ag)	Patient will increase awareness of food/liquid and utensils in the mouth to improve the ability to move a bolus to the back of the mouth in a coordinated fashion to reduce the risk of it falling into the airway.	

Speech-Language Pathologist	Date	Time	Procedure

Sample Narrative Summary 1 (Fred) _____

Note: The superscript numbers correspond to the Medicare Guidelines on page 45.

History

Patient is a 68-year-old male who suffered a left CVA with resultant right hemiparesis, aphasia, dysarthria, and dysphagia. His medical history also includes arteriosclerotic cardiovascular disease, hypertension, and diabetes.[3A] Patient is currently being fed via NG and is NPO except for ice chips.[3B] Referred by physician to rule out dysphagia before trying PO.[1]

Cognition/Communication

Patient is alert and responsive.[2A] Patient follows basic one-step commands when given gestural cues. Patient has basic yes/no response to simple questions.[2C] Patient is attempting some single-word responses but speech is very unintelligible. Patient indicates he wants to eat.[2B]

Oral Phase

Patient has poor lip closure which results in an inability to keep the food in his mouth once presented.[2E] When he tries to masticate a bolus, he has a lot of residue in the right oral cavity.[2D] When external pressure is provided to the right cheek, patient is able to form a much better bolus.[4C] Without intervention, patient will not be able to eat normal foods.[5]

Pharyngeal Phase

Patient presents what appears to be adequate laryngeal elevation on palpation, however he presents a wet vocal quality. This wet vocal quality was present before the exam began and throughout.[3C] Patient coughed intermittently during the assessment. The wet vocal quality and intermittent cough are clinical signs of aspiration and if further evaluation is not completed and treatment is not initiated, this patient would appear to have a higher risk for aspiration and possibly developing aspiration pneumonia.[5] When patient is placed in chin-down posture, he appears to cough less frequently.[4C]

Diagnosis: Patient presents oral and pharyngeal dysphagia with suspected aspiration.[3D,E]

Recommendations[3F]

1. modified barium swallow to rule out aspiration and determine appropriate intervention techniques

2. treatment for oral-motor disorder

3. pureed diet and honey-thick liquids with one soft vegetable pending MBS results

4. treatment at meals by SLP

5. positioning precautions as posted

Directions for Bedside Dysphagia Evaluation – Summary for Skilled Nursing Facilities – Form D ———

Identifying Information

Medical Diagnosis — List the diagnosis that is related to the dysphagia.

Medical History — Include any other pertinent diagnoses that may have an effect on the patient's ability to perform during the evaluation and treatment. This must also include a statement of the dysphagia symptoms that prompted the referral.

Medications — Note if the patient is currently on, or has been on in the past, any medications which might reduce the level of alertness, cause confusion, or cause dry mouth.

Current Method of Nutrition — Check if the patient is receiving a PO diet, and then indicate what that diet is. If the patient is NPO, check that box and then indicate if the patient is receiving nutrition via NG, PEG/PEJ, or total parenteral nutrition (TPN).

Precautions — List any precautions for the patient like diet restrictions or positioning precautions post-surgery.

History/Duration of Swallowing Problems/Recent Change — Describe the problems the patient is having. Try to include the following if appropriate:

- history of aspiration
- oral-motor disorders
- structural lesion
- neuromotor disturbances
- post-surgical reaction
- significant weight loss
- other conditions

Swallowing Function Prior to Onset/Recent Change — Describe how the patient was able to eat before this most recent change.

Previous Evaluation/Treatment — Describe any treatment the patient has previously received for dysphagia.

Evaluation Findings/Summary

Summarize your clinical observations about the patient's swallowing. You might use a more specific checklist like Form C on pages 56-57 and then provide a brief summary here. Describe your observations of the oral and oral voluntary phases and hypotheses about pharyngeal phase performance including laryngeal function.

Positive Expectation to Begin Service — Describe why you think this patient is a good candidate for intervention. Is the patient alert, motivated to eat, cooperative?

Need for Skilled Service — Document why this patient needs your level of intervention to improve his swallowing skills. List what would happen to the patient without your intervention.

Dysphagia Diagnosis

Specifically list the disorder related to the phase of the swallow (e.g., moderate oral dysphagia with suspected pharyngeal dysphagia).

Recommendations

Check all that are applicable.

> *Frequency and Duration of Service* — List number of minutes per week you want to see the patient. Give a prediction of how long service will continue.

Discharge Plan

Specify when you plan to discharge the patient. This might include statements such as:

- "When short-term goals achieved."
- "When staff and family trained in all techniques to safely feed patient."
- "When patient returns to full PO safely."

The type of reimbursement and the setting may determine how many sessions/minutes you can provide over what length of time. You should begin planning for discharge from the minute you begin your assessment.

Long-Term Goals

Circle the long-term goal(s) appropriate for the patient. Sometimes more than one long-term goal may be selected. These goals are set for a one-month period since services have to be recertified monthly.

Short-Term Goals/Treatment Objectives

Circle the appropriate oral phase short-term goal(s) and then write in the abbreviation codes for the treatment objectives you have chosen. (See Chapter 7, pages 182-197.) These should be objectives you expect can be achieved in 30 days. Pharyngeal phase goals are not included on this bedside screening since they cannot accurately be determined without an instrumental exam. You may write in some pharyngeal goals if you want to begin to work on them while you await the instrumental exam. For instance, if the patient presents with a very breathy vocal quality and weak cough, you might choose to begin work on laryngeal closure activities, or teach the super-supraglottic swallow so that the patient will be able to perform the technique if needed during the instrumental exam.

Bedside Dysphagia Evaluation – Summary Sheet for Skilled Nursing Facilities – Form D

Date _____

Patient _____ Birthdate _____ Age _____

Physician _____ Room # _____

Medical Diagnosis _____

Medical History _____

Medications _____

Current Method of Nutrition: ❐ PO _____ diet ❐ NPO NG/PEG/TPN

Precautions _____

History/Duration of Swallowing Problems/Recent Change _____

Swallowing Function Prior to Onset/Recent Change _____

Previous Evaluation/Treatment _____

Evaluation Findings/Summary _____

_____

Positive Expectation to Begin Service _____

_____

Need for Skilled Service _____

_____

Dysphagia Diagnosis _____

_____

_____

Recommendations

_____ NPO — consider alternative feeding: _____

_____ NPO until instrumental exam

_____ trial therapeutic feeding only (no meal trays)

_____ tube feedings will be held a minimum of two hours before each meal

_____ PO: _____

     liquids: _____ spoon / cup / straw

     meds: _____

_____ supplemental tube feedings

_____ SLP to treat _____ meals/day   OT to treat _____ meals/day

_____ no therapeutic feeding by SLP indicated   _____ no treatment at meals by OT

_____ instrumental exam   ❐ MBS   ❐ FEES®

_____ Speech/language eval

_____ OT eval

_____ ENT consult re: _____

_____ re-eval pending: _____

_____ positioning/feeding precautions as posted

    _____ chin-down   _____ upright 90°   _____ liquid wash

    _____ head rotation R/L   _____ multiple swallows

_____ reflux precautions

_____ Dietitian to interview patient/family to determine food preferences

_____ calorie count

_____ review chart for spiked temps

_____ feed with trach cuff   up / down

        Passy-Muir   off / on

_____ suction per trach after each meal

_____ other: _____

> *Recommendations marked with * are pending results of an instrumental exam revealing if patient is safe to eat.

Bedside Dysphagia Evaluation – Form D, *continued*

Recommendations, *continued*

_____ Treatment by SLP (See Treatment Plan)   _____ Treatment by OT (See Treatment Plan)

_____ functional maintenance   _____ rehab dining

Frequency of service _____   Duration of service _____

Discharge Plan _____

_____

Long-Term Goals (Circle goals to be addressed.) ━━━━━━━━━━━━━━━━━━━━━━━━━━
These goals are set for a one-month time period.
1. Patient will safely consume _____ diet with _____ liquids without complications such as aspiration pneumonia.
2. Patient will be able to eat foods and liquids with more normal consistency.
3. Patient will be able to complete a meal in less than _____ minutes.
4. Patient will maintain nutrition/hydration via alternative methods.
5. Patient's quality of life will be enhanced through eating and drinking small amounts of food and liquid.
6. Patient's caregivers and family will demonstrate understanding of compensatory techniques to feed patient safely.

Oral Phase Short-Term Goals/Treatment Objectives ━━━━━━━━━━━━━━━━━━
(Circle goals to be addressed.) These goals are for _____ days/weeks. For related treatment objectives, see SLP Treatment Plan.

1.	(AL/jc)	Patient will improve jaw closure to reduce anterior loss to keep food and liquid in the mouth while eating.	
2.	(AL/lc)	Patient will improve lip closure to reduce anterior loss to keep food and liquid in the mouth while eating.	
3.	(AL/os)	Patient's oral sensation will improve to reduce anterior loss to keep food in the mouth while eating.	
4.	(BF/os)	Patient's oral sensation will increase to improve the ability to put food/liquid into a cohesive bolus to reduce the risk of food residue falling into the airway.	
5.	(BF/tm)	Patient will increase tongue movement to improve the ability to put food and liquid into a cohesive bolus to reduce the risk of food falling into the airway.	
6.	(BF/tc)	The tone in patient's cheek(s) will increase to improve the ability to put food and liquid into a cohesive bolus to reduce the risk of food residue falling into the airway.	
7.	(BP/tm)	Patient will increase tongue movement to improve the ability to move a bolus to the back of the mouth in a coordinated fashion to reduce the risk of it falling into the airway.	
8.	(BP/oc)	Patient will increase oral coordination to improve the ability to move a bolus to the back of the mouth in a coordinated fashion to reduce the risk of it falling into the airway.	
9.	(BP/os)	Patient's oral sensation will increase to improve the ability to move a bolus to the back of the mouth in a coordinated fashion to reduce the risk of it falling into the airway.	
10.	(BP/ag)	Patient will increase awareness of food/liquid and utensils in the mouth to improve the ability to move a bolus to the back of the mouth in a coordinated fashion to reduce the risk of it falling into the airway.	

_____   _____   _____
Speech-Language Pathologist   License #   Date

I certify the above patient requires therapy services, is under a plan of care established or reviewed every 30 days by me, and requires the above treatment specified on a continuing basis with the following changes:

Physician Notice: (Circle one)   I do / do not find it necessary to see this patient within the next 30 days.

_____   _____
Physician   Date

Date _____

Patient ___Ethel_____ Birthdate _____ Age __78__

Physician _____ Room # _____

Medical Diagnosis _Alzheimer's_____

Medical History _Diabetes, CHF_____
_referred by Dr. Davis for oral dysphagia and weight loss_____

Medications _____

Current Method of Nutrition: ☑ PO __reg_ diet ☐ NPO NG/PEG/TPN

Precautions _____

History/Duration of Swallowing Problems/Recent Change _lost 15 pounds over last 6 months on regular diet at home_

Swallowing Function Prior to Onset/Recent Change _prior to last 6 months, she ate without difficulty_

Previous Evaluation/Treatment _n/a_____

Evaluation Findings/Summary _Difficulty forming bolus with masticated foods. Holds food in oral cavity up to_
15 seconds. With increased pressure and pureed foods, she swallows after 8 seconds. Coughs with thin liquids.

Positive Expectation to Begin Service _Patient is cooperative with caregivers. Patient is alert and pleasant and likes_
to eat.

Need for Skilled Service _If patient's diet and food presentation aren't modified, she is at risk for aspiration and_
continued weight loss.

Dysphagia Diagnosis _moderate oral dysphagia, suspected pharyngeal dysphagia_

Recommendations

____	NPO — consider alternative feeding: _____
____	NPO until instrumental exam
____	trial therapeutic feeding only (no meal trays)
____	tube feedings will be held a minimum of two hours before each meal
✓	PO: _____pureed_____
	liquids: _honey thick_____ (spoon)(cup)/ straw
	meds: _crushed and mixed_____
____	supplemental tube feedings
____	SLP to treat _____ meals/day OT to treat _____ meals/day
____	no therapeutic feeding by SLP indicated ____ no treatment at meals by OT
✓	instrumental exam ☑ MBS ☐ FEES®
____	Speech/language eval
____	OT eval
____	ENT consult re: _____
____	re-eval pending: _____
✓	positioning/feeding precautions as posted
	____ chin-down ✓ upright 90° ____ liquid wash
	____ head rotation R/L ____ multiple swallows
____	reflux precautions
____	Dietitian to interview patient/family to determine food preferences
✓	calorie count
____	review chart for spiked temps
____	feed with trach cuff up / down
	Passy-Muir off / on
	suction per trach after each meal
✓	other: _added tactile stim to mouth_____

*Recommendations marked with * are
pending results of an instrumental
exam revealing if patient is safe to eat.

Sample – Form D, *continued*

Recommendations, *continued*

_____ Treatment by SLP (See Treatment Plan)   _____ Treatment by OT (See Treatment Plan)

✓ functional maintenance   ✓ rehab dining

Frequency of service _____90 mins/wk_____   Duration of service _____2 weeks_____

Discharge Plan When MBS completed and staff trained on techniques to feed patient safely
_____

Long-Term Goals (Circle goals to be addressed.)
These goals are set for a one-month time period.
1. Patient will safely consume _____pureed_____ diet with _____honey_____ liquids without complications such as aspiration pneumonia.
2. Patient will be able to eat foods and liquids with more normal consistency.
3. Patient will be able to complete a meal in less than _____ minutes.
4. Patient will maintain nutrition/hydration via alternative methods.
5. Patient's quality of life will be enhanced through eating and drinking small amounts of food and liquid.
6. Patient's caregivers and family will demonstrate understanding of compensatory techniques to feed patient safely.

Oral Phase Short-Term Goals/Treatment Objectives
(Circle goals to be addressed.) These goals are for _____ days/weeks. For related treatment objectives, see SLP Treatment Plan.

1. (AL/jc)	Patient will improve jaw closure to reduce anterior loss to keep food and liquid in the mouth while eating.	
2. (AL/lc)	Patient will improve lip closure to reduce anterior loss to keep food and liquid in the mouth while eating.	
3. (AL/os)	Patient's oral sensation will improve to reduce anterior loss to keep food in the mouth while eating.	
4. (BF/os)	Patient's oral sensation will increase to improve the ability to put food/liquid into a cohesive bolus to reduce the risk of food residue falling into the airway.	Tx Obj 6, 8, 10
5. (BF/tm)	Patient will increase tongue movement to improve the ability to put food and liquid into a cohesive bolus to reduce the risk of food falling into the airway.	
6. (BF/tc)	The tone in patient's cheek(s) will increase to improve the ability to put food and liquid into a cohesive bolus to reduce the risk of food residue falling into the airway.	
7. (BP/tm)	Patient will increase tongue movement to improve the ability to move a bolus to the back of the mouth in a coordinated fashion to reduce the risk of it falling into the airway.	
8. (BP/oc)	Patient will increase oral coordination to improve the ability to move a bolus to the back of the mouth in a coordinated fashion to reduce the risk of it falling into the airway.	
9. (BP/os)	Patient's oral sensation will increase to improve the ability to move a bolus to the back of the mouth in a coordinated fashion to reduce the risk of it falling into the airway.	
10. (BP/ag)	Patient will increase awareness of food/liquid and utensils in the mouth to improve the ability to move a bolus to the back of the mouth in a coordinated fashion to reduce the risk of it falling into the airway.	Tx Obj 1, 2, 3

_____   _____   _____
Speech-Language Pathologist   License #   Date

I certify the above patient requires therapy services, is under a plan of care established or reviewed every 30 days by me, and requires the above treatment specified on a continuing basis with the following changes:

Physician Notice: (Circle one)   I do / do not find it necessary to see this patient within the next 30 days.

_____   _____
Physician   Date

Sample Narrative Summary 2 (Ethel) _____

Note: The superscript numbers correspond to the Medicare Guidelines on page 45.

History

Patient is 78-year-old female just admitted to this facility after four-day hospital stay for UTI. Prior to that, she lived at home where she had a personal caregiver. She presents a diagnosis of Alzheimer's disease.[3A] She also presents diagnoses of diabetes and congestive heart failure. Patient was admitted on a regular diet.[3B] She has had a 15-pound weight loss over the last six months.[2E] She reportedly eats less than 1/4 of the food presented to her. Referred by the physician for dysphagia evaluation due to suspected problems in oral phase.[1]

Cognition/Communication

Patient is pleasantly confused. She is not oriented to time or place but still recognizes family members.[2C] She cannot follow any commands even with maximal cues. She is cooperative with caregivers.[2A] She enjoys mealtimes[2B] but is not able to self-feed.

Oral Phase

Patient removes food from spoon adequately but has difficulty forming a bolus if it is food that requires manipulation. She tends to hold the food a long time in her oral cavity, sometimes up to 15 seconds. She does not respond to verbal cues to swallow.[3C] When patient is presented with pureed textures and given added tactile stimulation in the oral cavity, she will initiate a swallow in approximately eight seconds.[2D] If diet is not modified, she will continue to be unable to eat enough food.[5]

Pharyngeal Phase

Patient does not initiate any laryngeal elevation until 15-20 seconds after the bolus is placed in her mouth. It is difficult to determine if patient is exhibiting a delayed pharyngeal swallow or a delay in oral swallow. She coughed on presentation of thin liquids indicating that she may be aspirating this consistency.[4D] She did not cough with honey consistency. If further evaluation is not completed, she may be at high risk for aspiration.[5]

Diagnosis: Moderate oral dysphagia with suspected pharyngeal dysphagia[3D,E]

Recommendations[3F]

1. modified barium swallow to rule out aspiration, assess for pharyngeal vs. oral delay and for appropriate intervention techniques

2. pureed diet with honey-thick liquids per spoon

Chapter 4

Education: Patient/Family, Staff, Physicians, Administrators, and Payers

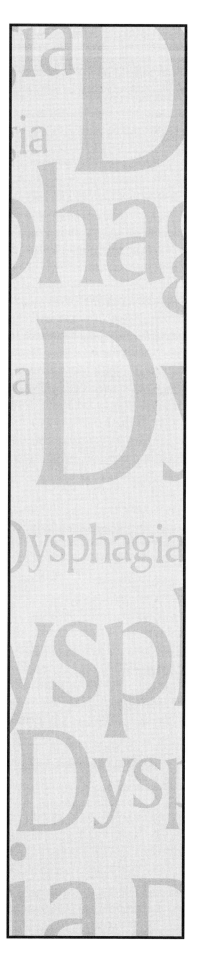

Education has always been an important part of the services provided by speech-language pathologists (SLPs). We educate patients and significant others whenever we have an opportunity to interact with them. We educate staff and physicians when we share information about specific patients and they use that information to plan the patient's care. Now, however, two new audiences have emerged who are in need of education about our services and the value of these services. It is critical that SLPs provide information to administrators about the value that dysphagia services add to the care of the patient. It is also important to share information about how dysphagia care can reduce the overall cost of treating patients. (For more information, see Chapter 10, pages 250-261.) Third-party payers are also very interested in the cost of the care provided as well as the results of that care. Education needs to be provided to payers to help them understand the importance of dysphagia management.

Why is it important to educate a patient's family about feeding precautions and compensatory techniques? You cannot be with a patient every time she is being given something to eat or drink. Very often when the family comes to visit, they give the patient some food or liquid. It is not unusual for them to bring homemade food or to buy something special for the patient to eat. It is also not unusual for this special treat to be unsafe for the patient, given dietary restrictions or feeding precautions.

It is important that the patient and family understand the recommendations you are making. If a patient is a silent aspirator, it will not be easy for the family to understand why the patient can't have thin liquid, for instance. However, if you are able to show a tape of the patient's modified barium swallow, or a sample modified barium swallow depicting aspiration, this may be an easier concept for them to understand.

Opportunities to Educate the Family

If you begin your education attempts with the family before the evaluation, work closely with them to discuss your findings, and enlist their help, you may have better allies in carrying out your recommendations.

Bedside Dysphagia Screening

Before the bedside evaluation:
If the family is present at the time of the evaluation, explain what you will be looking for during the assessment. Explain in detail why you're doing the evaluation. The handout on page 77 explains the purpose of the bedside evaluation. It also explains the difference between this screening procedure and other instrumental procedures that may be recommended. It's also helpful to use the time before the evaluation to obtain information from the patient and family. You may be the first staff member who has spent a considerable amount of time listening to their questions and concerns about the patient's swallowing skills. They may be able to tell you things about how the patient has swallowed in the past and how long the problem has been present. You may gain much more detailed information from the patient or family than from the patient's medical record.

During the bedside evaluation:
If the family is observing the bedside evaluation, point out some of the things you observe. For instance, if the patient is having trouble masticating a bolus and has a lot of pocketing in her cheek, you might point this out to the family. If the patient is losing liquids out the front of her mouth when trying to drink from a cup, you might demonstrate a compensatory technique.

After the bedside evaluation:
Discuss your findings and your recommendations. Depending on the physician(s) with whom you are working, you may need to explain that you will make recommendations to the physician who will then make the final determination about the need for other evaluations like an MBS study, FEES®, or a consult with another medical specialist. It's important that the patient and family understand that the physician will determine the patient's diet based upon your recommendations.

Modified Barium Swallow Studies

Before the modified barium swallow study:
You may want to send/give the patient the handout on page 81 when you schedule the study. Provide a diagram to the patient and her family. Point out the basic features of anatomy and what you will be watching for. (See illustrations on pages 79-80.)

During the modified barium swallow study:
If you have the opportunity, let family members observe the modified barium swallow study to help them understand the problem. Families are often surprised that they will be allowed to watch the study and will be told the results immediately.

After the modified barium swallow study:
Again you will have to make judgments based upon the physician(s) with whom you work as to how to phrase the information shared with the patient and family about the results of the study. You may want to review the videotape with the patient and family members after the study to point out the findings and explain the patient's response to any treatment techniques you attempted. Patients and families may have a particularly difficult time understanding silent aspiration. If the patient "looks" all right when swallowing, it is puzzling to hear that food or liquid is entering the airway. The information on the handout on pages 114-115 may be helpful.

Fiberoptic Endoscopic Evaluation of Swallowing (FEES®)

Before the procedure:
Provide a diagram to the patient and her family (page 78). Describe what you will be doing and what you will observe during the procedure.

During the FEES®:
If you are videotaping the evaluation, the family will be able to watch the monitor with you, so you can explain what you see.

After the FEES®:
If the family has been present during this procedure, you will have had the opportunity to explain what you are seeing. If the family was not available, you can review the videotape with them and the patient so they can see the problems. If aspiration was observed, you may find the handout on pages 114-115 to be helpful. It describes aspiration and silent aspiration.

Therapeutic Feeding Treatment

During a therapeutic feeding treatment:
If the patient is going to eat by mouth, it's very important to educate the patient and family on all the precautions and compensatory techniques they will need to know to help the patient eat safely. Explain what is happening during a therapeutic feeding session.

Not only should the family observe you using specific techniques with the patient, but they should try the technique themselves while you observe. For example, it's an effective teaching technique for family members to actually try to position the patient in bed at 90º. Postural changes and compensatory techniques may be second nature to you, but are new to the family and patient. Therefore, opportunities to practice these techniques will help family members become more efficient and effective.

Documenting Teaching

As with all services we provide, documenting what was done is as important as doing it. You may want to devise specific goals for the family. (See page 83.) In the acute care setting, patient and family education is critical since the average length of stay has significantly decreased. In skilled nursing facilities, you may see families less frequently, making it challenging to provide teaching. In home health, you usually have good access to families and caregivers. Each of these settings may have different requirements for documentation.

Staff Education

Staff also require patient-specific education. It's unlikely, however, that a staff member will have enough time to observe the modified barium swallow study and participate fully during a therapeutic treatment at mealtime as a family member might. However, it's just as important that you actually demonstrate techniques and share information with the nursing staff. Don't assume they know as much about swallowing as you do. Be specific in your recommendations. For instance, if a patient is not allowed to have thin liquids, be sure you mention that this applies to cups of ice chips as well.

You may want to teach the nursing staff how to complete a screening for possible dysphagia. (See page 93.) Review characteristics and behaviors that might indicate dysphagia. Be sure that the nursing staff understand that a patient may be aspirating without any clinical signs.

Patient-Specific In-services

Especially in skilled nursing facilities, it's possible to offer a patient-specific in-service for the staff providing care to the patient. In this in-service, you might review the results of the evaluation and show part of the taped modified barium swallow study. Take this opportunity to discuss in detail the specific recommendations for the patient. Have the staff practice positioning and compensatory techniques.

Case Conferences

In facilities like sub-acute care facilities and skilled nursing facilities, you may discuss some very specific recommendations for treatment of a patient's dysphagia during a case conference. This is a wonderful opportunity to make sure that all staff involved with the patient hear your recommendations. It's not only nursing staff who have the opportunity to provide food or liquid to the patient, but patients may ask the respiratory therapist, physical therapist, or occupational therapist to give them a drink of water. It's important that all staff in contact with the patient are aware of any precautions.

General In-services

It's often challenging to get members of nursing staff or nursing assistants to attend a general in-service. Such a general in-service is typically not a reimbursable service, but providing such in-services periodically is very helpful. The turnover of staff in many health care facilities is fairly high and it's important to repeat these in-services at periodic intervals. A sample outline for an in-service on dysphagia is provided on pages 103-104.

Physician Education

Educating physicians is a challenging proposition. It usually occurs slowly as you build rapport with physicians with whom you work. It's also usually patient-specific. Sometimes you'll have the opportunity to respond to a specific question from a physician. Two sample letters to physicians are provided which may be helpful to you when physicians raise specific questions about the cost and purpose of bedside screenings and instrumental examinations. (See pages 72-75.)

Physicians may also have questions about the predicted outcome of dysphagia intervention and the relationship of the outcome to the cost of the service. Chapter 10 provides detailed information about outcomes. Other handouts (pages 106-115) may be helpful to address specific questions raised by physicians. Make sure to add recent references to support the claims made in the handouts. As research in the area of dysphagia continues, some conclusions and practice patterns change as well.

Administrators and Payers

The questions raised by administrators and payers typically concern the cost of the service, predicted length of treatment, projected functional outcome, and the cost/benefit ratio. It is important that you be able to explain how dysphagia services can reduce the risk of medical complications and therefore save money for the facility or payer. You will also need to be able to describe the benefits of specific procedures (e.g., instrumental examinations) and to explain the role the examination plays in a comprehensive dysphagia management program. (See handout, page 106-108.) Chapter 10 provides more information on outcomes and efficacy that will be helpful to you as you prepare materials for education.

Sample Letter to Physician — A

Date _____

RE: Dysphagia management

Dear Dr. _____,

I understand you are interested in knowing the cost of a bedside screening for dysphagia as well as the cost of instrumental procedures such as a modified barium swallow study or Fiberoptic Endoscopic Evaluation of Swallowing (FEES®) because you are reluctant to order these without knowing the cost. The attached sheet details not only the cost, but provides the kind of information that can be gained from a bedside evaluation vs. a modified barium swallow study or FEES®.

In addition, I've included some references which confirm what we have seen in studies here — that up to 60% of patients are silent aspirators. The modified barium swallow study allows detection of aspiration and determination of techniques, diet changes, and postures which may prevent aspiration and allow the patient to eat safely. The FEES® provides similar information. Certainly you agree that the cost of an instrumental exam is less than the cost of treatment for aspiration pneumonia.

I would welcome the opportunity to discuss this information with you if you have further concerns about the cost of these evaluations. We provide a high quality, cost-effective service that is of great benefit to the patient, physician, and family.

Thank you for your interest.

Sincerely,

_____

Speech-Language Pathologist

Suggested readings

1. Linden, P. and A. Siebens. "Dysphagia: Predicting Laryngeal Penetration." *Archives of Physical Medicine and Rehabilitation*, Vol. 64, 1983, pp. 281-284.

2. Ott, D. J., R. G. Hodge, L. A. Pikna, M. Y. M. Chen, and D. W. Gelfand. "Modified Barium Swallow: Clinical and Radiographic Correlation and Relation to Feeding Recommendations." *Dysphagia*, Vol. 11, 1996, pp. 187-190.

3. Smith, C. H., J. A. Logemann, L. A. Colangelo, A. W. Rademaker, and B. R. Pauloski. "Incidence and Patient Characteristics Associated with Silent Aspiration in the Acute Care Setting." *Dysphagia*, Vol. 14, No. 1, 1999, pp.1-7.

4. Splaingard, M., B. Hutchins, L. Sulton, and G. Chaudhuri. "Aspiration in Rehabilitation Patients: Videofluoroscopy vs. Bedside Clinical Assessment." *Archives of Physical Medicine and Rehabilitation*, Vol. 69, August 1988, pp. 637-640.

Bedside Screening

Speech-language pathology and occupational therapy perform this screening together. Speech-language pathology's assessment of oral-motor skills provides information about how the patient can form, maintain, and manipulate a bolus. The speech-language pathologist (SLP) also assesses basic communication and cognitive skills, and makes judgments about laryngeal closure and elevation, essential for airway protection.

Occupational therapy assesses visual perceptual skills, fine motor skills, and head and neck control. The assessment of these functions helps determine the patient's ability to self-feed.

Cost: _____

Information obtained from bedside screening:

Bedside screenings provide the most information about type and texture of food a patient can handle in the oral phase and about a patient's ability to self-feed.

Modified Barium Swallow Study

Modified barium swallow studies are performed by radiology and speech-language pathology. The modified barium swallow study is the best way to assess whether a patient is aspirating. Of course, the main intent of the study is not to rule out or confirm aspiration, but to determine the type(s) or texture(s) of food a patient can take without aspiration. It also helps to determine any postural changes or compensatory techniques which might be needed to allow the patient to eat or drink without aspiration. It's much more a trial therapeutic study than a straight diagnostic study.

Cost: _____

Decisions typically made from information obtained from a modified barium swallow study are:

- whether the patient should eat by mouth
- which compensatory techniques the patient needs to prevent aspiration

Fiberoptic Endoscopic Evaluation of Swallowing (FEES®)

The SLP may utilize fiberoptic endoscopic evaluation during the bedside assessment of the patient. This procedure involves passing the endoscope transnasally so that the tip of the endoscope hangs in the hypopharynx. The SLP can then observe premature movement of the bolus of food over the back of the tongue and possibly into the airway before the swallow. Residue in the pharynx after the swallow can be observed to see if the residue is going to spill into the airway. The actual moment of swallowing is not visible as the scope is obliterated when the glottis closes. Use of this procedure does not preclude the need for a modified barium swallow, but does allow the SLP to determine at bedside which patients are candidates for videofluoroscopic assessment.

Cost: _____

Decisions typically made from information obtained utilizing FEES® at bedside:

- whether patient is aspirating and should be made NPO
- if texture changes can eliminate the aspiration
- if patient is swallowing safely and does not need further instrumental assessment

Sample Letter to Physician – B

Date _____

Dear Dr. _____,

Thank you for agreeing to meet with us to discuss protocols for clinical (bedside) screenings, fiberoptic endoscopic evaluation of swallowing (FEES®), and videofluoroscopic evaluations (modified barium swallow studies). As you know, dysphagia intervention has several goals.

1. To prevent or significantly decrease risk for aspiration pneumonia. A secondary benefit of this goal is to decrease length of stay and patient complications.

2. To return the patient to safe PO feeding status to obtain adequate nutrition and hydration.

3. For patients who cannot yet return safely to full PO, the goal is to allow the presentation of some foods and liquids by mouth therapeutically to help improve the patient's prognosis for returning to full PO.

4. In certain cases in which the prognosis is poor that the patient will return to full PO, dysphagia therapy may be designed to allow the patient to take some food or liquid safely by mouth to improve the quality of life.

Clinical (bedside) screening yields very important information about the oral preparatory and oral voluntary phases of the swallow. In addition, it provides important information such as the patient's level of alertness, appropriate positioning for feeding, and ability to self-feed.

However, aspiration cannot be confirmed nor ruled out with certainty using only a clinical (bedside) screening, even when the patient is tracheostomized. Several studies have indicated that as many as 60% of patients judged to be safe feeders on a clinical evaluation are actually found to be silent aspirators when an instrumental assessment is performed. (See suggested readings list at end of letter.)

A procedure called fiberoptic endoscopic evaluation (FEES®) may be utilized at bedside by the SLP. This procedure involves passing an endoscope transnasally into the hypopharynx so that the patient's airway can be observed before and after, but not during, the swallow. The procedure allows the clinician to determine if the patient is safe to eat or should not be eating at all. The procedure also allows for more selective referral of patients for modified barium swallow studies.

A videofluoroscopic evaluation of swallowing (modified barium swallow study) is the best way to know whether the patient is aspirating or is at significant risk for aspiration and to plan treatment. The intent of the study is not merely to confirm if the patient is aspirating. The main point of completing this study is to determine if there are compensatory or positioning techniques that can be used, or food consistency and texture changes that can be implemented which would allow the patient to eat some foods safely without aspirating. These determinations cannot be made on the basis of a clinical (bedside) evaluation.

Each of the assessments yields different information. When a clinical and instrumental exam are performed, a complete picture is obtained about the patient's abilities.

Some physicians don't want their patients to undergo a videofluoroscopic evaluation of swallowing because they might aspirate. However, these same patients are often fed on the floor where, of course, they also might aspirate. The difference is that a modified barium swallow study is a very controlled procedure where small amounts of a benign substance (barium sulfate) are presented and if aspiration occurs, it is immediately seen. In contrast, beginning trial feedings on the floor without a modified barium swallow study can mean that up to 60% of patients might be aspirating. This might not be known until sometime later when the patient develops aspiration pneumonia. (The safety of the medium used during the studies is explained in the fourth article in the suggested readings list.)

We would be happy to have you observe a procedure at any time or to discuss this information in more detail. Thank you so much for taking the time to read this information.

Sincerely,

_____

Speech-Language Pathology Department

Suggested readings:

1. Gelfand, D. W. and D. J. Ott. "Barium Sulfate Suspensions: An Evaluation of Available Products." *American Journal of Roentgenology*, Vol. 138, 1982, p. 935.

2. Leder, S. B., C. T. Sasaki, and M. I. Burrell. "Fiberoptic Endoscopic Evaluation of Dysphagia to Identify Silent Aspiration." *Dysphagia*, Vol. 13, No. 1, 1998, pp. 19-21.

3. Linden, P., K. Kuhlemeier, and C. Patterson. "The Probability of Correctly Predicting Subglottic Penetrations and Clinical Observations." *Dysphagia*, Vol. 8, 1993, pp. 170-179.

4. Ott, D. J. and D. W. Gelfand. "Gastrointestinal Contrast Agents: Indications, Uses, and Risks." *Journal of the American Medical Association,* Vol. 249, 1983, p. 2380.

5. Ott, D. J., R. G. Hodge, L. A. Pikna, M. Y. M. Chen, and D. W. Gelfand. "Modified Barium Swallow: Clinical and Radiographic Correlation and Relation to Feeding Recommendations." *Dysphagia*, Vol. 11, 1996, pp. 187-190.

6. Sorin, R., S. Somers, W. Austin, and S. Bester. "The Influence of Videofluoroscopy on the Management of the Dysphagic Patient." *Dysphagia*, Vol. 2, 1988, pp. 127-135.

7. Splaingard, M., B. Hutchins, L. Sulton, and G. Chaudhuri. "Aspiration in Rehabilitation Patients: Videofluoroscopy vs. Bedside Clinical Assessment." *Archives of Physical Medicine and Rehabilitation*, Vol. 69, August 1988, pp. 637-640.

Education Materials _____

The handouts on pages 77-115 may be helpful in patient, family, and staff education.

What Is Being Evaluated on a
Bedside Dysphagia Screening?

Patient: _____ Date: _____

A bedside dysphagia screening is performed by a speech-language pathologist (SLP). It assesses a patient's swallowing skills and determines if further in-depth testing is needed. A tray of food with different textures and temperatures is used during the screening. Liquids are presented from a spoon, a cup, and a straw.

Both the patient and the patient's family can provide valuable information about changes in the patient's eating habits. For instance, is the patient avoiding certain foods or drinks or complaining that certain things are hard to swallow?

The SLP will:

- ask questions about the patient's swallowing problems

- read the patient's medical history

- assess how well the patient can use his/her lips and tongue, as good lip and tongue movement are needed in order to eat and drink

- listen to the patient's voice (If the patient's voice is weak and breathy, it may mean that the patient's vocal cords aren't closing tightly. This might indicate that the patient can't close the vocal cords tightly to protect the airway during a swallow.)

- see how well the patient can follow directions (It may be necessary for the patient to learn some techniques to swallow safely.)

If an occupational therapist (OT) is participating in the evaluation, she will assess the following:

- strength and coordination of the arm and hand the patient will use to eat

- the patient's ability to see the utensils and food on all parts of the tray

- the patient's ability to sit and hold his/her head up, at midline

- the patient's ability to open packages, use utensils, and take food to his/her mouth

Using the tray of food, the SLP will determine how well the patient can use his/her lips, cheeks, and tongue to take food into his/her mouth, control and manipulate the food, and swallow. The SLP will watch for any possible signs of aspiration (which means food or liquid is entering the airway). Some of these signs are coughing and choking, wet sounding voice, throat clearing, swallowing multiple times for a small bite, or limited movement of the larynx in the neck (determined by feeling for movement).

The SLP and the OT may be able to make recommendations about how the patient should eat (e.g., types of food and liquid, position, kinds of utensils) at the end of the bedside screening. However, many patients who are aspirating show no signs (e.g., coughing). This is called silent aspiration, and as many as 60% of patients with dysphagia may be silent aspirators. For that reason, the SLP may recommend a more thorough evaluation of swallowing. This might be an x-ray procedure called a modified barium swallow (or videofluoroscopy) or a procedure performed at bedside with an endoscope. The SLP can explain the difference between the two procedures and why one might be recommended instead of the other.

What You'll See on Fiberoptic Endoscopic Evaluation (FEES®)

Patient: _____   Date: _____

The FEES® is performed by the speech-language pathologist (SLP), usually at bedside. A small endoscope is passed into the patient's nose and then down into the throat. A small amount of anesthetic may be placed in the nose to make the patient more comfortable during the procedure. The endoscope is attached to a light source and to a camera so that the study can be recorded. The tip of the endoscope hangs right above the larynx.

Once the endoscope is in place, the SLP can observe what is happening in the patient's throat before and after the swallow. At the moment of the swallow, the screen will go blank. This is because the larynx is lifting and closing. The camera's view is blocked until after the swallow when the patient releases his/her larynx and breathes.

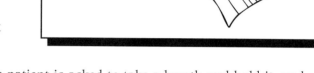

During the exam, the SLP will:

- assess how well the soft palate lifts to close off the opening into the nasal cavity

- observe the back of the tongue moving as the patient makes sounds like "k"

- observe the larynx: during quiet breathing, when the patient is asked to take a breath and hold it, and when the patient makes sounds

- give the patient small amounts of food and liquid (usually dyed blue or green so it is easier to see) to observe if any of the food or liquid is entering the airway

Special compensatory techniques may be tried during the exam, such as having the patient take a thicker liquid or hold his/her breath before swallowing. These techniques will allow the SLP to determine if such techniques can keep the food or liquid from getting into the airway.

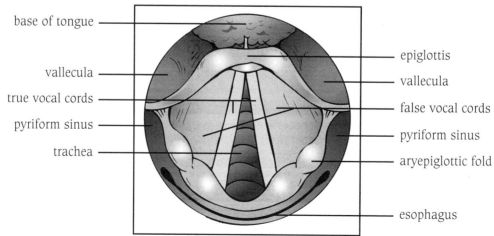

base of tongue

vallecula

true vocal cords

pyriform sinus

trachea

epiglottis

vallecula

false vocal cords

pyriform sinus

aryepiglottic fold

esophagus

What You'll See on a Modified Barium Swallow Study

A videofluoroscopic evaluation of swallowing is also called a modified barium swallow study.

The speech-language pathologist and radiologist will observe the patient's swallowing ability to see if any food or liquid enters the airway instead of going down the esophagus. They will also observe to see if there is any pooling, where material is left in the valleculae and the pyriform sinuses after the swallow. If material is left in these areas, there is a chance it can later fall into the airway.

The patient may be asked to try different techniques such as changes in posture or changes in food texture. For example, the patient may be asked to tuck his/her chin to see if that improves airway protection. The esophageal phase may be screened while the patient is sitting up or we may have the patient lie on the table on his/her side and/or back to observe how the food moves through the esophagus and into the stomach, and whether the patient has a hernia or gastroesophageal reflux.

The patient will also be observed from the front to determine:
- movement of the vocal folds to see if they're closing tightly to protect the airway
- if the barium material moves through the area symmetrically
- if the pooling in the valleculae and pyriform sinuses is symmetrical

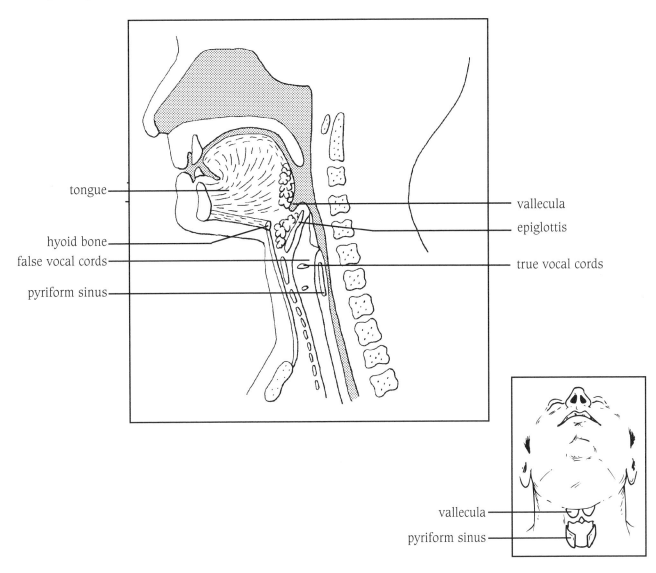

Stages of Swallow

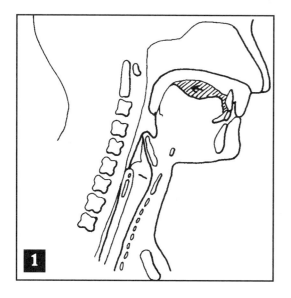

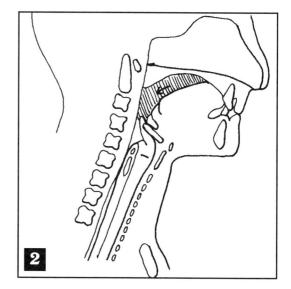

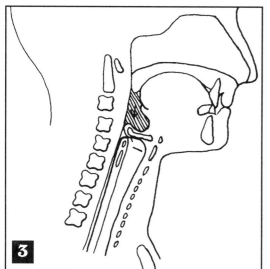

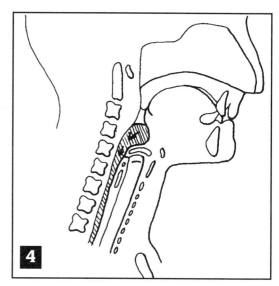

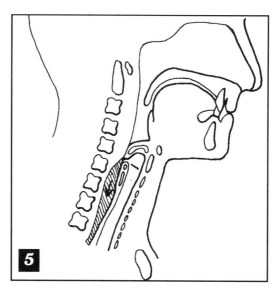

Questions & Answers About the Modified Barium Swallow

Patient_____

Your appointment is on _____ at _____ A.M. / P.M.

Your physician has referred you for a modified barium swallow study, a special x-ray of your swallowing skills. This study is performed in the Radiology/X-ray Department at _____.

Can I eat before I come?

Yes. You do not have to have an empty stomach for this test.

How long will the study take?

Once you are in the X-ray suite, the study should take no longer than 30 minutes, including discussing the results. We will make every effort to keep your waiting time to a minimum.

What does the study involve?

You'll be given small amounts of liquid to drink, a pudding-like texture to eat, and a cookie to swallow while video x-rays are taken. If there are particular foods that cause you difficulty like dry foods or pills, you may be asked to try to swallow them.

While you are seated, both a side view and a front view will likely be done. If you have problems with heartburn, you may also be asked to lie down and drink more liquid so that the esophagus can be assessed.

When will I know the results?

The speech-language pathologist or radiologist will talk with you immediately after the study to tell you what was seen and make recommendations. Your physician (and speech-language pathologist if you are already being treated by one) will be called and each will receive a detailed written report.

Can my family observe?

We are happy to have one member of your family accompany you and observe the study.

Who can I call if I have other questions?

Contact the Speech-Language Pathology Department at _____. We will be happy to answer any questions.

Teaching Fact Sheet for PO Feeding _____

1. Suggested techniques for positioning a patient for safe feeding may include:
   - sitting up as straight as possible at 90°
   - placing a pillow or towel roll behind the back and neck
   - tucking the chin
   - turning the head to one side

2. Compensatory techniques to assist in safe feeding may include the following. The SLP can provide detailed information about any appropriate techniques.

   To compensate for oral problems:
   - lip support
   - external pressure to cheek
   - reminding patient to sweep mouth with tongue

   To compensate for residue:
   - effort swallow
   - alternate sips of (thickened) liquids every few bites
   - swallowing twice for each bite/sip

   To compensate for decreased lifting of the larynx:
   - Mendelsohn maneuver

   To compensate for delayed swallow:
   - thermal/tactile stimulation
   - alternating bites of cold food

   To compensate for decreased closure of the larynx:
   - super-supraglottic swallow
   - periodic cough/throat clear

3. Signs and symptoms of aspiration:
   - coughing
   - choking
   - throat clearing
   - wet gurgling voice after swallowing
   - increased temperature
   - leakage of food or saliva around tracheostomy or mouth

Patients having silent aspiration DO NOT cough or choke, and may appear to swallow safely.

4. Signs and symptoms of difficulty with oral-phase swallowing:
   - pocketing of food
   - drooling
   - weak lip closure

5. If thickened liquids are ordered, all liquids should be made the same consistency by using _____. Follow the directions on the can. Thicken to _____ consistency.

6. Proper technique for administering medications will be posted on the Swallowing Guidelines sheet. Observe the patient while swallowing medications. Then check inside the mouth for pocketing or inability to swallow.

7. Oral care should be given after each meal. A lip moisturizer is suggested for dry lips. If the patient is on thickened liquids, make sure he/she doesn't swallow plain water during oral care.

Note: The "facts" on this page correspond directly to the family goals on page 83.

Family Goals for Safe Feeding ———————————

_____ 1. Family demonstrates the ability to safely position the patient.
- ❏ positioning the patient upright at 90°
- ❏ placing a pillow behind the back and neck if needed
- ❏ using other positioning changes recommended by the SLP:

_____

_____ 2. Family demonstrates the ability to help the patient use specific compensatory techniques for meals that have been taught to him/her.

To compensate for oral problems:
- ❏ lip support
- ❏ external pressure to cheek
- ❏ reminding patient to sweep mouth with tongue

To compensate for decreased lifting of the larynx:
- ❏ Mendelsohn maneuver

To compensate for decreased closure of the larynx:
- ❏ super-supraglottic swallow
- ❏ periodic cough/throat clear

To compensate for residue:
- ❏ effort swallow
- ❏ alternate sips of (thickened) liquids every few bites
- ❏ swallowing twice for each bite/sip

To compensate for delayed swallow:
- ❏ thermal/tactile stimulation
- ❏ alternating bites of cold food

_____ 3. Family is able to state signs and symptoms of aspiration.

_____ 4. Family is able to state signs and symptoms of difficulty with oral-phase swallowing.

_____ 5. Family demonstrates the ability to thicken liquids to appropriate consistency.

_____ 6. Family demonstrates the ability to administer medications.

_____ 7. Family demonstrates the ability to perform oral care.

Swallowing Exercises _____

Patient: _____ Date: _____

You need to work on specific exercises to strengthen certain muscles and improve coordination of your swallowing. The exercises you need to perform are checked on the list below. Step-by-step directions on how to perform the exercises can be found on pages 85-91.

I have indicated whether you should do the exercise with or without any liquid/food in your mouth. If you should practice with saliva only, saliva is circled. If you are to perform the exercise with a swallow of food or liquid, then food is circled and I have written in which food or liquid you can use.

Perform the exercises _____ times a day.

1. ❑ improve lip closure

2. ❑ improve tongue movement
   - ❑ forward/backward movement
   - ❑ side-to-side movement
   - ❑ lifting of back of tongue

3. ❑ improve lifting of the larynx
   - ❑ Mendelsohn maneuver   saliva/food: _____
   - ❑ falsetto

4. ❑ improve closure of the larynx
   - ❑ supraglottic swallow   saliva/food: _____
   - ❑ super-supraglottic swallow   saliva/food: _____
   - ❑ breath hold/Valsalva maneuver
   - ❑ push-pull with phonation
   - ❑ head rotation with phonation

5. ❑ improve base of tongue movement and strength
   - ❑ tongue base retraction
   - ❑ super-supraglottic swallow   saliva/food: _____
   - ❑ pretend to gargle
   - ❑ pretend to yawn
   - ❑ effort swallow   saliva/food: _____

6. ❑ improve movement of back wall of throat
   - ❑ tongue hold
   - ❑ pretend to gargle
   - ❑ pretend to yawn

7. ❑ improve timing, initiation, and overall coordination of swallow
   - ❑ thermal/tactile stimulation   saliva/food: _____
   - ❑ three-second prep   saliva/food: _____
   - ❑ suck-swallow
   - ❑ sour bolus   lemon swab/lemon ice
   - ❑ cold bolus   ❑ food: _____ ❑ liquid: _____
   - ❑ neurosensory stimulation
   - ❑ super-supraglottic swallow   saliva/food: _____
   - ❑ Mendelsohn maneuver   saliva/food: _____

8. ❑ improve forward movement of the larynx
   - ❑ head lift

How to Perform the Swallowing Exercises ────────

Patient: _____ Date: _____

1. Lip Closure

These exercises are used if you are having trouble keeping food from falling out of the front of your mouth, having trouble taking food off a spoon, or having trouble sucking from a straw.

❐ Purse your lips and protrude as far forward as possible and hold.
❐ Pull your lips back into a wide smile and hold.
❐ Smack your lips together forcefully.

2. Tongue Movement

These exercises are used to help you move the food around in your mouth and keep it from falling over the back of your tongue too soon.

❐ forward/backward movement

    ❐ Stick your tongue out of your mouth as far as possible and hold. Try to keep your tongue in the middle while you do this.

    ❐ Pull your tongue back as far as you can in your mouth, as if you are trying to scratch the back wall of your throat with the back of your tongue.

    ❐ Lift the tip of your tongue to the roof of your mouth. Move the tip back as far as you can, keeping the tip on the roof of your mouth.

❐ side-to-side movement

    ❐ Put the tip of your tongue in your right cheek as far back as you can and hold it. Repeat with tip of tongue in left cheek.

    ❐ Smile. Put the tip of your tongue in the corner of your lips on the right, then move it to the left.

❐ lifting back of tongue

Repeat these words ending with "k." Make a hard, forceful "k" each time you say a word.

walk	talk	work	pack	pike	peek
back	bake	bike	book	hike	jack
lake	look	like	lick	lark	make
mark	nick	pick	sick	shake	take
wake	black	truck	rake	rack	hawk

3. Lifting of Larynx

❐ Mendelsohn maneuver   saliva/food: _____

This technique is designed to keep the larynx, or voice box, at its highest point. It is used if you have food sticking in your throat which might fall into your airway.

Place your fingers lightly on your neck to feel how the larynx/voice box lifts as you swallow. You will notice that at the very peak of the swallow, the larynx is lifted to its highest point in the neck, and when the swallow is finished, the larynx falls down again.

1. Swallow with your fingers lightly on your larynx.

2. When you feel your larynx get to its highest point, hold it up by pushing your tongue hard against the roof of your mouth and keeping it there. (The base of the tongue is attached to the hyoid bone, which is attached to the larynx, and that is why pushing the tongue up keeps the larynx up.)

3. Keep the larynx lifted for _____ seconds.

❏ falsetto

This is designed to increase the amount of elevation of the larynx. Elevation is helpful if you have food residue in your throat which might fall into your airway.

1. Say "eee." Sing one continuous note while saying "eee" and go up into the falsetto range. Hold that high note.

4. Closure of the Larynx

❏ supraglottic swallow   saliva/food: _____

This technique is designed to close the airway at the level of the vocal cords. This is useful if food is getting into your airway during the swallow.

1. Take a breath.
2. Let a little out.
3. Hold your breath tightly.
4. Swallow.
5. Cough.
6. Swallow again.

❏ super-supraglottic swallow   saliva/food: _____

This technique is similar to the supraglottic swallow, but is designed to achieve closure of the airway not only at the vocal cords, but above the vocal cords too. It is useful if food or liquid is getting into the airway before or during the swallow. It can also help improve the timing of the swallow so that the larynx starts moving without a delay as well as helping the base of the tongue move.

1. Take a breath.
2. Let a little out.
3. Hold your breath as tightly as possible.
4. Swallow, squeezing as hard as you can.
5. Cough.
6. Swallow again.

❐ breath hold/Valsalva maneuver

This technique is designed to improve closure at the vocal cords. This is helpful if food or liquid is getting into the airway during the swallow.

1. Take a breath.

2. Bear down and hold your breath. You should not hold your breath with your lips, but in your throat, like you do if you are trying to lift something very heavy.

3. Hold for _____ seconds and then let go.

❐ push-pull with phonation

This technique gets the vocal cords closing together more tightly. This is helpful if food or liquid is getting into the airway during the swallow.

1. Place one or both hands under your chair, and pull as if you were trying to lift your chair up with you in it. (You can also do this by standing up and pushing against the wall, as if you were trying to move the wall.)

2. Hold your breath tightly.

3. Let go of your breath (still pulling) and say "ahh."

❐ head rotation with phonation

Head rotation brings the weaker vocal cord closer to the strong vocal cord. This is helpful if you have weakness on one side of the throat which lets food or liquid get into your airway. Your head should not be tipped, but turned to look over one shoulder.

1. Turn your head to the left/right.
2. Hold your breath tightly.
3. Let go of your breath and say "ahh."

5. Base of Tongue Movement and Strength

❐ tongue base retraction

This helps strengthen the base of the tongue. (Note: This part of the tongue is not visible when looking into the mouth as it is actually the "front wall" of your throat.) If the base of the tongue is weak, it lets food residue build up in the throat. This residue could then fall into your airway.

1. Pull the back of your tongue as far back as you can in your mouth. Pretend you are trying to scratch the back wall of your throat with the back of your tongue.

2. Hold the tongue in this position for several seconds. (Note: Do not lift the tip of your tongue. This exercise is for the very back of your tongue, not for the tip.)

87

❐ super-supraglottic swallow   saliva/food: _____

This technique is similar to the supraglottic swallow, but is designed to achieve closure of the airway not only at the vocal cords, but above the vocal cords too. It is useful if food or liquid is getting into the airway before or during the swallow. It can also help improve the timing of the swallow so that the larynx starts moving without a delay as well as helping the base of the tongue move.

1. Take a breath.
2. Let a little out.
3. Hold your breath as tightly as possible.
4. Swallow, squeezing as hard as you can.
5. Cough.
6. Swallow again.

❐ pretend to gargle

This is designed to increase movement of the back wall of the throat and the base of the tongue. It is helpful if you have food residue sticking high in your throat.

1. Look up toward the ceiling.
2. Pretend you have liquid in your mouth.
3. Pretend to gargle.

❐ pretend to yawn

This technique is designed to increase movement of the back wall of the throat and the base of the tongue. This helps reduce the amount of food residue in the upper throat.

1. Open your mouth wide.
2. Start to yawn. You will feel all the muscles open wide in your throat and mouth.

❐ effort swallow   saliva/food: _____

The effort swallow is designed to get more movement of the base of the tongue and to help push the food down so there is not as much left in pockets in your throat.

1. Squeeze all of your mouth and throat muscles as hard as possible (as if trying to swallow a ping-pong ball).
2. Swallow.

6. Movement of Back Wall of Throat

❐ tongue hold

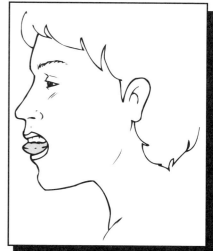

This technique is designed to help the back wall of the throat move forward to meet the base of the tongue. This helps reduce the amount of food residue high in the throat.

1. Protrude your tongue slightly from your mouth.
2. Hold it gently with your teeth.
3. Swallow while keeping your tongue protruded.

❏ pretend to gargle

This is designed to increase movement of the back wall of the throat and the base of the tongue. It is helpful if you have food residue sticking high in your throat.

1. Look up toward the ceiling.
2. Pretend you have liquid in your mouth.
3. Gargle.

❏ pretend to yawn

This technique is designed to increase movement of the back wall of the throat and the base of the tongue. This helps reduce the amount of food residue in the upper throat.

1. Open your mouth wide.
2. Start to yawn. You will feel all the muscles open wide in your throat and mouth.

7. Timing, Initiation, and Overall Coordination of Swallow

If your swallowing reflex doesn't start as soon as food enters your throat, the delay can cause the food or liquid to fall into your airway.

❏ thermal/tactile stimulation   saliva/food: _____

This technique is performed using a size 00 laryngeal mirror.

1. Hold the mirror like a pencil so you can easily rotate it in your hand.
2. Dip it in ice.
3. Rub it up and down five times on one of the anterior faucial arches.
4. Dip the mirror back into the ice quickly.
5. Rotate it so the flat head of the mirror is facing the other direction.
6. Rub it on the other faucial arch.
7. Swallow. (Note: If you are to use food, put the food in your mouth after Step 6.)

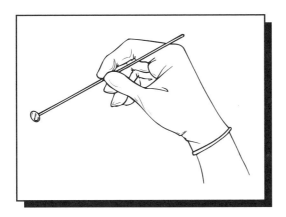
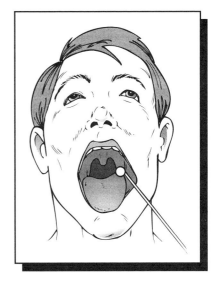

How to Perform the Swallowing Exercises, *continued*

❑ three-second prep   saliva/food: _____

    1. Think about getting ready to swallow while someone counts to three or you count to three in your head.

    2. When you get to three, swallow.

❑ suck-swallow

    1. Using exaggerated movements of the tongue and jaw, pretend you are noisily sucking a really thick milkshake through a very thin straw.

    2. Suck for several seconds, and then swallow.

❑ sour bolus

Foods that are sour can help the swallow reflex start sooner.

    ❑ lemon swab (to be used if you are not allowed to have thin liquids)

        1. Suck on a lemon swab for several seconds.
        2. Swallow.

    ❑ lemon ice (to be used if you are allowed to have thin liquids)

        1. Take a small amount (about 1/4 teaspoon) of lemon ice into your mouth.
        2. Suck the lemon ice for about one second.
        3. Swallow.

❑ cold bolus

Alternate bites or sips of very cold food/liquid. (Note: Your SLP may also ask that you eat only cold foods.)

❑ neurosensory stimulation

    1. Fill a finger of a latex glove with water or crushed ice.
    2. Tie it off.
    3. Freeze it.
    4. Suck on it.
    5. Swallow.

❑ super-supraglottic swallow   saliva/food: _____

This technique is similar to the supraglottic swallow, but is designed to achieve closure of the airway not only at the vocal cords, but above the vocal cords too. It can also help improve the timing of the swallow so that the larynx starts moving without a delay as well as helping the base of the tongue move.

    1. Take a breath.
    2. Let a little out.
    3. Hold your breath as tightly as possible.
    4. Swallow, squeezing as hard as you can.
    5. Cough.
    6. Swallow again.

❐ Mendelsohn maneuver   saliva/food: _____

This technique is designed to keep the larynx, or voice box, at its highest point. It is used if you have food sticking in your throat which might fall into your airway.

Place your fingers lightly on your neck to feel how the larynx/voice box lifts as you swallow. You will notice that at the very peak of the swallow, the larynx is lifted to its highest point in the neck, and when the swallow is finished, the larynx falls down again.

1. Swallow with your fingers lightly on your larynx.

2. When you feel your larynx get to its highest point, hold it up by pushing your tongue hard against the roof of your mouth and keeping it there. (The base of the tongue is attached to the hyoid bone, which is attached to the larynx, and that is why pushing the tongue up keeps the larynx up.)

3. Keep the larynx lifted for _____ seconds.

8. Forward Movement of the Larynx

❐ head lift

In order to reduce the amount of food residue in the pockets in the throat called pyriform sinuses, the larynx has to lift up and move forward in the neck. This helps a muscle at the top of the esophagus open so that food can enter the esophagus and travel to the stomach. If you have problems with your neck (e.g., arthritis), you may not be able to do this exercise. There are two parts to this exercise, sustained and repetitive.

Sustained
1. Lie flat on your back with no pillow under your head.
2. Lift your head to look at your toes.
3. Keep your shoulders flat on the floor/bed.
4. Hold that position for 60 seconds.
5. Release.
6. Repeat twice.

Repetitive
1. Lift your head.
2. Look at your toes.
3. Let your head go back down.
4. Repeat 30 times (almost like sit-ups for the neck).
5. Rest a minute.
6. Repeat twice (total of 90 "sit-ups").

Lifestyle Modifications for Patients with Gastroesophageal Reflux Disease

Discuss these recommendations with your physician. The following are changes which provide relief to some patients who suffer from reflux, or what is commonly called heartburn. Ask your physician about any medications you're taking that could reduce esophageal pressure, as this could contribute to your symptoms.

1. Always eat in a relaxed setting.

2. Eat small meals throughout the day rather than one large meal.

3. Try separating solids and liquids. Don't drink during your meals.

4. Always include some protein foods like lean meat, poultry, cottage cheese, or low-fat cheese in each meal.

5. Keep fat content of meals low.

6. You might avoid the following items as some people report that certain foods irritate the reflux:
    - caffeine (found in coffee, tea, cola)
    - mint
    - alcohol
    - chocolate or cocoa
    - chili powder and other spices
    - cured and spiced meats like sausages and hot dogs
    - pepper
    - citrus juices (orange, lemon)
    - pickled items
    - acidic foods (tomato)

7. Don't eat right before you lie down to rest, go to sleep at night, or recline in a chair. Allow about 30-45 minutes after eating before lying down. (Note: This also applies to drinking a glass of water before bed or taking pills before bed.)

8. Elevate the head of your bed six inches. This is best done with blocks under the legs at the head of the bed. It's not effective to add extra pillows.

Other Things You Can Change

1. If overweight, lose weight.

2. Avoid tight clothing.

3. Stoop. Don't bend over.

4. Avoid lifting heavy objects.

5. Stop smoking.

Dysphagia Screening Tool for Nursing _____

Patient: _____ Date: _____

Check any of the following symptoms which you may observe or find documented in the chart or learn in discussions with patient or family:

- ❐ recent unexplained weight loss

- ❐ patient avoids certain foods or consistencies

- ❐ patient coughs or chokes

- ❐ patient has food left in mouth after meal

- ❐ patient shows some drooling

- ❐ history of pneumonia, which may not necessarily have been specified as aspiration pneumonia

- ❐ wet, gurgly vocal quality

- ❐ patient swallows multiple times for a single bite/sip

Check for any of the following problems noted in your assessment of the patient or in the chart:

- ❐ spiking temperatures

- ❐ unclear lung sounds, particularly at the base (not necessarily only in the right lower lobe)

If any of these symptoms exist, consider referral for assessment of swallowing.
Contact SLP at _____.

Return to _____ by _____.

Swallowing Guidelines

Patient _____

Room _____ Date _____

This patient has been evaluated by the Speech-Language Pathologist and the following guidelines are necessary to assure safe intake of food and liquids.

Sit upright at 90°.

Stay upright for at least 30 minutes after taking anything by mouth.

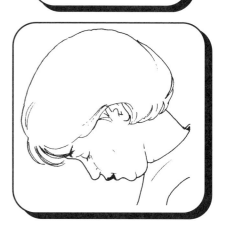

Put chin on chest for swallowing. An extra pillow behind the head is a good reminder.

If voice becomes wet or gurgly, ask patient to cough or clear his/her throat.

Diet: _____

Liquids: Thin liquids are okay. Patient can have ice chips, water, juice, coffee, etc. Use a:

        straw   cup   spoon   cut-out cup

Medicine: _____

Additional Recommendations:

_____

_____

_____

Swallowing Guidelines ─────────────────────

Patient _____

Room _____ Date _____

This patient has been evaluated by the Speech-Language Pathologist and the following guidelines are necessary to assure safe intake of food and liquids.

Sit upright at 90°.

Stay upright for at least 30 minutes after taking anything by mouth.

Put chin on chest for swallowing. An extra pillow behind the head is a good reminder.

If voice becomes wet or gurgly, ask patient to cough or clear his/her throat.

Diet: _____

Liquids: NO THIN LIQUIDS. NO ICE CHIPS.

All liquids must be thickened to syrup consistency. Nutra-Thik can be used to thicken water, juices, coffee, etc. Mix one tablespoon into 6 fluid ounces. Stir well or shake to eliminate lumps. Use a:

  straw   cup   spoon   cut-out cup

Medicine: _____

Additional Recommendations:

_____

_____

_____

Swallowing Guidelines

Patient _____

Room _____ Date _____

This patient has been evaluated by the Speech-Language Pathologist and the following guidelines are necessary to assure safe intake of food and liquids.

Sit upright at 90°.

Stay upright for at least 30 minutes after taking anything by mouth.

Put chin on chest for swallowing. An extra pillow behind the head is a good reminder.

If voice becomes wet or gurgly, ask patient to cough or clear his/her throat.

Diet: _____

Liquids: NO THIN LIQUIDS. NO ICE CHIPS.

All liquids must be thickened to honey consistency. Nutra-Thik can be used to thicken water, juices, coffee, etc. Mix one and a half tablespoons per 6 fluid ounces. Stir well or shake to eliminate lumps. Use a:

straw   cup   spoon   cut-out cup

Medicine: _____

Additional Recommendations:

_____

_____

_____

Swallowing Guidelines ————————————

Patient _____

Room _____ Date _____

This patient has been evaluated by the Speech-Language Pathologist and the following guidelines are necessary to assure safe intake of food and liquids.

Sit upright at 90°.

Stay upright for at least 30 minutes after taking anything by mouth.

Put chin on chest for swallowing. An extra pillow behind the head is a good reminder.

If voice becomes wet or gurgly, ask patient to cough or clear his/her throat.

Diet: _____

Liquids: NO THIN LIQUIDS. NO ICE CHIPS.

All liquids must be thickened to pudding consistency. Nutra-Thik can be used to thicken water, juices, coffee, etc. Mix two tablespoons per 6 fluid ounces. Stir well or shake to eliminate lumps. Use a:

        straw   cup   spoon   cut-out cup

Medicine: _____

Additional Recommendations:

_____

_____

_____

Patient _____

Room _____ Date _____

NPO

This patient has been evaluated by the Dysphagia Team and is not safe to take anything by mouth.

Patient should **NOT** have:
- water
- ice chips
- anything else by mouth

Please call the Speech-Language Pathologist if you have any questions.

Patient _____

Room _____ Date _____

Patient must sit upright at 90° when taking PO medications.

AND ALL FOODS.

Patient _____

Room _____ Date _____

Patient is at risk for aspiration.

If patient chokes, clears throat, or has a wet voice, STOP FEEDING and talk to a nurse who will contact the Speech-Language Pathologist.

Chapter 4
The Source for Dysphagia   100

Patient _____

Room _____ Date _____

PATIENT IS A SILENT ASPIRATOR.

Patient does not cough or choke when food/ liquid enters airway.

To promote safe feedings, strictly follow swallowing guidelines.

Reflux Precautions

Patient _____

Room _____ Date _____

- Sleep with head of bed elevated 30°.

- Don't lie down for 30-45 minutes after eating or drinking.

- Eat smaller meals throughout the day.

- Avoid coffee, spicy foods, citrus fruits, tomatoes, chocolate, and peppermint.

- Avoid late evening snacks.

General In-service on Dysphagia

Note: Provide snacks for staff members. Have them chew to see if they can tell when the three phases of swallowing occur.

Mix up fruit juice in syrup, honey, and pudding thicknesses in small medicine cups so staff can try it. Usually most staff members are surprised that the taste of the thickened liquid is not changed, but only the texture.

I. Information about normal swallowing

Three phases of swallowing:

- oral phase to prepare the bolus

- oral voluntary phase to move the bolus back

- pharyngeal phase as soon as the swallowing reflex is triggered

II. Importance of positioning

Have each person take a small sip of water and swallow it while sitting upright. Then have each person lie flat, take a small sip of water, and try to swallow it.

- Discuss how a person uses the back of her tongue to keep a bolus in her mouth until she's ready to swallow.

- Discuss how putting a person in a reclined position may cause a bolus to move too quickly over the base of the tongue.

- Demonstrate a chin-down posture and how to achieve this with a towel roll or extra pillow behind the patient's head.

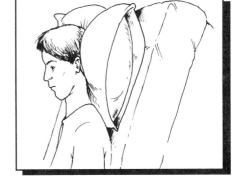

III. Textures of foods

- Explain why thin liquids are often hard for patients to swallow. Remind the attendees of how they felt leaning back with thin liquid in their mouths. Be sure to mention that things like ice cream, sherbet, Jell-O, and ice chips turn into thin liquids in the mouth.

- Have participants try some of the thicker liquids.

- Explain different thicknesses of liquids which the patient can control more easily in the mouth.

- Discuss why pureed foods are easier for patients to handle if they have trouble forming a bolus.

- Discuss why we make recommendations for foods to be one texture only, as it's harder to manipulate something in the mouth with two textures (like milk and cereal).

IV. Aspiration

• Describe what aspiration is. If possible, show a videotape with an example of aspiration.

• Explain silent aspiration, including the fact that 60% of patients with dysphagia are silent aspirators.

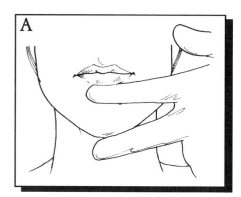

After you explain these techniques, have staff members try them on each other.

• Demonstrate the way to provide jaw and lip support. (See picture A.)

• Demonstrate how to monitor for a swallow by placing fingers lightly on the larynx. (See picture B.)

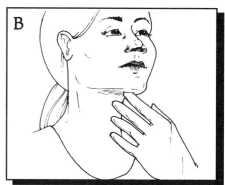

• Demonstrate how to give external pressure to the cheek to decrease pocketing. (See picture C.)

• Describe multiple swallows and explain how they help clear oral residue or residue in the valleculae and pyriform sinuses.

• Describe a liquid wash. Some patients can safely use a liquid wash to clear their mouths, but some may aspirate a liquid wash.

• If the staff is interested, you might demonstrate some more specialized techniques like the supraglottic swallow and the Mendelsohn maneuver. (See Chapter 7, pages 206 and 207.)

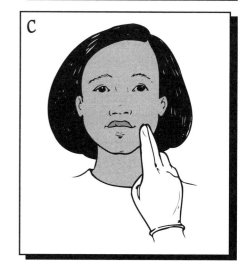

V. Share all precaution signs with staff members. (See pages 94-102.)

Pre- and Post-Test for Staff Education on Dysphagia ___

Name _____

1. There are five phases of swallowing.   True   False

2. Tipping a patient's head back will help her swallow.   True   False

3. If a patient aspirates, she will always cough.   True   False

4. Patients sometimes get food caught in their
   cheeks because they can't feel it there.   True   False

5. Adding thickener to juice changes the taste.   True   False

6. If a patient is NPO, she can't have water but
   she can have ice chips.   True   False

7. One of the most common positions to help prevent aspiration is:
   a. leaning forward
   b. tipping head back
   c. lying on right side
   d. tucking chin down to chest

8. Which of the following are considered thin liquids?
   a. water
   b. mashed potatoes
   c. ice cream
   d. a and c

9. Which of the following is easiest to form into a ball before swallowing?
   a. water
   b. cereal in milk
   c. pudding
   d. rice

10. Aspiration means that food:
    a. is spit out
    b. goes into the lungs
    c. gets caught in the throat
    d. is swallowed

ANSWERS			
1. False	6. False		
2. False	7. d		
3. False	8. d		
4. True	9. c		
5. False	10. b		

Why Is an Instrumental Examination of Swallowing Needed?

Patient: _____   Date: _____

Can a bedside/clinical screening of swallowing tell as much as an instrumental examination?

No. The bedside/clinical evaluation is a thorough assessment of oral-phase disorders such as weak lip closure resulting in anterior loss, or reduced tongue control which interferes with the patient's ability to form a bolus. However, for disorders of the pharyngeal phase (e.g., reduced laryngeal closure with aspiration, reduced base of tongue strength with pharyngeal residue), the bedside/clinical exam is really a screening tool.

Management of dysphagia has followed a medical model, identifying patients at risk through a screening, and then completing a more thorough diagnostic evaluation on patients identified as at risk for pharyngeal disorders. The instrumental diagnostic evaluation is crucial in determining which treatment techniques are needed. (Note: A medical analogy is that a cardiac stress test is considered a screening. Another diagnostic procedure, such as cardiac catheterization, would be performed before determining the kind of treatment the patient needs [e.g., medical management, surgery, balloon dilation].)

Similarly, a bedside screening might reveal some symptoms of pharyngeal dysphagia. But each symptom can have multiple causes. For example, if the patient coughs during the assessment, aspiration might be strongly suspected. However, this cough might be due to aspiration during the swallow secondary to poor vocal fold closure, or because of mistiming of laryngeal elevation/closure, or might even be due to aspiration after the swallow from residue in the pyriform sinuses caused by reduced laryngeal elevation. Each of these physiological causes of the symptom of coughing requires a very different treatment technique.

What are the instrumental procedures used?

The most frequently used procedure is the modified barium swallow study, a videofluoroscopic procedure performed by the radiologist and speech-language pathologist. Lateral and anterior/posterior (A-P) views are obtained of the oral and pharyngeal regions while the patient swallows a variety of textures of liquids and foods impregnated with barium.

A second instrumental procedure is the Fiberoptic Endoscopic Evaluation of Swallowing (FEES®). This procedure is performed by the speech-language pathologist, who places the endoscope transnasally for a view of the pharynx while the patient swallows saliva or food and liquid (usually dyed blue or green for better visualization).

Is one instrumental procedure better than another?

The modified barium swallow is considered by most practitioners to be the gold standard evaluation for the pharyngeal phase of the swallow. It allows for analysis of the structures and movements of the oral, pharyngeal, and esophageal anatomy before, during, and after the act of swallowing.

The FEES® allows direct visualization of the upper airway before the swallow and after the swallow. At the moment of the swallow, the view from the scope is obliterated as the larynx closes. After the swallow, the airway can again be visualized to determine if any material has entered the airway. The FEES® can be performed at bedside, and is probably best used as an adjunct to the bedside screening.

How does an instrumental exam help determine appropriate treatment?

Particularly during the modified barium swallow, different compensatory postures and other maneuvers can be tried to observe the effect on swallowing safety. For instance, if a patient is observed to aspirate thin liquids during the swallow, the patient can be presented with thicker liquids to see if the slower movement of the bolus allows time for airway closure. The patient might also be asked to use a maneuver called the super-supraglottic swallow to establish voluntary closure of the airway. Some of these compensations can be assessed with the FEES® as well. FEES® can also be used during treatment as a biofeedback tool.

How well do screening procedures at the bedside predict who is at risk for aspiration?

There are different procedures which have been used at bedside to determine if the patient is aspirating. DePippo et al. (1992) described a procedure called the *3-oz. Water Swallow Test for Aspiration Following Stroke*. They report a 76% sensitivity and conclude that their test is sensitive enough to be useful as a screening tool for MBS referral. However, the authors recommend that the 3-oz. Water Swallow Test be used in conjunction with a clinical symptom checklist when determining which patients should be referred for further study. However, Garon et al. (1995) tested the reliability of the 3-oz. Water Swallow Test utilizing the cough reflex as the sole indicator of aspiration and found that only 35% of patients who were found to be aspirating on the modified barium swallow had coughed at bedside, for a silent aspiration rate of 65%.

Research studies designed to identify which symptoms/behaviors exhibited at bedside can accurately predict aspiration continue. For example, Logemann et al. (1999) report on a 28-item screening test designed to identify patients who aspirate, have an oral stage disorder, a pharyngeal delay, or a pharyngeal stage disorder. Their results identified variables that could classify patients as having or not having aspiration 71% of the time, pharyngeal delay 72% of the time, and pharyngeal stage swallowing problems 70% of the time. This is important work, as it will provide speech-language pathologists the information they need to avoid over- or under-referral for instrumental exams. However, as stated above, identifying which patients are or are not aspirating is only a small part of dysphagia management. The more important component is determining appropriate treatment strategies.

What is the cost/benefit ratio of instrumental exams?

The most obvious cost benefit of instrumental exams is that patients who are aspirating can be identified and an appropriate management plan determined. In this way, the chances of these patients developing aspiration pneumonia is reduced. The cost of treating an aspiration pneumonia is estimated to be approximately $15,000. This makes the cost of evaluation and treatment of dysphagia very cost effective. In addition, the instrumental exam often reveals that the patient's diet can be upgraded (Martin-Harris et al., 1998), eliminating the extra cost of tube feeding. The instrumental exam also allows for precise identification of the physiologic cause of the symptoms, which allows the speech-language pathologist to select the appropriate treatment techniques. In this way, guesswork is avoided and no time is wasted in therapy on unnecessary or inappropriate techniques.

References

DePippo, K., M. Holas, and M. Reding. "Validation of the 3-Oz Water Swallow Test for Aspiration Following Stroke." *Archives of Neurology*, Vol. 49, 1992, pp. 1259-1261.

Garon, B. R., M. Engle, and C. Ormiston. "Reliability of the 3-oz. Water Swallow Test Utilizing Cough Reflex as Sole Indicator of Aspiration." *Journal of Neurological Rehabilitation*, Vol. 9, No. 3, 1995, pp. 139-143.

Kidder, T. M., S. E. Langmore, and B. J. W. Martin. "Indications and Techniques of Endoscopy in Evaluation of Cervical Dysphagia: Comparison with Radiographic Techniques." *Dysphagia*, Vol. 9, No. 4, 1994, pp. 256-261.

Langmore, S. E. and T. M. McCulloch. "Examination of the Pharynx and Larynx and Endoscopic Examination of Pharyngeal Swallowing." In A. Perlman and K. Schultz (eds.). *Deglutition and Its Disorders*. San Diego: Singular Press, 1996, pp. 201-226.

Logemann, J. *Evaluation and Treatment of Swallowing Disorders*. Austin, TX: Pro-Ed, 1998, pp. 54-62, 168-185.

Logemann, J., S. Veis, and L. Colangelo. "A Screening Procedure for Oropharyngeal Dysphagia." *Dysphagia*, Vol. 14, No. 1, 1999, pp. 44-51.

Martin-Harris, B., S. I. McMahon, and R. Haynes. "Aspiration and Dysphagia: Pathophysiology and Outcome." *Phonoscope*, Vol. 1, No. 2, 1998, pp. 123-132.

Chapter 4
The Source for Dysphagia

108

Answers to Frequently Asked Questions About Dysphagia

Patient: _____   Date: _____

Why no ice chips?

Patients are placed on a diet with no thin liquids because they are aspirating thin liquids. When ice chips are placed in the patient's mouth, they turn into liquid and are aspirated.

What good are thickened liquids?

Thin liquids are the hardest thing to control in the mouth and keep together in a bolus. As the liquids travel through the throat past the larynx, it is easier to aspirate thin liquids because they break apart and some of it can fall into the larynx. Thickened liquids are easier to keep together in one piece. Thick liquids also move more slowly through the pharynx, giving the larynx more time to close and protect the airway.

Why can't I tell if a patient is aspirating at bedside?

Studies confirm that up to 60% of patients who aspirate are silent aspirators. That means that food or liquid may enter the airway through the larynx with absolutely no reaction by the patient.

What good are postural changes?

Some postural changes can provide increased airway protection. Others can direct the food down the stronger side of the throat.

How is a modified barium swallow different from a barium swallow?

Barium Swallow	*Modified Barium Swallow*
Patient lying down	Patient sitting up
Patient given whole bottle of liquid barium to drink	Patient given small controlled amounts of a variety of textures
Assesses esophagus and stomach	Assesses oral and pharyngeal stages of the swallow; may screen esophagus
Diagnostic in nature only	Trial therapy as much as diagnostic

How would I know if my patient is at risk for aspiration?

If you have a patient who is debilitated secondary to lengthy illness or disease, a patient with a tracheostomy tube, a patient who is bedridden, and/or a patient with any type of neurological diagnosis, he or she may be at risk for aspiration.

What are some signs of dysphagia?

Signs of oral phase dysphagia include pocketing of food in the cheeks, losing food or liquid out the front of the mouth, or residue of food long after the patient has finished eating. Signs of pharyngeal dysphagia are coughing or choking during a meal or a wet, gurgly vocal quality.

If my patient has a gag reflex, doesn't that mean he/she is swallowing fine?

The gag is a protective reflex, but is totally unrelated to swallowing. Recent studies confirm that many people who swallow normally have no gag reflex. The studies have also found that individuals with intact gag reflexes can have significant pharyngeal dysphagia with aspiration.

Why is oral care so important?

Some patients who are aspirating are also at risk for aspirating their own secretions. Many patients have gram negative bacilli and such secretions are one of the worst things that can be aspirated. Aggressive oral care, particularly in patients who are NPO because of aspiration, is critical.

Why is it important for patients to sit at 90° when eating?

Many patients with dysphagia have decreased back of tongue control. This allows food or liquid to fall over the back of the tongue with risk of it entering the airway. If the patient is even slightly reclined when eating, it greatly increases the risk of premature loss of food over the back of the tongue.

Why do patients need to sit up for 30 minutes after eating?

Patients may have residue of food left in the valleculae (formed between the base of the tongue and the epiglottis) and/or the pyriform sinuses (formed by the cricopharyngeus muscle at the base of the larynx, very near the entrance to the airway). This is usually caused by reduced laryngeal elevation or reduced strength of the base of the tongue as the person swallows. When food remains in the valleculae and pyriform sinuses, patients are at risk for the food falling into the airway. Therefore, it is important that they sit up until they are able to clear this residue.

How do I make a referral if I think my patient has some problems with swallowing?

A referral to speech-language pathology to assess swallowing requires a physician's order. You can contact the physician directly to ask for the order or you can ask the SLP to screen the patient (this is a no charge service) and contact the physician for you. Most SLPs prefer that the physician write an order that states "Dysphagia evaluation with modified barium swallow if indicated." This eliminates the need to contact the physician a second time for the order for the modified barium swallow study if one is indicated.

If a patient is NPO, can I give him/her medication(s) by mouth?

No. If patients are made NPO it is because they are considered at very high risk for aspiration. Therefore, giving them pills by mouth places them at risk for aspirating those pills. Most patients who are made NPO have an alternative feeding source placed (e.g., NG tube).

How can I give patients medication(s) if they can't take thin liquids?

If the patient can still manipulate the whole pill within his/her mouth, you may try placing the whole pill in a spoonful of yogurt, applesauce, pudding, or other slippery material.

However, some patients may need to have the pill crushed and mixed with the spoonful of slippery material. Be sure to check the patient's mouth after you've given him/her the pill to make sure it has been swallowed and not pocketed in the cheek or on the tongue.

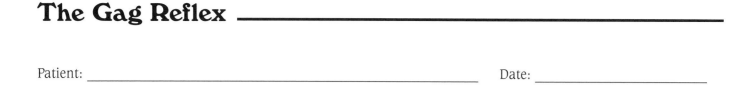

The Gag Reflex

Patient: _____   Date: _____

What does the gag reflex have to do with swallowing?

The short answer is . . . NOTHING. The gag reflex is not elicited during a normal swallow.

What is a gag reflex?

The gag reflex is a protective response. It is designed to keep foreign material from entering the pharynx and airway.

What happens physically when a person gags?

The mandible lowers, the tongue moves down and forward, the pharynx constricts, and the velum lifts.

Doesn't the velum lift during swallowing?

Yes. It lifts to keep food and liquid from entering the nasopharynx. However, one study (Leder, 1996) demonstrated the physiologic differences between the velum lifting during phonation and the lifting of the velum during the gag reflex. There may also be physiologic differences in the lifting of the velum during the gag and swallowing.

Can a patient without a gag reflex swallow safely?

Yes. The Leder study found that 86% of patients referred for dysphagia evaluations because they did not have a gag reflex were able to eat at least a pureed diet.

Do all normal individuals have a gag reflex?

One study assessed the gag reflex in 140 healthy subjects (half elderly and half young). They found the reflex to be absent in 37% (Davies et al.,1995).

References

Davies, A. E., D. Kidd, and S. P. Stone. "Pharyngeal Sensation and Gag Reflex in Healthy Subjects." *The Lancet*, Vol. 345, 1995, pp. 487-488.

Leder, S. B. "Gag Reflex and Dysphagia." *Head & Neck*. March/April 1996, pp. 138-141.

Leder, S. B. "Videofluoroscopic Evaluation of Aspiration with Visual Examination of the Gag Reflex and Velar Movement." *Dysphagia*, Vol. 12, 1997, pp. 21-23.

Selley, W. G. "A Comment on 'Videofluoroscopic Evaluation of Aspiration with Visual Examination of the Gag Reflex and Velar Movement.'" *Dysphagia*, Vol 13, No. 4, 1998, pp. 228-230.

The Fallacy of the Inflated Cuff _____

Patient: _____ Date: _____

It is a misperception that an inflated cuff protects a patient from aspiration. Aspiration is defined as food or liquid passing below the vocal cords. In fact, if food reaches the cuff, the patient has aspirated.

- The tracheostomy tube is placed below the larynx, which means the cuff is well below the larynx too.

- If food reaches the cuff, it has already passed the following natural protective mechanisms:

  > true vocal fold closure
  > false vocal fold closure
  > arytenoid tipping
  > laryngeal elevation which results in tipping of the epiglottis

- If food reaches the cuff, it will move further into the trachea around the cuff. The width of the trachea expands slightly with each inhalation, allowing some leakage around the cuff. If the cuff is deflated, any material on top of the cuff will fall into the lungs.

- If food or liquid passes all of the body's natural protective mechanisms to keep food and liquid out of the lungs, and it reaches the cuff, then that patient is not safe to eat/drink anything by mouth.

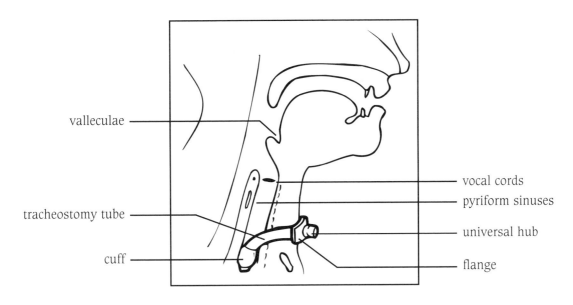

References

Bonnano, P. C. "Swallowing Dysfunction After Tracheostomy." *Annals of Surgery*, Vol. 174, 1971, pp. 29-33.

Cameron, J. L., J. Reynolds, and G. D. Zuidema. "Aspiration in Patients with Tracheostomies." *Surgery, Gynecology, and Obstetrics*, Vol. 136, 1973, pp. 68-70.

Eibling, D. E., G. Bacon, and C. H. Snyderman. "Surgical Management of Chronic Aspiration." In *Advances in Otolaryngology: Head and Neck Surgery*. Chicago: Mosby Yearbook, 1992, pp. 93-113.

Muz, J. M., R. H. Mathog, R. Nelson, and L. A. Jones. "Aspiration in Patients with Head and Neck Cancer and Tracheostomy." *American Journal of Otolaryngology*, Vol. 10, 1989, pp. 282-286.

Nash, M. "Swallowing Problems in the Tracheotomized Patient." *Otolaryngology Clinics of North America*, Vol. 21, 1988, pp. 701-709.

Questions & Answers About Aspiration and Aspiration Pneumonia

Patient: _____   Date: _____

Is aspirating food or liquid always the cause of aspiration pneumonia?

Most pneumonia in institutionalized elderly is believed to be secondary to microaspiration of oral pharyngeal secretions that have been pathologically colonized.

How does aspirating cause pneumonia?

Aspirated materials entering the airway can cause atelectasis (i.e., incomplete expansion or collapse of pulmonary alveoli, or of a segment, lobe, or lobes of a lung) and can alter mucociliary clearing action. Both of these predispose a patient to pneumonia.

Will I know that the patient has aspirated?

You may not. Some patients cough and choke when they aspirate, but up to 60% of patients may be silent aspirators. That is, they don't cough or even clear their throats when they aspirate.

Do patients who are tube fed get pneumonia?

Studies of artificially-fed nursing home patients have shown that neither jejunostomy nor gastrostomy tubes help protect against aspiration in those who are known to aspirate.

Are all infiltrates secondary to aspiration pneumonia?

No. Infiltrates can occur secondary to pneumonia, atelectasis, pulmonary infection, drug reaction, or even neoplasm.

Is pneumonia easy to diagnose?

No. Pneumonia is often hard to diagnose because the classic symptoms of cough, dyspnea, sputum production, and chest pain are often lacking in the elderly. Fever may not be present, or if it is, may be attributed to more common causes such as a urinary tract infection or decubitus ulcers.

Can patients aspirate without developing aspiration pneumonia?

Yes. One study identified shifting and fleeting lung infiltrates in both oral and artificially-fed major aspirators. These radiographic abnormalities lasted only hours or a few days and were sometimes associated with a low-grade fever or upper respiratory illness. They suspect these infiltrates represented aspirated materials that filled subsegmental airways and were subsequently cleared.

How long after an occurrence of aspiration before a temperature spike is noted?

There is no definitive answer. It depends on what and how much is aspirated, overall pulmonary health of the patient, and whether they are taking antibiotics that might mask an infection. Pneumonia can develop quickly or gradually over several weeks.

Of what benefit is a chest x-ray to the diagnosis of pneumonia?

Chest films are often suboptimal and portable rather than standard, which makes it more difficult to judge. The chest x-ray of a patient with aspiration may not look different than a chest x-ray of a patient with a community acquired pneumonia.

Pneumonia in the elderly will continue to be visible on chest x-rays, with infiltrates lasting a mean of five weeks.

References

Cogan, R. and J. Weinryb. "Aspiration Pneumonia in Nursing Home Patients Fed Via Gastrostomy Tube." *American Journal of Gastroenterology*, Vol. 84, 1989, pp. 1509-1519.

Cogan, R. J., Weinryb, C. Pomerantz, and P. Senstemacker. "Complications of Jajunostomy Tube Feedings in Nursing Facility Patients." *American Journal of Gastroenterology*, Vol. 86, 1991, pp. 610-613.

Fineburg, M. F., J. Knebl, and J. Tully. "Prandial Aspiration in Pneumonia and in Elderly Population Followed Over Three Years." *Dysphagia*, Vol. 11, 1996, pp. 104-109.

Garb, J. R., B. Brown, and R. W. Tuthill. "Differences in Etiology of Pneumonia in Nursing Home and Community Patients." *Journal of the American Medical Association*, Vol. 240, 1978, pp. 2169-2172.

Gleckman, R. and M. M. Burgman. "Bacterial Pneumonia: Specific Diagnosis and Treatment of the Elderly." *Geriatrics*, Vol. 42, 1987, pp. 29-41.

Niederman, M. S. and A. M. Fine. "Pneumonia in the Elderly." *Geriatric Clinics of North America*, Vol. 2, 1986, pp. 241-268.

Chapter 5

Ethical Dilemmas and Challenging Case Management Decisions

SLPs involved in dysphagia treatment will frequently find themselves faced with a dilemma that requires them to carefully assess the ethics of the situation. For instance, you may determine from your assessment that it's not safe for the patient to eat. However, the patient or perhaps the patient's physician, may decide that tube feeding isn't appropriate. In these situations, you'll have to decide whether to continue treating the patient. In other situations, you may have to counsel patients and family members concerning prognosis, and may even become involved in end-of-life discussions.

The Code of Ethics of the American Speech-Language-Hearing Association (ASHA, 1995) provides some guidance. Principle of Ethics I states "Individuals shall honor their responsibility to hold paramount the welfare of persons they serve professionally."

Two specific rules of ethics give some guidance when dealing with the cases described in the following pages.

Rule D   "Individuals shall fully inform the persons they serve
          of the nature and possible effects of services rendered
          and products dispensed."

Rule F   "Individuals shall not guarantee the results of any
          treatment or procedure, directly or by implication;
          however, they may make a reasonable statement
          of prognosis."

Principle of Ethics II states that "Individuals shall honor their responsibility to achieve and maintain the highest level of professional competence." Most of the rules provide helpful information about not providing services unless you are competent to do so, but Rule D may help if you are asked to teach someone else to provide dysphagia services.

Rule D   "Individuals shall delegate the provision of clinical ser-
          vices only to persons who are certified or to persons in
          the education or certification process who are appropri-
          ately supervised. The provision of support services may
          be delegated to persons who are neither certified nor in
          the certification process only when a certificate holder
          provides appropriate supervision."

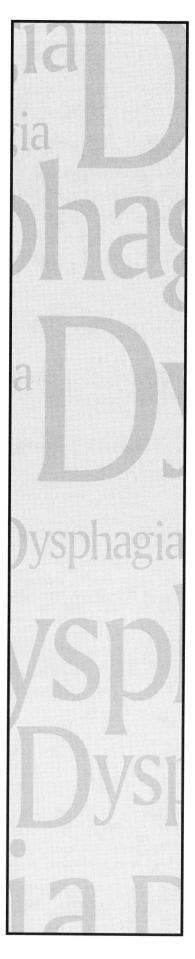

Some decisions you're called upon to make may not necessarily be guided by the ASHA Code of Ethics, but may require an understanding of the principles of biomedical ethics. These principles may help you relate to the family and physician in making difficult decisions.

Principles of Biomedical Ethics

The field of biomedical ethics provides guidance about principles that guide decision making in our culture. A brief summary of some of the major principles is provided here, drawn from the text *Principles of Biomedical Ethics* by Beauchamp and Childress (1994).

Respect for Autonomy

Patients have the right to make independent choices about their care. In order for patients to make autonomous choices, they should be free from controlling influences and actually have the capacity to make independent decisions. Often patients with dysphagia have had strokes with concomitant aphasia, making it difficult for them to make independent choices. When that is the case, you need to involve the patient to the extent he is able to participate, and then rely on the family member(s) to assist in decision making. Beauchamp and Childress call these individuals "surrogate decision makers." Several important court cases have involved decisions made by surrogate decision makers concerning continuing tube feeding (e.g., Karen Ann Quinlan, Claire Conroy, Paul Brophy).

Your evaluation of receptive and expressive language provides crucial information about the patient's ability to participate in decision-making. Medical professionals must not assume that patients and family members cannot make complex decisions about their health. You must provide enough information and education to the patient and family to allow them to make an informed decision, rather than deferring the decision to a physician, nurse, or other medical professional.

Nonmaleficence

This principle asserts a primary principle of medical ethics: "Above all, do no harm." Nonmaleficence means that one should not cause harm or impose risk of harm. It is closely tied to the next principle discussed, beneficence. Some ethicists consider them to be one principle.

Several concepts that provide more specific guidance about doing no harm are related to patients with dysphagia. One is the discussion of a distinction between withholding (i.e., never beginning) and withdrawing (i.e., stopping once it is started) medical treatment. Some argue that withholding is not maleficence, but withdrawing is. Family members may question the difference in removing a feeding tube once it is placed and never putting a tube in to begin with. The more commonly-held belief now is that there is no distinction between withholding and withdrawing treatment.

Another concept discusses the difference between sustenance technologies and medical technologies (Beauchamp and Childress). This is directly related to dysphagia regarding withdrawing artificial feeding vs. withdrawing other life-sustaining technology (e.g., ventilator). The Quinlan and Brophy cases were two early cases which declared that medically administered nutrition and hydration are not significantly different from other life-support techniques. This view is increasingly upheld by courts.

Also related to not doing harm is the issue of whether you should feed a patient suspected of having a significant pharyngeal dysphagia if you cannot obtain an instrumental examination which will allow you to plan appropriate treatment. The principle of nonmaleficence would argue that feeding a patient at risk for aspiration without all necessary information would indeed be placing him at risk for harm.

Beneficence

This principle requires us to not only avoid harming a patient, but to provide positive benefits to them as well. Beauchamp and Childress define beneficence as an "action done for the benefit of others." It implies an obligation to help others. Prevention and education activities might be viewed as beneficent. For example, observing a nursing assistant feeding a patient (not one you are actively treating) too quickly and with the patient in an unsafe position, you, acting in a beneficent manner, would suggest changes in the feeding techniques to the nursing assistant. This would be providing a positive benefit to the patient. Providing general in-services to the staff on appropriate feeding techniques to reduce the risk of aspiration might also be viewed as beneficent acts since positive benefit to all patients in the facility might be the result.

Sometimes professionals must exercise paternalism in order to provide benefit to the patient, or avoid doing harm to the patient. Paternalism is an attitude that, as the professional, you know what is best for the patient. When paternalism is employed, there is a conflict with autonomy. In medicine, an example of paternalism is a physician choosing not to fully disclose a medical diagnosis to a patient based on the belief that the patient will not be able to handle the information and might harm himself. Paternalism involves overriding the patient's right to make autonomous decisions. A common example in dysphagia might occur when a patient who has had a right hemisphere CVA declares that he certainly can remember to take small sips and leave his chin down when taking thin liquids, and therefore does not need supervision to do so. You may know very well that the patient cannot consistently follow this precaution due to impulsivity, and therefore make the paternalistic decision that the patient can have thin liquids only with supervision. This paternalistic decision is a beneficent one.

Justice

The final principle to be discussed is that of justice, which refers to fairness. There is much discussion at the present time about justice, or fairness, related to access to health care. Studies have demonstrated differences in access to care depending on age, race, gender, and ability to pay. The debate over national health care reform centered on providing access to health care for all Americans. The implementation of the Balanced Budget Act of 1997 invoked renewed discussion among SLPs about justice and access to care, as patients in settings like long-term care now have their access to care limited by prospective payment methods and caps on services.

Understanding Patients' Rights

The Patient Self Determination Act (Omnibus Budget Reconciliation Act of 1990) requires all hospitals and nursing homes receiving federal Medicare or Medicaid funding to inform patients of their rights to provide advance directives like living wills, health care surrogates, and durable power of attorney.

An *advance directive* is a legal, written statement of medical choices or the way the patient wants medical choices to be determined. This is written prior to the need for such decisions. Anyone age 18 or over who is of sound mind may write an advance directive. It only goes into effect when the patient can no longer decide for himself or can no longer tell others of his decision. A patient cannot be required to have an advance directive.

Laws about living wills may vary from state to state, but typically a living will directive may include one or more, or all of the following:

- directions that life-prolonging treatment not be provided, or once started, that such treatment be stopped (Life-long prolonging treatment is generally considered to be medical care used to keep a vital body function going after it fails because of illness or injury.)

- directions that food (nutrition) and water (hydration) not be provided through artificial means like tubes, or once started, that they be stopped

- a choice of one or more persons to act as your surrogate(s) and make decisions for you

A health care surrogate is a person you appoint in your living will or in another written document to make medical decisions for you if you're not able to speak for yourself.

The durable power of attorney is an advance directive that lets you name someone (known as your attorney-in-fact) to make medical decisions for you if you're unable to speak for yourself. It's similar to having a health care surrogate, but you might also give your attorney-in-fact power to make decisions about personal and financial affairs.

Familiarize yourself with articles that discuss issues of ethics related to feeding. It appears that U.S. law is ever-increasing in support of the fact that food and liquid should be considered as any other sort of medical treatment which could be refused by a competent patient or on behalf of the patient by a family member or other surrogate. As one of the members of the health care team providing the most information about a patient's ability to eat and prognosis for recovery, you may be asked by family members to help them make a decision.

It can be very effective to help family members make decisions regarding a loved one's care by meeting with family members and:

- patient (when appropriate)
- primary physician
- nurses
- social worker
- spiritual, ethical, and/or legal advisors
- representatives of the institutions involved

Case Examples _____

The following ten case examples may help you think through some ethical dilemmas and challenging case management decisions.

| Case 1 | "I know it takes a long time to feed her, but Mom really enjoys eating." |

The patient is a 75-year-old with advanced dementia. Her daughter thinks that the patient still understands everything going on around her and has chosen not to talk.

The daughter tells you the patient always loved to eat. The patient won't routinely open her mouth for the spoon. Food has to be forced between her lips and it's almost impossible to tell when the patient has swallowed. In an hour and a half, the patient may take 15 bites and a few sips. She has had a modified barium swallow which was fairly inconclusive due to this behavior, but did not show any aspiration on the few swallows of liquid which were poured into her mouth.

1. The physician talks to you because she's concerned that the patient is losing weight and is experiencing some skin breakdown related to poor nutrition. She wants to know your recommendation.

    Discuss your impression that the patient's daughter thinks it's still a pleasurable event for her mother to eat but that in your observation this isn't the case. Ask the physician if the patient had ever expressed her wishes regarding whether she would like to have a feeding tube. Ask if a calorie count might substantiate the impression that the patient isn't able to eat enough by mouth and provide factual information to share with the daughter.

2. The physician wants you to observe the daughter feed the patient a meal and then discuss your observations with the daughter. What will you say to the daughter?

    Try to help the daughter understand that although feeding was a pleasurable event for her mother in the past, having food forced between her lips for an hour and a half three times a day is probably not a pleasurable experience anymore. Also mention your concerns about her mother's weight loss and skin breakdown and discuss the fact that tube feeding and oral feeding can occur together.

3. In the course of the discussion the daughter asks, "If it were your mother, what would you do?" What do you say?

    Try to guide the conversation back to the fact that the daughter has to make the decision about her mother. You might tell her that if you were in this position, you would want to consider all the information available, consider your mother's wishes, and determine what is providing the patient with the most comfort at this time.

Case 2 "I have to ask for a modified barium swallow from Dr. Idon'tthinkso."

You have completed a bedside evaluation on a patient who showed several clinical signs of aspiration, including coughing immediately after thin liquids and wet vocal quality. The patient is also spiking temperatures. The patient did not show clinical signs of aspiration with pudding-thick liquids. Dr. Idon'tthinkso notoriously refuses requests for modified barium swallows, saying they're a waste of money.

1. How do you word your request to Dr. Idon'tthinkso?

   It might be best to sit down with Dr. Idon'tthinkso to discuss the actual cost of a procedure of a modified barium swallow study compared to the cost of treating an aspiration pneumonia. You might also see if you can find a physician who is your ally who would agree to talk with Dr. Idon'tthinkso. Perhaps a radiologist who performs modified barium swallow studies or another specialist who frequently refers for these studies can help you with this discussion. Physicians often listen to one another more readily than they will to other professionals. You may find some useful information in the handout in Chapter 4, pages 106-108.

2. Should you try to find another physician who treats this patient to get the order without consulting Dr. Idon'tthinkso?

   Every facility and physician is different in terms of who will order special studies. Most often, unless the physician is the attending physician, he won't order any special studies without consulting the attending physician.

3. Do you tell the family that it's not safe to feed the patient without the modified barium swallow study and ask them to talk to Dr. Idon'tthinkso?

   Sharing the results of your evaluation including your diagnosis and prognosis with the patient and family is very appropriate. You can even share with them the fact that you're suggesting a modified barium swallow study. However, if you're trying to build a working relationship with the physician, it probably would be best to work through the problem with the physician directly rather than indirectly through the family.

Case 3 "Does the doctor think I have x-ray vision?"

You have recommended a modified barium swallow study on a patient after a bedside evaluation and have also recommended that the patient be made NPO until the study is completed. However, Dr. Goaheadandfeed refuses the modified and writes an order: "SLP to feed whatever diet seems easiest and safest for this patient."

1. Do you begin trial feedings with this patient?

   It's presumed that if you made a recommendation for NPO, you were unable to find any textures the patient could eat safely or any positions or compensatory techniques that would allow the patient to eat safely. If that's the case, it wouldn't make sense to begin trial feedings. However, if you found one texture that the patient seemed to be fairly safe on, like pudding-thick materials, you might begin trial feedings.

2. If you decide not to feed the patient, what do you say to the doctor?

   Either in person or in writing, communicate to the physician that you don't think it's safe for the patient to eat any textures and that no compensatory techniques are effective in eliminating what you consider to be significant clinical signs of aspiration. Indicate that you're declining to participate in further treatment of the patient.

3. If you decide not to feed the patient, what do you say to the patient and/or family?

   This must be carefully worded. You definitely do not want to complain about the physician in front of them. If you had already counseled the patient and family about the results of the evaluation, you might tell them the physician has decided that he or she does not want the patient to have the special x-ray study and wants the patient to eat.

   Suggest some techniques you know which could reduce, but not totally eliminate the risk of aspiration. For instance, you might show them how to position the patient at 90° and discuss other positioning or compensatory techniques. Be sure the family understands why you are uncomfortable participating in therapeutic feeding.

4. If you decide not to feed the patient, what do you say to the staff?

   Explain that you don't think there are any textures the patient can safely take and that your involvement wouldn't be therapeutic at this time. You may want to convey to the staff your concern about the risk for aspiration, and ask that they carefully observe the patient for any further clinical signs of aspiration like spiking temperatures or decreased lung sounds.

Case 4 "But he never wanted a tube . . ."

This 87-year-old patient with advanced dementia and in frail health has returned from a stay in an acute facility for aspiration pneumonia. While there, a modified barium swallow study demonstrated frank aspiration of all textures. No compensatory techniques were found which reduced or eliminated this aspiration.

The patient's family states that years ago the patient expressed that he "never wanted to have to eat my food through no tube in my nose." The patient cries "I want water" throughout the day. The doctor and family have decided against a tube and the doctor writes an order for pureed diet and thick liquids. Staff wants you to feed the patient because you "will know how to do it."

1. Do you agree to feed the patient?

   Consider whether feeding the patient at this point would be a skilled treatment service. It most likely is not, but you might decide to feed the patient for a short period of time to complete patient and family education about techniques which might reduce the risk of aspiration.

2. If you decide to feed the patient, how will you reduce the risk of aspiration?

   Be sure to position the patient at 90° and use other general precautions such as having the patient take small bites and sips and making sure his mouth is empty before presenting the next bite or sip.

3. Why might you decide not to feed the patient?

   You may choose not to become involved if you decide the assessment completed at the acute care facility contains all the information needed for staff to begin to feed the patient.

4. What will you tell the doctor and the family?

   Communicate to the doctor that the assessment completed at the acute care facility provides all necessary information for staff to feed the patient and that there is no need for skilled services at this time.

   Discuss with the family that you understand their careful consideration of the issues and respect their decision to feed the patient. In this type of case, it appears that the physician and family have carefully considered the prognosis for this patient and that they're respecting the wishes of a statement the patient made at a time in his life when he was alert and able to make such decisions.

   Explain that you'll be happy to show them positioning techniques which might help, but there really is no need for you to be involved further because they will be able to feed the patient based on your recommendations.

5. Do you or the family give the patient sips of water per his request?

   You definitely do **not** want to give patient sips of water since the order by the physician is for pureed diet and thick liquids. The family might decide to give water to the patient, but you should recommend against it.

   You may want to discuss with the physician the fact that free water between meals is used with some dysphagia patients in some facilities.

   Many patients state that thickened liquids don't satisfy their feelings of being thirsty. This issue becomes a consideration of patient comfort because if the patient is taking enough thickened liquids, he's getting enough hydration.

6. What other considerations should be discussed?

   It's likely this patient will continue to acquire aspiration pneumonia. The physician and family should discuss whether to treat the aspiration pneumonia.

Case 5	"What is it like to starve to death?"

This patient is an 80-year-old in declining physical health (chronic obstructive pulmonary disease, diabetes mellitus, heart failure) but is cognitively alert. She has had a recent

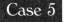

brain stem CVA with resultant profound pharyngeal dysphagia and she is aspirating everything. You have mentioned aspiration pneumonia to her as a probable consequence of eating. She asks you to sit down to discuss her options.

1. She asks what it's like to die of aspiration pneumonia and what it's like to starve to death. What do you tell her?

   Explain to the patient that these questions are probably premature since her dysphagia is the result of an acute event and that you expect some recovery. Suggest that she try some alternatives like therapy and non-oral feedings. Mention that she could choose a time-limited trial of tube feeding and could decide at any point in the future to have the tube feeding removed.

2. She wants to continue to eat and work with you on "exercises to improve my throat." Do you agree to treat her?

   If you have every reasonable expectation that she can achieve some significant improvement in function, you might agree to work with her on exercises, but you probably wouldn't want to work with her in presenting food.

3. The patient's son asks you to talk his mother into a feeding tube. What do you say to him?

   Invite him to sit down in a discussion with the patient, the physician, and any other applicable individuals to discuss the situation. Based on the information provided, a short trial of the feeding tube is probably the most appropriate at this time.

Case 6   "Why are Dad's hands tied down?"

A patient you're seeing through home health has advancing dementia. During a recent inpatient hospitalization, it was determined the patient could eat safely but couldn't eat enough to maintain adequate nutrition and hydration by mouth. Therefore, an NG tube was placed. His hands are restrained because when they aren't restrained, he keeps pulling out the NG tube.

1. The patient's family asks why it's necessary to restrain the patient's hands.

   One consideration is whether the patient's pulling on the tube is a nonverbal expression that he wants the tube out. Sometimes the only thing left in a patient's life over which he has any control is whether or not to agree to tube feeding. Discuss with the family that if the decision is made to keep the NG tube in place, it probably is best to restrain the patient's hands because of the significant discomfort of having to reinsert the tube.

2. The family asks about other available options.

   Explain that a PEG tube is more comfortable for a patient than an NG tube. You might also suggest that another assessment by the clinical nutritionist be completed.

Perhaps the patient wasn't eating well in the hospital because he was away from familiar surroundings. An analysis of how much he takes by mouth in more familiar home surroundings might indicate that he's able to maintain adequate nutrition and hydration.

Case 7 "What's the rush?"

You're called in to consult on a patient in the acute care hospital who has had a right hemisphere CVA two days ago and has an NG tube in place. Patient is believed to have aspiration pneumonia at this time. Physician states she wants to change the NG tube to a G-tube to prevent further development of the aspiration pneumonia.

1. What do you say to the physician about the patient's risk of aspiration pneumonia?

   Discuss that complete bedside and modified barium swallow assessments should give you enough information to make a prognosis for the length of time it might take the patient to return to full PO. If it's a short period of time, keeping the NG tube in place might be a better alternative. Also mention to the physician that many studies indicate that aspiration pneumonia occurs just as frequently with the G-tube and even with the J-tube. Also discuss whether the aspiration could have occurred at the time of the CVA vs. aspiration from the tube feeding.

Case 8 "But a G-tube seems so permanent."

You have recently begun working at a skilled nursing facility and have evaluated a patient who has been fed only by NG tube for the last 10 weeks since his stroke. The patient's receptive and expressive language skills are so impaired that he cannot participate in discussions about his feeding. After your evaluation, you think that the patient will be able to return to eating some things by mouth and possibly even to full PO. However, you estimate that the patient will not reach this level for at least 8 to 12 weeks. You discuss the results of your evaluation with the family and suggest that they discuss a G-tube with the physician.

1. When you explain that you're recommending a change to a G-tube, the family is upset because it sounds like a permanent recommendation. What do you say?

   Discuss that patient comfort is a concern and that 10 weeks is a long time for an NG tube to be in place. Explain that a G-tube is not permanent and that patients can have G-tubes removed if they return to eating safely by mouth.

2. The physician asks on what basis you're making a prognosis for return to PO in 8 to 12 weeks. What do you say?

   You can consult the outcomes information provided by ASHA's National Outcomes Measurement System (NOMS). This report will tell you, on average, how many sessions over what period of time it takes to move a patient from a level requiring tube feeding to a level where the patient can maintain nutrition and hydration by mouth. If your facility is participating in NOMS, you can use your facility's data to answer this question.

| Case 9 | "My facility won't let me ask the doctor for an order for an instrumental exam." |

You provide services in a long-term care facility functioning under the prospective payment system (PPS). The administrator has told you that sending patients out for instrumental assessment of swallowing is too costly and that you will need to plan dysphagia management without any instrumental exams.

1. What can you say to the administrator to convince her that this is not a good decision, either in terms of patient care or fiscal management?

   Discuss what bedside examinations can and cannot tell you about the pharyngeal phase of the swallow. Share statistics about silent aspiration and the risk of aspiration pneumonia associated with patients who aspirate. Volunteer to find out what it costs to treat the patient if pneumonia develops (even if the patient is sent to a hospital, when he returns there will likely be costly medication that needs to continue). You may find some useful information in the handout on pages 106-108. Discuss the legal liability the facility is exposing itself to if they are not providing all the care a patient needs and the patient ends up getting sick because of the facility's policy.

2. How can you show that you aren't over-referring for instrumental exams?

   Review your records and show the administrator how many bedside screenings you have performed and how many times you have asked for instrumental exams in the past (e.g., 6 months, one year). If you have a protocol for determining which risk factors indicate the need for an instrumental exam, share those too.

3. What do you say when the administrator states that the cost of instrumental exams are not covered in the PPS payment?

   Remind her that the Health Care Finance Administration (HCFA) states it did indeed consider the cost of instrumental exams when determining the reimbursement rates for each Resource Utilization Group (RUG) category.

| Case 10 | "My boss wants me to teach the OT how to treat dysphagia." |

You work in a small rural hospital and are only there three days a week. The rehab director wants you to teach the OT on staff (who is there daily and has extra time) how to perform bedside dysphagia evaluations, modified barium swallow studies, and how to treat dysphagia.

1. How do you prepare for the meeting you have asked for to discuss this with the rehab director?

   Prepare for the meeting by obtaining a copy of your state licensure law with your scope of practice and the OT law and their scope. See if anything in the OT scope mentions pharyngeal phase of swallowing. Many OT laws talk about self-feeding or oral-motor skills, but many do not mention pharyngeal phase skills. Obtain a copy of your transcripts from graduate school showing your dysphagia classwork (and related classwork like anatomy and physiology of the respiratory system, head, and neck) as well as documentation of continuing education in the area of dysphagia.

Review your Code of Ethics, specifically Principle of Ethics II, Rule D concerning delegating provision of clinical services only to individuals who are qualified. Review the latest national report card from ASHA's National Outcomes Measurement System (NOMS) to see how much progress patients with dysphagia make when service is provided by a certified SLP (although this is not a comparison of progress patients make when seen by an SLP vs. an OT, OT has no similar national data to combat your outcomes statement). Better yet, if your facility participates in NOMS, you will have your own data to share.

2. What do you say to the rehab director?

Begin by acknowledging that it is problematic that there is not daily coverage for patients with dysphagia. Suggest an arrangement where you (or another SLP) can be on call on the days you are not working at the facility. Perhaps some of the OT "extra" hours could be reduced to pay for the needed SLP hours. If this alternative isn't immediately acceptable, review the documents you have brought with you which clearly indicate that your education and training prepares you to work with patients with dysphagia, while the OT's probably does not, particularly in the area of pharyngeal dysphagia. Discuss how a team approach, with each professional evaluating and treating different components of the patient's problem, will yield the very best care for the patient. Summarize that your Code of Ethics prohibits you from delegating the provision of clinical services to persons who are not qualified.

3. What if the rehab director is not swayed by any of these arguments?

Then you must decide if you can ethically agree to her demands.

Chapter 6

Instrumental Assessment of Swallowing

A bedside, or clinical, evaluation of swallowing has significant limitations. In fact, it should probably be considered a screening. Regardless of how astute your observation skills are at bedside, one can only hypothesize about possible pharyngeal problems. If there is reason to suspect a pharyngeal problem, you should complete an instrumental assessment of swallowing on the patient or refer her for such an assessment.

Currently Medicare regulations state that medical workup and professional assessments must document history, current eating status, and clinical observations. This information is used to determine necessity for further medical testing such as videofluoroscopy. Medicare regulations do not require an instrumental exam, but some intermediaries have decided that they will not reimburse for treatment of pharyngeal dysphagia unless an instrumental examination is done. In at least one state, the intermediary will not reimburse for treatment of any type of dysphagia (i.e., oral and/or pharyngeal) until a modified barium swallow has been done.

When Is an Instrumental Exam Needed?

If the payer does not dictate when you should perform an instrumental examination, how do you decide if one is needed? The overriding consideration is that you suspect a pharyngeal dysphagia. (See Chapter 3, page 41 for information on indicators of pharyngeal problems.) In addition, you may want to recommend an instrumental examination if:

- the patient's pulmonary status or nutritional status is compromised, and dysphagia might be part of the cause of the problem

- you cannot develop an appropriate treatment plan without information obtained on the instrumental examination

- the patient continues to show signs and symptoms of aspiration (e.g., temperature spikes, lung congestion), even though the initial bedside evaluation did not indicate a pharyngeal problem

- the patient has had a previous instrumental examination with specific diet and compensatory techniques recommended to maintain a safe swallow, but you think the patient has changed (improved or declined) and the recommendations need to be adjusted

- the bedside screening is inconclusive (e.g., patient can't vocalize, so you can't tell if a wet vocal quality is present)

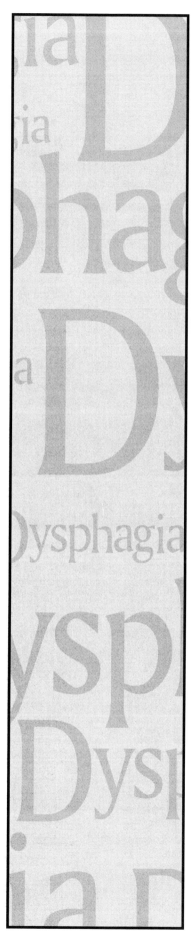

Options for Instrumental Assessment

At the present time, two procedures are widely used by SLPs to assess the pharyngeal phase of the swallow: the videofluoroscopic evaluation (modified barium swallow [MBS]) and fiberoptic endoscopic evaluation of swallowing (FEES®). The majority of this chapter focuses on the MBS and the FEES®. (Note: A derivation of the FEES® includes sensory testing and is known as the FEESST.)

There are four other instrumental techniques that are often used by physicians to assess other aspects of swallowing (e.g., those related to the esophageal phase). These four techniques are not clinically applicable, and therefore are not generally used by SLPs. Brief information about these four techniques follows:

1. *Electromyography*
   This technique uses surface electrodes, or hooked wire electrodes, to provide information about the contraction of a muscle or muscle group. The surface electrodes are usually placed under the patient's chin to measure activity of the floor of mouth muscles which contribute to anterior and superior movement of the hyolaryngeal complex. Hooked wire electrodes have been used to study pharyngeal constrictors. At the present time, such procedures are not easily applied outside the laboratory for diagnosis of swallowing disorders (although surface EMG is used as a biofeedback technique in treatment as described in Chapter 7, page 203).

2. *Pharyngeal Manometry*
   This technique measures the pressure in the upper and lower esophageal sphincters. A flexible tube containing sensors is passed transnasally into the pharynx where the sensors measure pressure at specific points (e.g., base of tongue and cricopharyngeus). This procedure is often done in conjunction with a videofluoroscopic study so that the material passing through the pharynx can be viewed at the same time as the manometric readings are taken. This is still largely an experimental technique.

3. *Scintigraphy*
   This test, completed by nuclear medicine, allows for measurement of the amount of material aspirated. It is the only test which accurately measures the amount of aspiration. It can also determine when aspiration is occurring. For instance, if aspiration of reflux material is suspected, the patient can be scanned at intervals over a period of time, and the amount of aspirated material measured at each interval. This is also considered more of a research tool than a clinical procedure.

4. *Ultrasound*
   Ultrasound uses high frequency sounds to produce dynamic images of soft tissues. It is considered a totally non-invasive procedure. The study is completed by holding a transducer under the chin. This procedure is useful in studying the oral and oral preparatory phases of swallowing. Ultrasound does not allow for observation of aspiration or for thorough analysis of the pharyngeal phase.

Competencies for Performing Instrumental Assessment Procedures

In a position statement entitled "Instrumental Diagnostic Procedures for Swallowing" (1991), ASHA states its position that "clinical (observational) and instrumental assessment of oral, pharyngeal, and upper esophageal function for the purpose of diagnosing and treating patients with swallowing disorders is within the scope of practice of the speech-language pathologist." This helpful document lists precautions or circumstances to consider before beginning to use these procedures. They include:

- Check with your state licensure board to make sure they agree that the procedure is within your scope of practice.

- Check with your institution to see if there are any credentialing steps you must complete before performing the procedure.

- Discuss the procedure with the risk manager at the institution to assure that appropriate policies and procedures are developed.

- Check your professional liability insurance to make sure the procedure is not excluded.

- Use universal precautions for infection control.

- Obtain informed consent of the patient or guardian

- Working with a physician, determine guidelines for when the procedure should and should not be used, and when it needs to be terminated to assure patient safety.

It is also important to assure that staff who are to perform these procedures have demonstrated competence before performing the procedure independently. Arsenault and Atwood (1991) describe a competency-based training model for dysphagia management that can serve as a model for developing your own competency-based training. The ASHA document also provides some information about knowledge and skills needed. You should determine what basic knowledge and skills are needed, how many procedures the staff member will need to perform under direct supervision (of another competent speech-language pathologist and/or a physician), and what specific competencies need to be demonstrated before the staff person can perform the procedure independently. After demonstrating competency, it is important that continued competency be measured. For example, if staff members do not perform the procedure on a routine basis, they may need a refresher training session. It is always a good idea to do periodic checks of staff competencies.

Procedures Routinely Performed by SLPs

The FEES®, FEESST, and the MBS are performed by an SLP to assess the pharyngeal phase of the swallow. Although the MBS has long been considered the gold standard for pharyngeal assessment, the FEES® is being used more frequently now than in the past. ASHA recognizes all of the instrumental procedures listed in "Instrumental Diagnostic Procedures for Swallowing" as being within the scope of SLPs.

Another document which provides information about SLPs performing FEES® is the joint position statement of ASHA and AAO-HNS (American Academy of Otolaryngology-Head and Neck Surgery) entitled: "Roles of the Speech-Language Pathologist and Otolaryngologist in the Performance and Interpretation of Endoscopic Examinations of Swallowing" (ASHA, 2000). This document states in part: "fiberoptic endoscopy is an imaging procedure that may be utilized by SLPs, otolaryngologists, and other qualified health care providers to evaluate velopharyngeal, phonatory, and swallowing functions in adults and children. Physicians are the only professionals qualified and licensed to render medical diagnoses related to the identification of pathology affecting swallowing functions. The assessment and management of dysphagia falls within the scope of practice of speech-language pathology. SLPs with expertise in dysphagia and specialized training in fiberoptic endoscopy are professionals qualified to use this procedure for the purpose of assessing swallowing function and related functions of structures within the upper aerodigestive tract."

There are advantages and disadvantages to both the FEES® and the MBS. Some facilities utilize both procedures. For example, the FEES® may be used as a part of the bedside evaluation to determine if a patient is or is not aspirating. If there is no aspiration, then the FEES® may be the only instrumental examination needed. But for other patients, the FEES® may be used initially to help determine whether the patient is safe to eat and an MBS may be done later for more thorough evaluation of compensatory techniques in order to determine a comprehensive treatment plan.

When performing either the MBS or the FEES®, you should first obtain a complete history (see Chapter 1, pages 7-23 for information on history taking) and find out what the diagnostic question is. For example, does the referring SLP want to know if the patient can upgrade the diet to allow for safe swallowing of thin liquids? Does the physician want to know what the safest diet is for the patient? Knowing the referring question will help you determine the information you need to obtain in the history and help you focus your instrumental examination.

It is not the purpose of this chapter to teach you how to perform and interpret these procedures. Rather, information about each of the procedures is provided, as well as forms that may be useful when performing these procedures.

Modified Barium Swallow (MBS) (Videofluoroscopy)

The MBS is the most frequently used procedure to assess the pharyngeal phase of the swallow. Logemann (1993a; 1993b) was the leader in the development of this procedure and in training SLPs in its use, resulting in widespread acceptance of the MBS. The procedure is performed by an SLP and a radiologist, with a radiology technologist presenting the barium materials to the patient. The MBS allows for visualization of all phases of the swallow, from the oral preparatory phase through the esophageal phase. This dynamic view is captured on videotape for later review (frame by frame if necessary).

The materials needed to perform the study include:

- barium sulfate powder mixed into a liquid form

- thickener (to be mixed with the barium to derive syrup, honey, and pudding-thick consistencies; a smoother liquid will be obtained if the dry thickener and dry barium powder are mixed together before adding the water)

- barium paste (e.g., Esophatrast)

- barium cookies (These are preferred over cookies with barium paste spread on them

as the patient often sucks the paste off a cookie and swallows it. Then when the cookie is masticated and swallowed, it is hard to visualize. [Barium Cookie Recipe, page 161])

- empty capsules which can be filled with barium powder (If the patient particularly complains about inability to swallow pills, use these to see why the patient is having trouble.)

Barium paste or liquid can also be mixed with or applied to specific foods (e.g., particulate matter like rice) if the patient presents with a very specific complaint about difficulty with certain foods. When assessing children, it is often helpful to mix the barium with strongly flavored juices and foods to mask the taste of the barium (e.g., grape juice).

Typically, two views are obtained: lateral and anterior-posterior (A-P). The study typically begins in the lateral view with thin liquids given in small amounts (3cc, 5cc, 10cc) and progresses to uncontrolled amounts if the patient is swallowing safely. Some examiners begin with 1cc, but we have found that such a small bolus is often absorbed into the dry oral cavity and is not enough for the patient to manipulate posteriorly. Liquids are tried from both a cup and a straw (the initial small boluses are often presented on a spoon). The sequence of thick liquids (e.g., syrup, honey, pudding) should be pre-mixed and ready to use in case the patient aspirates on thin liquids and you want to try texture changes. The patient is also given paste bolus (though this material is stickier than many "real" foods, with the possible exception of peanut butter), so a pudding-thick liquid may give a more accurate representation of what the patient will be able to do with pureed foods. If the patient is able to masticate, he is presented with a barium cookie.

The lateral view allows visualization of the oral preparatory and oral (voluntary) phases as the patient manipulates the bolus. You can see problems such as anterior loss, material falling to the floor of the mouth or anterior or lateral sulci, residue on the hard palate, and premature spill of the bolus over the back of the tongue. Be sure the radiologist opens the frame of the fluoroscopy view so that you can see the oral cavity and the pharynx in the same view. The camera should not move to "follow the bolus" if the picture is framed appropriately. The lateral view also allows you to assess the pharyngeal phase where you can observe problems such as: delay in initiation of the pharyngeal swallow; penetration into the upper laryngeal vestibule; aspiration before, during, or after the swallow; residue in valleculae and/or pyriforms, etc. It is crucial to determine what physiological impairment is causing the problem(s).

The lateral view also allows for screening of the esophageal phase of the swallow. Since many esophageal problems have symptoms which are manifested in the pharyngeal region, it is important to screen this phase.

The A-P view provides a way to visualize symmetry of residue in the valleculae and pyriforms, shows whether the bolus moves symmetrically through the hypopharynx, and provides a view of the movement of the vocal cords toward midline. It is very difficult to visualize aspiration in this view because the trachea is immediately in front of the esophagus.

The most important part of the MBS is not the determination of whether or not the patient is aspirating, but rather to figure out why she is and if there is a way to prevent it. Therefore, as soon as the patient begins to exhibit difficulty, you must try compensatory techniques (e.g., posture changes, changes in texture, techniques such as the supraglottic swallow). The charts in Appendix A, pages 162-169, will help you choose compensatory techniques which can be attempted during the study based on the symptom you see as well as the impaired physiology causing that symptom. The chart also lists other facilitation techniques you might try in therapy, but are not appropriate as compensations during the study.

Efficacy of the MBS

There are many studies in the literature which show that the MBS study allows the SLP to identify specific problems in anatomy and physiology of the swallow and to try appropriate treatment or compensatory techniques. For example, Welch et al. (1993) demonstrated that with the chin tucked, there was a posterior shift of anterior pharyngeal structures and a narrowing of the laryngeal entrance and the distance from the epiglottis to the pharyngeal wall and the laryngeal entrance, therefore widening the angle of the epiglottis to the anterior tracheal wall. This provided better airway protection. Logemann et al. (1994) demonstrated that postural techniques are effective in eliminating aspiration of liquids. Postural techniques were successful in eliminating aspiration on at least one volume of liquid in 81% of head and neck surgical patients.

There are also several studies which indicate that the MBS study is more accurate than the bedside exam in identifying whether or not aspiration is occurring as well as identifying the cause of the aspiration (Martin-Harris et al., 1998). Some studies attempt to demonstrate that the use of the MBS changes the number of patients who ultimately get aspiration pneumonia (Daniels et al., 1998; Odderson et al., 1995; Nilsson et al., 1998). The problem with these studies is that the patients got treatment between the assessment and the follow-up to determine if they acquired pneumonia. This made it difficult to determine what role the MBS played in prevention of pneumonia.

By determining which patients are safe to eat, the MBS can prevent unneeded or trial-and-error therapy for patients who do not really need it. Such trial-and-error therapy can be more costly in the long run. In an interesting study with head and neck cancer patients, Logemann et al. (1992) found that patients who had initially been assessed with videofluoroscopy (as compared to bedside assessment alone) had better swallow times and more efficient swallows. The authors conclude that this occurred "because the patient's swallowing therapy was more accurately directed at the nature of the physiologic impairment." Martin-Harris et al. (1998) found that swallowing therapy was only warranted in 37% of 608 patients seen for videofluoroscopic evaluations. Strategies that improved the safety of the swallow and/or efficiency of the swallow were identified on 48% of the exams and diet modifications were determined on 45% of the patients, with most of the patients being upgraded.

Although not exactly comparable, data collected at Central Baptist Hospital in Lexington, Kentucky, an acute care facility, revealed that approximately 17% of outpatients who were not eating by mouth prior to the study could return to some oral intake after the study. We have found that approximately 15% of inpatients who were NPO before the study were able to begin taking some consistencies safely after the MBS study. In addition, 10% of inpatients who had been on a diet were made NPO as a result of the MBS.

Fiberoptic Endoscopic Evaluation of Swallowing (FEES®)

Fiberoptic Endoscopic Evaluation of Swallowing (FEES®) is a procedure initially developed by Susan Langmore, Ph.D. (1988). The FEES® requires a flexible endoscope which is passed transnasally into the pharynx where the tip of the scope hangs just above the epiglottis so that the hypopharynx and larynx can be seen. The scope is left in this position most of the time, but after each swallow it is moved lower into the laryngeal vestibule so you can see the vocal cords and into the subglottic region to see if any material has been aspirated.

The FEES® examination has two basic parts. The first part of the procedure is an examination of the structures and function of the pharynx and larynx. During this part of the exam, the patient's ability to manage secretions can be observed.

Murray et al. (1996) developed a rating scale to predict which patients are at risk for aspiration based on the location of secretions:

0 = no excess secretions
1 = secretions in valleculae, pyriform, lateral channels
2 = transitional rating (changed from a 1 to a 3 during the observation)
3 = secretions in laryngeal vestibule, not cleared

The Murray et al. study involved 49 patients. The authors concluded that using the FEES® to visualize excess secretions and the place of secretions could predict aspiration. They found that 100% of patients rated a 2 or 3 aspirated food or liquid and 53% of patients rated a 1 aspirated food or liquid. However, 21% of patients rated 0 also aspirated. Therefore, visualization of secretions alone cannot be used to determine if the patient will aspirate. Certainly patients rated a 2 or 3 would be considered at high risk to aspirate food or liquid, but those rated a 1 or 2 also have to be considered at risk. As a result, the FEES® should not be stopped after this part of the exam (unless the patient is aspirating her own secretions and does not appear to be able to follow compensatory techniques) because you would have no information about how the patient might do with different textures.

During the second part of the exam, the patient is presented with a variety of textures and bolus sizes of food and liquid to assess swallowing. These materials are dyed green or blue so that they are easy to see in contrast to the mucosal tissue. Some of the problems which may be observed include premature spilling of the bolus over the back of the tongue, penetration of the material into the upper laryngeal vestibule, residue in the valleculae or pyriforms, delay in initiation of swallow, and timing of airway closure.

When the patient demonstrates a problem, compensatory strategies can be attempted (e.g., changes in the texture of food being presented or postural changes). The patient's response to these compensatory strategies yields important information to help make recommendations and develop a treatment plan. A copy of the FEES® Examination Protocol (Karnell and Langmore, 1998) is in Appendix B, page 170-171.

One significant drawback to the FEES® is that at the moment of swallow when the larynx closes, the tip of the scope is obliterated. This is called white-out.

After the swallow when the patient opens her larynx to breathe, the area can again be visualized. Aviv et al. (1998a, 1998b) describe the FEESST. This combines the two stages described above with a technique to determine laryngopharyngeal sensory discrimination thresholds by endoscopically delivering a pulse of air to the anterior wall of the pyriform sinus or to the aryepiglottic folds (innervated by superior laryngeal nerve). Karnell and Langmore (1998) perform sensory testing by touching the tip of the scope lightly to the pharyngeal mucosa, the base of the tongue, or the tip of the epiglottis.

The risks of any endoscopic procedure include discomfort, possible laryngeal spasm and vasovagal response, nose bleed, and allergic reaction to the topical anesthesia used. Endoscopic procedures are typically contraindicated for patients with:

- cardiac arrhythmias
- recent respiratory distress or arrest
- bleeding disorders
- severe arthritis or cervical osteophytes

In addition, endoscopic procedures may be difficult to use with patients who are agitated, aggressive, or hostile, as well with patients with movement disorders, septal deviations, or hypertrophy or reflection (turns back on itself) of the epiglottis.

Efficacy of the FEES®

Leder et al. (1998) and Leder (1998) have contributed two articles to the research base supporting the effectiveness of the FEES® in the evaluation and management of patients with dysphagia. Leder et al. performed the FEES® on 400 consecutive patients referred because of their dysphagia. On the first 56 patients, both the FEES® and the MBS were performed, and a 96% agreement was reached on identifying patients with silent aspiration. Leder detailed the advantages of using FEES® multiple times during a patient's admission to help make decisions about changes in the management of the patient. Specifically, 47% of the subjects received FEES® 3 to 5 times within 6 to 22 days. Leder

stated that "Timely serial FEES® allowed 22 of 32 (69%) subjects to resume an oral diet as early and safely as possible."

Comparison of MBS and FEES®

These two procedures yield similar, but not identical information. There are times when one procedure may be more appropriate than the other. Kidder et al. (1994) summarize some findings that may be better revealed with one or the other technique. Their information has been modified and included below:

Things which are more easily observed with MBS:

- oral phase, with specifics such as tongue movement for formulation and manipulation of the bolus

- tongue base retraction to posterior pharyngeal wall

- forward movement of posterior pharyngeal wall

- anterior and superior movement of hyoid

- laryngeal elevation

- opening of cricopharyngeus

- closure at entrance to the airway between arytenoids and epiglottis

- tipping of the epiglottis

- movement of the bolus during the swallow, including aspiration during the swallow

- movement of bolus through esophageal phase

- effect of the Mendelsohn maneuver

Things which are more easily observed with the FEES®:

- airway closure by true vocal cords, false vocal cords, arytenoid movement

- amount and location of secretions

- pharyngeal/laryngeal sensitivity

- residue in lateral channels, valleculae, and pyriforms

- coordination of breathing and swallowing

- fatigue over the course of a meal

- altered anatomy

Several studies provide comparative information about these two procedures. Briani et al. (1998) examined 23 patients with motor neuron disease using three instrumental procedures: video-fluoroscopy, videopharyngolaryngoscopy, and pharyngo-esophageal manometry. They concluded that "videofluoroscopy was the most sensitive technique in identifying oropharyngeal alterations of swallowing." They also stated "videofluoroscopy was also capable of detecting preclinical abnormalities in non-dysphagic patients who later developed dysphagia."

Périé et al. (1998) evaluated the ability of videoendoscopic swallowing studies to assess pharyngeal propulsion and aspiration episodes when compared with videofluoroscopy and manometry. They examined 34 patients with each of the procedures and found total agreement between videoendoscopy and videofluoroscopy in 76.4% of the patients for pharyngeal propulsion and 82.3% agreement for aspiration.

Langmore et al. (1991) tested 21 subjects with both FEES® and MBS within a 48-hour period. The FEES® was found to be reliable for detecting some of the major pharyngeal symptoms. They found that 75% of subjects who had penetration on FEES® also had penetration on the MBS. Eighty-eight percent of subjects who aspirated on the FEES® also aspirated on the MBS.

Questions and Answers About Instrumental Procedures

When should you refer for an instrumental exam?

Any time you suspect the patient is presenting with a pharyngeal disorder, you should refer for an instrumental exam. Medicare fiscal intermediaries vary greatly in their interpretation of whether or not a patient needs an instrumental exam before they will pay for treatment of that patient. In addition, some facilities are requiring that an instrumental exam be done before they will proceed with a recommendation for the placement of a PEG tube.

Before you refer a patient for an instrumental exam, carefully assess whether the patient will be able to fully participate. Physicians are sometimes reluctant to order repeated studies, so if your patient is being fed by an alternative means and is not very alert or did not participate well on the bedside evaluation, it may not be the best time to refer her for an instrumental exam. It may be more beneficial for the patient to remain NPO with the alternative feeding source until she is more alert and fully able to participate in the study.

An exception to the above might be a patient for whom you do not expect to see improvement in the swallow, but for whom the payer or facility is requiring an instrumental exam to document your prognosis. If that is the case, referral for the exam may be appropriate while the patient is still less than optimally alert.

In addition, if you have a patient for whom a specific technique may be helpful, you may want to defer the study until you can teach the patient that technique (only if the patient is not in any danger of aspiration from PO feeding in the meantime). For example:

1. Your patient presents with a very breathy vocal quality and a wet voice, so you suspect decreased laryngeal closure. You begin working on laryngeal adduction exercises and teaching the patient the supraglottic and super-supraglottic swallow.

2. Your patient shows reduced laryngeal elevation on palpation with a wet vocal quality and delayed cough, so you suspect some aspiration after the swallow coming from residue in the pyriform sinuses. You begin to teach the patient the Mendelsohn maneuver.

It's much better if the patient has begun to learn these techniques before she arrives for the instrumental exam than to try to learn a very difficult maneuver in the span of a few minutes.

What information should you supply about the patient you are referring for an instrumental exam? or If you are performing the study, what kind of information do you want to have?

The *Outpatient Instrumental Exam Referral Form* on page 140 will help you gather the following information:

Medical History: Pertinent information about the patient's medical history may include any diagnoses that might be the etiology for the dysphagia, weight loss that may signal dysphagia, and any recent hospitalizations.

Code Status: It's not likely that a patient will experience cardiac arrest during the exam, but it is critical that you know what to do should this occur. This information is provided in an advance directive.

Tracheostomy: If the patient has a tracheostomy, note which type of tracheostomy tube the patient has and whether it has a cuff. It's also important to know if the cuff can be deflated and whether the patient is routinely fed with the cuff up or down. If the patient is fed with the cuff down, find out if the patient has a tracheostomy speaking valve.

Medications: Some medications can alter the patient's level of alertness during the study. In addition, strong antibiotics might mask temperature spikes related to aspiration.

Present/History of Pneumonia/Aspiration: Temperature spikes, decreased lung sounds, or any recent hospitalizations for pneumonia may indicate aspiration.

Present Complaint: The patient's or referring clinician's description of the problem in the oral phase and suspicions about pharyngeal problems provide diagnostic clues. In addition, although the esophageal phase can't be assessed at bedside, valuable information can be gained about the possible interaction with the esophageal stage through observation and patient report.

Esophageal Symptoms: The patient may complain of a fullness or feeling like there's a lump in her throat. This is a more common symptom of GERD than heartburn. The patient may burp a lot or state that food "comes back up." The patient may cough when lying down or complain of feeling like she's smothering at night. If the patient is experiencing any of these symptoms, you may want to complete an esophageal screening at the same time the MBS study is completed.

Onset of Dysphagia: Information about the onset of dysphagia as sudden versus gradual and about any other related medical problems noted around the same time as onset are important.

Previous Instrumental Exam or Bedside Evaluation Results: Note the results of any previous instrumental exams or bedside evaluations of swallowing. Specify the dates, locations, and results.

Current Diet/Intake: Note which kinds of food and liquids the patient is eating and any special techniques or positions the patient has to use. If the patient is receiving alternative feeding, note whether this feeding is occurring continuously or via bolus feeding.

Independent Sitting Balance/Transfers: Information about the patient's ability to sit and maintain balance and difficulty of transfer is crucial so appropriate seating for the study can be determined. Note whether specialized seating is needed. Also, note whether the patient is wearing any restraints and the reason for the restraints.

What do you tell the patient who is coming in for a study?

You might use fact sheets like the ones on page 78 and 79-81 to provide the patient with information before she comes in for the study. Answer all questions the patient has about the procedure.

What should an instrumental exam report include?

Again relying on Medicare guidelines to provide structure to the discussion, the necessary components of a report on an evaluation should include the following information. A *Modified Barium Swallow Report* is provided on pages 141-144 to collect the information. Two completed sample reports are also included (pages 145-152) to provide further explanation. A *FEES® Report* form is included on pages 153-156. A completed sample *FEES® Report* is provided on pages 157-160.

History: This section should include some information about the patient's prior level of function. Medicare in particular will not pay for therapy designed to take a patient above her prior level of function.

The history should also include any information about the results of previous treatment or evaluations. If a patient showed little progress with previous therapy, a claims reviewer will probably not see the need for further intervention. However, if you can determine why the patient made limited progress, your chances of continuing therapy are improved. For example, you might find that the patient's level of alertness changed due to a medication change or that a previous therapist neglected to try an appropriate technique.

Need for service: The report should clearly indicate why this particular evaluation is needed.

Effects of any strategies attempted: The report should describe any compensatory techniques, facilitation strategies, or diet changes tried during the exam and the patient's response.

Positive expectation: The report should indicate your belief that the patient will be able to change swallowing behaviors. This might be information about some skills the patient exhibited on the modified barium swallow study, her level of cooperation, or her alertness. Conversely, if the patient showed extremely poor performance on the modified barium swallow study, was not alert, or had many complicating diagnoses, it would be difficult to justify intensive therapeutic intervention which requires a lot of cooperation on the patient's part.

Reports should provide information about each of the phases of the swallow assessed. For the MBS, this will include oral preparatory, oral (voluntary), pharyngeal, and esophageal. For the FEES®, only the pharyngeal phase is assessed.

An objective rating scale may be used to provide more information. Duke University (Horner et al., 1992) has developed a *Rating of Radiologic Swallowing Abnormalities* which uses a 5-point (0-4) scale to rate oral preparatory phase, reflex initiation phase, pharyngeal phase residue, pharyngeal appearance in A-P view, aspiration, and pharyngeal-esophageal phase screening.

Rosenbek et al. (1996) developed an 8-point scale to describe penetration and aspiration during videofluoroscopic studies. These scores describe the depth to which material enters the airway and indicates whether or not the material was expelled and swallowed with the rest of the bolus. These objective rating scales provide detailed information about different aspects of the physiology of the swallow, and are particularly useful for patients who receive repeat studies so that changes in physiology can be compared against the scale. These scales are found in Appendix C, pages 172-174.

Specific recommendations: The report should include recommendations about: (See page 144.)

- diet
- food presentation
- food placement
- positioning
- status
- presentation of medications
- nutrition
- charting/monitoring
- compensatory techniques to use during meals
- facilitation/treatment techniques
- re-evaluation

Diagnosis: The report also must identify a specific diagnosis and the phase(s) of swallow affected.

Need for re-evaluation: The report must indicate whether the patient needs to come back for a repeat exam before any changes can be made in the recommendations. For example, if the patient was aspirating, it will almost certainly be necessary for the patient to have another study before the recommendations can be altered.

It's apparent that a silent aspirator will need a repeat exam before trying any food. Some people think that a patient who coughs with aspiration on a study can be upgraded at bedside because a cough can be used to judge whether aspiration is occurring. Unfortunately, the patient's larynx may become desensitized so she no longer coughs with aspiration. In addition, patients are often inconsistent with coughing on aspiration.

What can you do if you aren't getting a report on the studies completed on your patients?

If you are sending a patient to another facility for an instrumental study and do not receive reports or verbal indications concerning the results of the evaluation, make an effort to establish contact with the person who is performing the study. Document your conversation. You might also consider:

a. telephoning the facility and requesting their records

b. sending a signed medical release form requesting their records

c. indicating that you will expect a complete written report by a certain date

If your schedule permits, you may also want to attend the study so you can actually see what is going on with your patient. In addition, you may want to request a videotape of the study so you have a permanent record at your facility. It is impossible to plan effective treatment for the patient if you don't know the complete results of the study. Some facilities will write out a short consult on a form to give to the patient. (See page 139.)

How do you document if you are not following the recommendations from the report?

Once you've received a report from the instrumental exam and are implementing intervention, it is important to document any changes which occur in the patient's status and whether they are positive or negative changes. For example, you may send a patient for a study and within a week of that study, the patient experiences a neurological event such as a CVA or TIA. This may render the recommendations of the study invalid. Make sure you note this in your documentation and indicate why you're changing the treatment plan from that which was recommended based on the instrumental exam.

Instrumental Exam Consult ━━━━━━━━━━━━━━━━━━

Patient _____ Date _____

Patient # _____

On _____, a special evaluation of this patient's swallowing was completed. The patient received a:

    ❏ modified barium swallow

    ❏ fiberoptic endoscopic evaluation of swallowing

Special instructions based on the results of that evaluation include:

_____

_____

_____

_____

_____

_____

You can call us at _____ any time if you have any questions.

_____
    Speech-Language Pathologist

Outpatient Instrumental Exam Referral Form _____

Patient _____ Birthdate _____ Age _____

Address (if patient lives at home) _____

_____

Patient's Phone _____ Physician _____

Physician Address _____

Facility _____

Facility Address _____

Facility Phone _____

Person Making Referral _____ Relationship to Patient _____

A. **Medical History** _____

_____

B. **Code Status** _____

C. **Tracheostomy**   type _____
        cuffed / uncuffed   fed with cuff up / down
        If cuff is down, speaking valve used?   yes / no

D. **Medications** _____

_____

E. **Presence/History of Pneumonia/Aspiration** _____

F. **Present Complaint** _____

_____

G. **Esophageal Symptoms** _____

H. **Onset of Dysphagia** _____

I. **Previous Instrumental Exam or Bedside Evaluation Results** _____

_____

J. **Current Diet/Intake** _____

_____

K. **Independent Sitting Balance/Transfers** _____

_____

Referral Information taken by _____ Date _____

Modified Barium Swallow Report

History_____

_____

_____

_____

Why Study Is Needed _____

_____

_____

Procedure

The patient was seen for a modified barium swallow/videofluoroscopic evaluation with radiology and speech-language pathology. _____ consistencies (_____) were presented for analyses of three / four phases of the swallow.

Oral Preparatory Phase

This phase involves oral movements immediately before initiation of the voluntary stage of the swallow.

thin liquids _____

thick liquids _____

pudding _____

cookie _____

Oral Voluntary Phase

This phase begins when the tongue initiates posterior movement of the bolus. It typically takes less than one second to complete.

thin liquids _____

thick liquids _____

pudding _____

cookie _____

Pharyngeal Phase

This phase begins with the triggering of the swallow reflex. Normally the swallowing reflex is triggered as the bolus contacts the anterior faucial arches. Normal transit time from anterior faucial arches to cricopharyngeal juncture is one second or less.

thin liquids _____

_____

thick liquids _____

_____

pudding _____

_____

cookie _____

_____

A-P View _____

_____

_____

Cervical Esophageal Phase _____

_____

_____

Effects of Treatment Strategies Attempted _____

_____

_____

_____

Duke Ratings Oral Prep: _____   Reflex Initiation: _____   Pharyngeal Phase: _____

A-P View: _____   Aspiration: _____   Pharyngeal-Esophageal Screening: _____

Penetration-Aspiration Rating _____

Summary and Need for Service _____

_____

_____

_____

_____

_____

Diagnosis _____

Positive Expectation to Begin Service _____

_____

_____

Patient/Caregiver Teaching _____

_____

_____

Short-Term Goals

These goals reflect disordered physiology related to the pharyngeal phase. (Goals for the oral phase are found on the bedside evaluation form, page 57.)

_____ Patient will improve back of tongue control to keep food from falling over the back of the tongue and into the airway.

_____ Patient will decrease delay in initiation of pharyngeal swallow to reduce food falling into the airway during the delay before the swallow.

_____ Patient will increase closure of the true vocal folds to keep food from falling into the airway during the swallow.

_____ Patient will improve rate of laryngeal elevation/timing of closure to keep food from falling into the airway during the swallow.

_____ Patient will increase laryngeal elevation to reduce residue in the pyriform sinus(es) and reduce risk of the residue falling into the airway after the swallow.

_____ Patient will increase anterior movement of the hyolaryngeal complex to reduce residue in the pyriform sinuses and reduce the risk of the residue falling into the airway after the swallow.

_____ Patient will improve laryngeal elevation to reduce penetration into the upper laryngeal vestibule to reduce the risk of the penetrated material being aspirated after the swallow.

_____ Patient will improve arytenoid tipping/closure at entrance to the airway to reduce penetration into the upper laryngeal vestibule to reduce the risk of the penetrated material being aspirated after the swallow.

_____ Patient will improve the rate of laryngeal elevation/timing of closure to reduce penetration into the upper laryngeal vestibule to reduce the risk of the penetrated material being aspirated after the swallow.

_____ Patient will increase base of tongue movement to reduce vallecular residue (unilateral or bilateral) to reduce the risk of the residue being aspirated after the swallow.

_____ Patient will increase movement of the posterior pharyngeal wall to reduce vallecular residue to reduce the risk of the residue being aspirated after the swallow.

_____ Patient will increase laryngeal elevation to reduce vallecular residue to reduce the risk of the residue being aspirated after the swallow.

_____ Patient will increase movement of pharyngeal wall(s) to reduce residue on pharyngeal wall(s) (unilateral or bilateral) to reduce the risk of the residue being aspirated after the swallow.

_____ Patient will increase movement of the tongue base to reduce bilateral residue on pharyngeal walls to reduce the risk of the residue being aspirated after the swallow.

_____ No skilled treatment indicated.   Comments:_____

Recommendations _____

Patient _____ Date _____ Patient # _____

❏ NPO

❏ PO Diet Recommendations

Dysphagia Diet
❏ Level I (runny pureed)
❏ Level II (thick pureed, pudding liquids)
❏ Level III (pureed and some soft;
   liquids: syrup/honey/pudding)
❏ Level IV (soft cohesive;
   liquids: syrup/honey/pudding)
❏ Level V (mech. soft; regular liquids)

Food Presentation
❏ bolus size: ½ tsp/1 tsp
❏ cut-out cup
❏ cup
❏ straw
❏ spoon only
❏ no straw
❏ no syringe

Food Placement
❏ left side mouth/visual field
❏ right side mouth/visual field
❏ present food from front to increase sensory input

Positioning
❏ sitting up at 90°
❏ head turned to _____
❏ chin tuck _____
❏ stay seated upright ___ minutes after meals

Status
❏ patient can self-feed without supervision
❏ verbal cues/standby assistance
❏ dependent to be fed by SLP only/staff/family

Presentation of Meds
❏ pills/tablets whole followed by liquids/applesauce/
   thick liquid
❏ pills/tablets must be crushed and mixed with applesauce
❏ no liquid meds
❏ meds via tube

Nutrition
❏ primary nutrition by tube
❏ trial PO during therapy only
❏ hold tube feedings _____ prior to oral feeding

Charting/Monitoring
❏ weekly heights
❏ calorie count
❏ monitor temperature _____
❏ listen for vocal quality throughout meal

Other
❏ reflux precautions—see attached
_____
_____
_____

c = compensatory techniques to use during meal
f = facilitation/treatment techniques

Selected treatment techniques to begin.
Others can be chosen to achieve short-term goals.

Oral Dysphagia
❏ labial closure (c, f)
❏ lingual elevation exercises (f)
❏ lingual lateralization exercises (f)
❏ lingual A-P exercises (f)
❏ lingual back of tongue exercises (f)
❏ compensations for oral residue (c)
   ❏ sweep mouth with tongue
   ❏ sweep mouth with finger
   ❏ external pressure to cheek
   ❏ rinse mouth/expel after meal

Decreased Laryngeal Elevation
❏ Mendelsohn maneuver/SEMG (c, f)
❏ falsetto/laryngeal elevation exercises (f)

Decreased Laryngeal Closure
❏ supraglottic (safe) swallow (c, f)
❏ super-supraglottic swallow (c, f)
❏ laryngeal closure exercises (f)
❏ encourage cough (c)

Decreased Base of Tongue Strength/ Posterior Pharyngeal Wall
❏ tongue hold (f)
❏ tongue base retraction (f)
❏ pretend to gargle (f)
❏ pretend to yawn (f)
❏ effort swallow (c, f)

Delayed Swallow
❏ thermal/tactile stimulation (c, f)
❏ three-second prep (c, f)
❏ slurp swallow (c, f)
❏ sour bolus (c, f)
❏ cold bolus (c, f)
❏ neurosensory stimulation (f)

Decreased Anterior Movement of Hyolaryngeal Complex
❏ head lift (f)

Misc. Compensation for Oral/Pharyngeal Dysphagia
❏ alternate (thick) liquid swallow every bite/PRN (c)
❏ discourage liquid wash between bites (c)
❏ multiple swallows
   (patient does/does not need cues) (c)
❏ empty mouth before next bite (c)
❏ cue patient to slow down (c)

Re-evaluation
❏ if condition changes
❏ before discontinuing any of these recommendations
❏ can advance food only at bedside
❏ can advance food and liquids at bedside
❏ other _____

Signature _____

Sample Modified Barium Swallow Report A _____

Patient _Fred_____	Date _____
Birthdate _____ Age _68_____	Patient # _____
Referral Physician _____	
Patient's Address _____	Phone _____

History _Fred is a 68-year-old male who is currently an in-patient at this acute care facility. He suffered a left_
CVA with resulting right hemiparesis, aphasia, dysarthria, and dysphagia. His medical history also includes
arteriosclerotic cardiovascular disease, hypertension, and diabetes. Patient currently has an NG tube and is
NPO except for ice chips.

Why Study Is Needed _Physician referral for an MBS study based on recommendations from the Dysphagia_
Team. Patient was seen at bedside and demonstrated wet vocal quality with all textures presented. He also had
an intermittent cough throughout the study.

Procedure

The patient was seen for a modified barium swallow/videofluoroscopic evaluation with radiology and
speech-language pathology. _____Four_____ consistencies (_thin liquid, syrup thick, pudding, cookie_____)
were presented for analyses of three /(four)phases of the swallow.

Oral Preparatory Phase

This phase involves oral movements immediately before initiation of the voluntary stage of the swallow.

thin liquids	_shows anterior loss_
thick liquids	_shows anterior loss, better able to form bolus_
pudding	_no anterior loss, able to form fairly adequate bolus_
cookie	_residue in lateral sulcus, difficulty getting entire bolus on top of tongue_

Oral Voluntary Phase

This phase begins when the tongue initiates posterior movement of the bolus. It typically takes less than
one second to complete.

thin liquids	_trickle over back of tongue in a premature fashion to valleculae; no penetration or aspiration before the swallow_
thick liquids	_able to propel bolus posteriorly with minimal difficulty_
pudding	_able to propel bolus posteriorly with minimal difficulty_
cookie	_very piecemeal in his approach to propelling the cookie posteriorly, residue on tongue and in sulcus_

Pharyngeal Phase

This phase begins with the triggering of the swallow reflex. Normally the swallowing reflex is triggered as the bolus contacts the anterior faucial arches. Normal transit time from anterior faucial arches to cricopharyngeal juncture is one second or less.

thin liquids — *b/c of decreased closure at entrance to airway, there is penetration into the upper laryngeal vestibule during the swallow w/boluses, trace aspiration after the swallow, consistent cough reaction to aspiration*

thick liquids — *reflex initiates adequately, occasional minimal penetration into upper laryngeal vestibule but never aspirated, minimal residue in valleculae and pyriform sinuses*

pudding — *no penetration/aspiration, adequate laryngeal elevation, vallecular residue after the swallow indicating reduced base of tongue pressure, decreased movement of posterior pharyngeal wall*

cookie — *no penetration or aspiration, some vallecular residue*

A-P View *reveals symmetrical pooling in valleculae, appears to reveal adequate movement of vocal folds to midline*

Cervical Esophageal Phase *screened only with patient in upright, does not present with any complaints related to esophageal phase, shows adequate esophageal motility*

Effects of Treatment Strategies Attempted *Thin liquids — Patient placed in chin-down posture. This position eliminates penetration on 3cc & 5cc boluses. At 10cc, patient has some penetration, but no aspiration. Honey & pudding — Patient asked to try an effort swallow to reduce amount of vallecular residue. It appears to help, but patient can only maintain this for several trials.*

Duke Ratings Oral Prep: *2 moderate* Reflex Initiation: *3 mild* Pharyngeal Phase: *3 mild residue*

A-P View: *4* Aspiration: *3* Pharyngeal-Esophageal Screening: *3 mild trace audible*

Penetration-Aspiration Rating *7*

Summary and Need for Service *Fred, age 68, presents with moderately impaired oral preparatory phase with difficulty forming a bolus with masticated materials. In addition, he shows decreased back of tongue control which results in thin liquids trickling over the back of the tongue. This can be decreased somewhat w/chin-down posture. Patient penetrated and then aspirated thin liquids. Penetration eliminated w/chin-down posture on smaller boluses and aspiration totally eliminated. Still had some penetration w/larger liquid boluses w/chin-down. Patient has vallecular residue secondary to reduced base of tongue and posterior pharyngeal wall movement. Patient needs intervention if he is to return to a more normal diet and avoid risk of aspiration.*

Diagnosis *oral and pharyngeal dysphagia w/audible trace aspiration of thin liquids*

Positive Expectation to Begin Service *Patient is alert and cooperative and follows basic one-step commands. He wants to have NG tube removed and eat by mouth.*

Patient/Caregiver Teaching *The results of the eval were discussed in detail w/patient. He appeared to*
understand that some modifications in his eating are necessary. His wife appeared to understand the
recommendations as well.

Short-Term Goals

These goals reflect disordered physiology related to the pharyngeal phase. (Goals for the oral phase are
found on the bedside evaluation form, page 57.)

✓ Patient will improve back of tongue control to keep food from falling over the back of the tongue
and into the airway.

_____ Patient will decrease delay in initiation of pharyngeal swallow to reduce food falling into the airway
during the delay before the swallow.

_____ Patient will increase closure of the true vocal folds to keep food from falling into the airway during
the swallow.

_____ Patient will improve rate of laryngeal elevation/timing of closure to keep food from falling into the
airway during the swallow.

_____ Patient will increase laryngeal elevation to reduce residue in the pyriform sinus(es) and reduce risk
of the residue falling into the airway after the swallow.

_____ Patient will increase anterior movement of the hyolaryngeal complex to reduce residue in the
pyriform sinuses and reduce the risk of the residue falling into the airway after the swallow.

_____ Patient will improve laryngeal elevation to reduce penetration into the upper laryngeal vestibule
to reduce the risk of the penetrated material being aspirated after the swallow.

✓ Patient will improve arytenoid tipping/closure at entrance to the airway to reduce penetration into
the upper laryngeal vestibule to reduce the risk of the penetrated material being aspirated after the
swallow.

_____ Patient will improve the rate of laryngeal elevation/timing of closure to reduce penetration into the
upper laryngeal vestibule to reduce the risk of the penetrated material being aspirated after the
swallow.

_____ Patient will increase base of tongue movement to reduce vallecular residue (unilateral or bilateral)
to reduce the risk of the residue being aspirated after the swallow.

_____ Patient will increase movement of the posterior pharyngeal wall to reduce vallecular residue to
reduce the risk of the residue being aspirated after the swallow.

_____ Patient will increase laryngeal elevation to reduce vallecular residue to reduce the risk of the residue
being aspirated after the swallow.

✓ Patient will increase movement of pharyngeal wall(s) to reduce residue on pharyngeal wall(s)
(unilateral or bilateral) to reduce the risk of the residue being aspirated after the swallow.

✓ Patient will increase movement of the tongue base to reduce bilateral residue on pharyngeal
walls to reduce the risk of the residue being aspirated after the swallow.

_____ No skilled treatment indicated.   Comments:_____

Sample Recommendations _____

Patient _Fred_____   Date _____   Patient # _____

❏ NPO

☒ PO Diet Recommendations

Dysphagia Diet
- ❏ Level I (runny pureed)
- ❏ Level II (thick pureed, pudding liquids)
- ☒ Level III (pureed and some soft;
  liquids: (syrup)/honey/pudding)
- ❏ Level IV (soft cohesive;
  liquids: syrup/honey/pudding)
- ❏ Level V (mech. soft; regular liquids)

Food Presentation
- ☒ bolus size: ½ tsp/(1 tsp)
- ☒ cut-out cup
- ❏ cup
- ❏ straw
- ❏ spoon only
- ❏ no straw
- ❏ no syringe

Food Placement
- ☒ left side mouth/visual field
- ❏ right side mouth/visual field
- ❏ present food from front to increase sensory input

Positioning
- ❏ sitting up at 90°
- ❏ head turned to _____
- ☒ chin tuck _for liquids_
- ☒ stay seated upright _30_ minutes after meals

Status
- ❏ patient can self-feed without supervision
- ☒ verbal cues/standby assistance
- ❏ dependent to be fed by SLP only/staff/family

Presentation of Meds
- ❏ pills/tablets whole followed by liquids/applesauce/
  thick liquid
- ☒ pills/tablets must be crushed and mixed with applesauce
- ❏ no liquid meds
- ❏ meds via tube

Nutrition
- ❏ primary nutrition by tube
- ❏ trial PO during therapy only
- ☒ hold tube feedings _2 hours_ prior to oral feeding

Charting/Monitoring
- ❏ weekly heights
- ☒ calorie count
- ❏ monitor temperature _____
- ❏ listen for vocal quality throughout meal

Other
- ❏ reflux precautions—see attached
  _thin liquids 5 cc only w/SLP_____
  _not at meals_____
  _____

c = compensatory techniques to use during meal
f = facilitation/treatment techniques

Selected treatment techniques to begin.
Others can be chosen to achieve short-term goals.

Oral Dysphagia
- ☒ labial closure (c)(f)
- ❏ lingual elevation exercises (f)
- ❏ lingual lateralization exercises (f)
- ❏ lingual A-P exercises (f)
- ☒ lingual back of tongue exercises (f)
- ☒ compensations for oral residue (c)
  - ☒ sweep mouth with tongue
  - ☒ sweep mouth with finger
  - ☒ external pressure to cheek (R)
  - ❏ rinse mouth/expel after meal

Decreased Laryngeal Elevation
- ❏ Mendelsohn maneuver/SEMG (c, f)
- ❏ falsetto/laryngeal elevation exercises (f)

Decreased Laryngeal Closure
- ❏ supraglottic (safe) swallow (c, f)
- ☒ super-supraglottic swallow (c,(f))
- ❏ laryngeal closure exercises (f)
- ❏ encourage cough (c)

Decreased Base of Tongue Strength/ Posterior Pharyngeal Wall
- ☒ tongue hold (f)
- ❏ tongue base retraction (f)
- ❏ pretend to gargle (f)
- ❏ pretend to yawn (f)
- ☒ effort swallow (c)(f)

Delayed Swallow
- ❏ thermal/tactile stimulation (c, f)
- ❏ three-second prep (c, f)
- ❏ slurp swallow (c, f)
- ❏ sour bolus (c, f)
- ❏ cold bolus (c, f)
- ❏ neurosensory stimulation (f)

Decreased Anterior Movement of Hyolaryngeal Complex
- ❏ head lift (f)

Misc. Compensation for Oral/Pharyngeal Dysphagia
- ☒ alternate (thick) liquid swallow every bite (PRN) (c)
- ❏ discourage liquid wash between bites (c)
- ☒ multiple swallows
  (patient (does)/does not need cues) (c)
- ❏ empty mouth before next bite (c)
- ❏ cue patient to slow down (c)

Re-evaluation
- ❏ if condition changes
- ❏ before discontinuing any of these recommendations
- ☒ can advance food only at bedside
- ❏ can advance food and liquids at bedside
- ❏ other _____

Signature _____

Sample Modified Barium Swallow Report B _____

Patient _Ethel_____	Date _____
Birthdate _____ Age _78_____	Patient # _____
Referral Physician _____	
Patient's Address _____	Phone _____

History _Referred for MBS by SLP at Happy Hills SNF where patient is a recent admit. Patient lived at home_
w/a caregiver, but over past 6 months, she has lost 15 lbs. on a regular diet. Diagnosed w/Alzheimer's disease,
insulin-dependent diabetes mellitus, and congestive heart failure. She was reportedly eating less than 1/4 of the
food presented to her at home. On admit, SLP eval revealed a delay in the oral phase of up to 15 secs which could
be reduced with extra stimulation in the oral cavity. Patient placed on a pureed diet and honey-thick liquids.

Why Study Is Needed _Patient shows coughing with thin liquids and was considered at risk for aspiration._

Procedure

The patient was seen for a modified barium swallow/videofluoroscopic evaluation with radiology and
speech-language pathology. ____Four_____ consistencies (_thin liquids, honey thick, pudding, cookie_____)
were presented for analyses of three /(four) phases of the swallow.

Oral Preparatory Phase

This phase involves oral movements immediately before initiation of the voluntary stage of the swallow.

thin liquids	_holds bolus in oral phase up to 10-15 seconds despite repeated verbal cues to swallow_
thick liquids	_holds bolus in oral phase up to 10-15 seconds despite repeated verbal cues to swallow_
pudding	_holds bolus in oral phase up to 10-15 seconds despite repeated verbal cues to swallow_
cookie	_chews bolus for up to 60 secs.; bolus then must be removed from oral cavity_

Oral Voluntary Phase

This phase begins when the tongue initiates posterior movement of the bolus. It typically takes less than
one second to complete.

thin liquids	_When patient finally initiates posterior movement, this phase is functional._
thick liquids	_When patient finally initiates posterior movement, this phase is functional._
pudding	_When patient finally initiates posterior movement, this phase is functional._
cookie	_not observed_

Pharyngeal Phase

This phase begins with the triggering of the swallow reflex. Normally the swallowing reflex is triggered as the bolus contacts the anterior faucial arches. Normal transit time from anterior faucial arches to cricopharyngeal juncture is one second or less.

thin liquids — presented w/graduated sizes: 3 and 5cc from spoon, 10cc from cup, then uncontrolled amounts from cup and straw; shows minimal penetration into upper laryngeal vestibule w/large boluses w/straw; coughs w/penetration; no aspiration

thick liquids — functional (patient in reclined position for thin/thick liquid presentations; aspiration occurred before the swallow)

pudding — functional

cookie — not observed

A-P View no residue and apparently adequate movements of vocal folds to midline

Cervical Esophageal Phase This stage was screened in sidelying and supine. Radiology reports the presence of dismotility and gastroesophageal reflux which could account for some of the patient's coughing.

Effects of Treatment Strategies Attempted Added pressure was provided in the oral cavity via spoon on the tongue, and it helped improve the patient's ability to move the bolus posteriorly. If the patient still didn't swallow, an empty spoon was touched to her lips. This seemed to initiate posterior movement.

Duke Ratings Oral Prep: 2 moderate   Reflex Initiation: 4   Pharyngeal Phase: 4
A-P View: 4   Aspiration: 4   Pharyngeal-Esophageal Screening: 4

Penetration-Aspiration Rating 2

Summary and Need for Service Ethel, age 78, presents with moderate oral dysphagia typically seen in patients w/Alzheimer's disease. She holds the bolus in her oral cavity for up to 15 seconds, but can reduce the time when added pressure and verbal cues are provided. She chews masticated foods for up to 1 minute and never initiates the voluntary phase. The foods then must be removed from the oral cavity. Because it had been reported that the patient is sometimes fed in a reclined position, she was presented with thin & honey-thick liquids in this position. Patient begins to aspirate boluses before the swallow in this position. This patient should need only diet changes and supervision during meals, but not skilled service from an SLP. Control bolus sizes w/thin liquids; honey-thick liquids can be taken in uncontrolled amounts.

Diagnosis moderate oral dysphagia, mild pharyngeal dysphagia

Positive Expectation to Begin Service Patient is alert and cooperative and should work well with caregivers who are modifying her diet.

Patient/Caregiver Teaching <u>This study was observed by a Nursing Assistant from the facility. Results</u>
<u>discussed w/her and w/patient to the extent that patient could understand. Results also discussed by phone</u>
<u>w/SLP from the facility.</u>

Short-Term Goals

These goals reflect disordered physiology related to the pharyngeal phase. (Goals for the oral phase are
found on the bedside evaluation form, page 57.)

_____ Patient will improve back of tongue control to keep food from falling over the back of the tongue
and into the airway.

_____ Patient will decrease delay in initiation of pharyngeal swallow to reduce food falling into the airway
during the delay before the swallow.

_____ Patient will increase closure of the true vocal folds to keep food from falling into the airway during
the swallow.

_____ Patient will improve rate of laryngeal elevation/timing of closure to keep food from falling into the
airway during the swallow.

_____ Patient will increase laryngeal elevation to reduce residue in the pyriform sinus(es) and reduce risk
of the residue falling into the airway after the swallow.

_____ Patient will increase anterior movement of the hyolaryngeal complex to reduce residue in the
pyriform sinuses and reduce the risk of the residue falling into the airway after the swallow.

_____ Patient will improve laryngeal elevation to reduce penetration into the upper laryngeal vestibule
to reduce the risk of the penetrated material being aspirated after the swallow.

_____ Patient will improve arytenoid tipping/closure at entrance to the airway to reduce penetration into
the upper laryngeal vestibule to reduce the risk of the penetrated material being aspirated after the
swallow.

_____ Patient will improve the rate of laryngeal elevation/timing of closure to reduce penetration into the
upper laryngeal vestibule to reduce the risk of the penetrated material being aspirated after the
swallow.

_____ Patient will increase base of tongue movement to reduce vallecular residue (unilateral or bilateral)
to reduce the risk of the residue being aspirated after the swallow.

_____ Patient will increase movement of the posterior pharyngeal wall to reduce vallecular residue to
reduce the risk of the residue being aspirated after the swallow.

_____ Patient will increase laryngeal elevation to reduce vallecular residue to reduce the risk of the residue
being aspirated after the swallow.

_____ Patient will increase movement of pharyngeal wall(s) to reduce residue on pharyngeal wall(s)
(unilateral or bilateral) to reduce the risk of the residue being aspirated after the swallow.

_____ Patient will increase movement of the tongue base to reduce bilateral residue on pharyngeal
walls to reduce the risk of the residue being aspirated after the swallow.

✓ No skilled treatment indicated. Comments:_____

Sample Recommendations

Patient _Ethel_   Date _____   Patient # _____

❏ NPO

❏ PO Diet Recommendations

Dysphagia Diet
  ❏ Level I (runny pureed)   _thin_
  ☒ Level II (thick pureed, ~~pudding~~ liquids)
  ❏ Level III (pureed and some soft;
       liquids: syrup/honey/pudding)
  ❏ Level IV (soft cohesive;
       liquids: syrup/honey/pudding)
  ❏ Level V (mech. soft; regular liquids)

Food Presentation
  ☒ bolus size: ½ tsp (1 tsp)
  ❏ cut-out cup
  ☒ cup
  ❏ straw
  ❏ spoon only
  ☒ no straw
  ☒ no syringe

Food Placement
  ❏ left side mouth/visual field
  ❏ right side mouth/visual field
  ☒ present food from front to increase sensory input

Positioning
  ☒ sitting up at 90°
  ❏ head turned to _____
  ❏ chin tuck _____
  ❏ stay seated upright ___ minutes after meals

Status
  ❏ patient can self-feed without supervision
  ❏ verbal cues/standby assistance
  ☒ dependent to be fed by SLP only/(staff) (family)

Presentation of Meds
  ❏ pills/tablets whole followed by liquids/applesauce/
       thick liquid
  ☒ pills/tablets must be crushed and mixed with applesauce
  ❏ no liquid meds
  ❏ meds via tube

Nutrition
  ❏ primary nutrition by tube
  ❏ trial PO during therapy only
  ❏ hold tube feedings _____ prior to oral feeding

Charting/Monitoring
  ☒ weekly heights
  ❏ calorie count
  ❏ monitor temperature _____
  ❏ listen for vocal quality throughout meal

Other
  ❏ reflux precautions—see attached
  added pressure to tongue or present empty spoon
  to touch lips to cue swallow; verbal cues to swallows

c = compensatory techniques to use during meal
f = facilitation/treatment techniques

Selected treatment techniques to begin.
Others can be chosen to achieve short-term goals.

Oral Dysphagia
  ❏ labial closure (c, f)
  ❏ lingual elevation exercises (f)
  ❏ lingual lateralization exercises (f)
  ❏ lingual A-P exercises (f)
  ❏ lingual back of tongue exercises (f)
  ❏ compensations for oral residue (c)
      ❏ sweep mouth with tongue
      ❏ sweep mouth with finger
      ❏ external pressure to cheek
      ❏ rinse mouth/expel after meal

Decreased Laryngeal Elevation
  ❏ Mendelsohn maneuver/SEMG (c, f)
  ❏ falsetto/laryngeal elevation exercises (f)

Decreased Laryngeal Closure
  ❏ supraglottic (safe) swallow (c, f)
  ❏ super-supraglottic swallow (c, f)
  ❏ laryngeal closure exercises (f)
  ❏ encourage cough (c)

Decreased Base of Tongue Strength/ Posterior Pharyngeal Wall
  ❏ tongue hold (f)
  ❏ tongue base retraction (f)
  ❏ pretend to gargle (f)
  ❏ pretend to yawn (f)
  ❏ effort swallow (c, f)

Delayed Swallow
  ❏ thermal/tactile stimulation (c, f)
  ❏ three-second prep (c, f)
  ❏ slurp swallow (c, f)
  ❏ sour bolus (c, f)
  ❏ cold bolus (c, f)
  ❏ neurosensory stimulation (f)

Decreased Anterior Movement of Hyolaryngeal Complex
  ❏ head lift (f)

Misc. Compensation for Oral/Pharyngeal Dysphagia
  ❏ alternate thick liquid swallow every bite/PRN (c)
  ❏ discourage liquid wash between bites (c)
  ❏ multiple swallows
       (patient does/does not need cues) (c)
  ❏ empty mouth before next bite (c)
  ❏ cue patient to slow down (c)

Re-evaluation
  ☒ if condition changes
  ❏ before discontinuing any of these recommendations
  ❏ can advance food only at bedside
  ❏ can advance food and liquids at bedside
  ❏ other _____

Signature _____

FEES® Report ———————————————————

Patient _____	Date _____
Birthdate _____ Age _____	Patient # _____
Referral Physician _____	
Patient's Address _____	Phone _____

History _____

_____

_____

_____

Why Study Is Needed _____

_____

_____

Procedure

The patient was seen for fiberoptic endoscopic evaluation of swallowing _____. The patient was positioned in (bed, chair) for the exam. _____ assisted in positioning the patient and presenting test materials. The procedure examined anatomy and physiology of the swallowing mechanism. The scope was passed transnasally through the R/L nostril with/without topical anesthetic.

Anatomy and Physiology

Velopharyngeal Closure _____

Secretion Management _____

Swallow Frequency _____

Back of Tongue Movement _____

Laryngeal Structure During Respiration _____

Airway Closure _____

Phonation _____

Pharyngeal Musculature _____

_____

Swallowing

ice chips _____

_____

pureed foods _____

_____

soft solid foods _____

_____

hard, chewy, crunchy foods _____

_____

thin liquids _____

_____

_____

thick liquids _____

_____

Effects of Treatment Strategies Attempted _____

_____

_____

_____

Sensory Testing _____

Summary and Need for Service _____

_____

_____

_____

_____

_____

_____

_____

Diagnosis _____

Positive Expectation to Begin Service _____

_____

_____

Patient/Caregiver Teaching _____

_____

_____

Short-Term Goals

These goals reflect disordered physiology related to the pharyngeal phase. (Goals for the oral phase are found on the bedside evaluation form, page 57.)

_____ Patient will improve back of tongue control to keep food from falling over the back of the tongue and into the airway.

_____ Patient will decrease delay in initiation of pharyngeal swallow to reduce food falling into the airway during the delay before the swallow.

_____ Patient will increase closure of the true vocal folds to keep food from falling into the airway during the swallow.

_____ Patient will increase laryngeal elevation to reduce residue in the pyriform sinus(es) and reduce risk of the residue falling into the airway after the swallow.

_____ Patient will improve laryngeal elevation to reduce penetration into the upper laryngeal vestibule to reduce the risk of the penetrated material being aspirated after the swallow.

_____ Patient will improve the rate of laryngeal elevation/timing of closure to reduce penetration into the upper laryngeal vestibule to reduce the risk of the penetrated material being aspirated after the swallow.

_____ Patient will increase laryngeal elevation to reduce vallecular residue to reduce the risk of the residue being aspirated after the swallow.

_____ Patient will increase movement of pharyngeal wall(s) to reduce residue on pharyngeal wall(s) (unilateral or bilateral) to reduce the risk of the residue being aspirated after the swallow.

_____ No skilled treatment indicated.   Comments: _____

Recommendations

Food Presentation _____

_____

Food Placement _____

_____

Positioning _____

_____

Status _____

_____

Presentation of Meds _____

_____

Schedule _____

_____

_____

Charting/Monitoring _____

_____

Other _____

_____

FEES® Report, *continued*

Compensatory Techniques to Use During Meal
_____

Facilitation/Treatment Techniques
_____

Re-evaluation
_____

_____
Speech-Language Pathologist

Sample FEES® Report _____

Patient _Fred_	Date _____
Birthdate _____ Age _68_	Patient # _____
Referral Physician _____	
Patient's Address _____	Phone _____

History _Fred is a 68-year-old male who is currently an inpatient at this acute care facility. He suffered a left CVA with resulting right hemiparesis, aphasia, dysarthria, and dysphagia. His medical history also includes arteriosclerotic cardiovascular disease, hypertension, and diabetes. Patient currently has an NG tube in and is NPO except for ice chips._

Why Study Is Needed _The dysphagia team determined he needed an instrumental exam because a bedside screening revealed wet vocal quality with all textures presented. He also had intermittent cough throughout the screening._

Procedure

The patient was seen for fiberoptic endoscopic evaluation of swallowing _at bedside_ . The patient was positioned in (bed,) chair) for the exam. _Nursing Assistant_ assisted in positioning the patient and presenting test materials. The procedure examined anatomy and physiology of the swallowing mechanism. The scope was passed transnasally through the (R)/L nostril (with)/without topical anesthetic.

Anatomy and Physiology

Velopharyngeal Closure _appears adequate_

Secretion Management _some secretions noted in vallecullae and pyriforms, but none in airway_

Swallow Frequency _appears adequate_

Back of Tongue Movement _appears to exhibit weak touch of back of tongue to velum_

Laryngeal Structure During Respiration _no abnormalities noted_

Airway Closure _vocal cords close symmetrically for breath hold_

Phonation _vocal cords close symmetrically on phonation_

Pharyngeal Musculature _soft palate elevates and contacts posterior pharyngeal wall; pharyngeal constrictors move on phonation of /i/, but movement seems diminished; laryngeal elevation on phonation seems decreased_

Swallowing

ice chips _____

pureed foods _pudding: no premature trickle observed; no material observed in airway; minimal residue in valleculae; none in pyriforms_

soft solid foods _solids: no premature loss, other than that expected w/masticated material; no residue in valleculae, pyriforms, or channels_ hard, chewy, crunchy foods _____

thin liquids   *exhibits trickle over back of tongue before initiating swallow; material rests in valleculae (w/larger boluses, it falls to pyriforms), but not aspirated before the swallow; when airway is visible again, there is a trace amount of material in airway; consistent cough*

thick liquids   *no premature trickle observed; no material observed in airway; no minimal residue in valleculae; none in pyriforms*

Effects of Treatment Strategies Attempted *Patient tried in chin-down posture to see if this would increase airway protection. After swallowing thin liquids in this position, no material was noted in the airway, though a very small amount remained in the upper laryngeal vestibule when patient was given more than 5cc at once.*

Sensory Testing *strong cough reaction to scope touching pharyngeal wall*

Summary and Need for Service *Fred shows some decreased control of the back of his tongue which lets thin liquids trickle over the back of the tongue. He does not aspirate before the swallow. After the swallow, thin liquids are observed in the upper laryngeal vestibule and/or airway (depending on size of bolus), leading to the conclusion that there is decreased closure at the entrance to the airway (given that cords close tightly on breath hold). The chin-down posture eliminates the aspiration, but not penetration if given large boluses. With some of the stickier materials, he has vallecular residue, indicating probable reduced base of tongue strength.*

Diagnosis *oral and pharyngeal dysphagia with audible trace aspiration of thin liquids*

Positive Expectation to Begin Service *Patient is alert and cooperative and follows basic one-step commands. He wants to have NG tube removed and eat by mouth.*

Patient/Caregiver Teaching *The results of the evaluation were discussed in detail w/patient. He appeared to understand that some modifications in his eating would be necessary. His wife appeared to understand the recommendations as well.*

Short-Term Goals

These goals reflect disordered physiology related to the pharyngeal phase. (Goals for the oral phase are found on the bedside evaluation form, page 57.)

✓   Patient will improve back of tongue control to keep food from falling over the back of the tongue and into the airway.

_____ Patient will decrease delay in initiation of pharyngeal swallow to reduce food falling into the airway during the delay before the swallow.

_____ Patient will increase closure of the true vocal folds to keep food from falling into the airway during the swallow.

_____ Patient will increase laryngeal elevation to reduce residue in the pyriform sinus(es) and reduce risk of the residue falling into the airway after the swallow.

✓ Patient will improve laryngeal elevation to reduce penetration into the upper laryngeal vestibule to reduce the risk of the penetrated material being aspirated after the swallow.

_____ Patient will improve the rate of laryngeal elevation/timing of closure to reduce penetration into the upper laryngeal vestibule to reduce the risk of the penetrated material being aspirated after the swallow.

_____ Patient will increase laryngeal elevation to reduce vallecular residue to reduce the risk of the residue being aspirated after the swallow.

✓ Patient will increase movement of pharyngeal wall(s) to reduce residue on pharyngeal wall(s) (unilateral or bilateral) to reduce the risk of the residue being aspirated after the swallow.

_____ No skilled treatment indicated.   Comments: _____

Recommendations

Diet — thin liquids in 5cc amounts with SLP only and not at meals, mildly thick liquids okay at meals, pureed plus one soft vegetable at each meal

Food Presentation — 1 tsp. bolus size, cut-out cup for honey-thick liquids

Food Placement — left side of mouth

Positioning — sitting at 90°, stay seated upright 30 minutes after meals, chin tuck for liquids

Status — verbal cues/standby assist

Presentation of Meds — pills should be crushed and mixed w/applesauce

Schedule — breakfast fed by SLP
lunch fed by OT
dinner fed by staff/family
hold tube feedings 3 hours prior to oral feeding

Charting/Monitoring — calorie count (if adequate, remove NG)

Other _____
_____

Compensatory Techniques   compensation for pocketing: sweep w/tongue and external pressure to right cheek
to Use During Meal   alternate thickened liquid swallows every several bites
                           multiple swallows (offer cues w/masticated foods)
                           encourage/stimulate lip closure
                           _____

Facilitation/Treatment   effort swallow
Techniques   oral-motor exercises: labial closure, back of tongue and lingual A-P
                           tongue retraction and tongue hold; super-supraglottic swallow
                           _____

Re-evaluation   before advancing to thin liquids
                           _____

_____

Speech-Language Pathologist

Barium Cookie Recipe

Ingredients

1 c. granulated sugar
4 T. butter
1 egg
¼ c. milk
1 t. vanilla
2 c. flour (all-purpose, sifted)
1 t. baking soda
¼ t. salt
10 T. (about ¾ c.) barium powder (You can get this from the Radiology Dept.)

Directions

Preheat the oven to 375°.

Beat the butter in a large bowl until soft, adding the sugar gradually. Blend until creamy.
In another bowl, combine the egg, milk, and vanilla. Beat and set aside.

In a third bowl, combine the flour, baking soda, salt, and barium powder. Mix well. Add the flour mixture and the milk mixture to the butter and sugar in three parts, alternating small amounts of each. Beat the batter after each addition. You may need to add extra milk if the batter is too sticky, so add gradually.

Using a teaspoon, place ½-inch portions of dough onto a greased baking sheet. You might want to sprinkle each cookie with sugar before baking.

Bake for about nine minutes. Cool before eating. These cookies freeze well.

Yield: approximately 75 cookies

Appendix A: Cue Sheets for Choosing Compensatory Strategies During a Modified Barium Swallow

If You See This	What Might Be Causing It?	Techniques To Try During the Study	Why?	Additional Therapy Techniques
diffuse falling of bolus over back of tongue with or without aspiration	poor back of tongue control	chin-down posture	to widen the valleculae and catch more of the material and protect the airway by positioning trachea under tongue	oral-motor exercises for back of tongue • hard /k, g/ • exert pressure on tongue blade with back of tongue
		smaller bolus size	will allow the valleculae to hold the amount better without it spilling over with chance of aspiration	
		thicker consistency	patient may have better control of thicker consistency with the tongue	
		different utensil (e.g., cup, cut-out cup, spoon, straw)	some patients are more coordinated when drinking from one or the other	
bolus moves over the back of the tongue with delayed pharyngeal swallow with or without aspiration	delayed pharyngeal swallow*	thermal/tactile stimulation	to stimulate the reflex	cold bolus/neurosensory stimulation suck-swallow oral gestures help facilitate the swallow (and also help with saliva management)
		sour bolus	to stimulate the reflex	
		chin-down posture	to widen the valleculae and provide better protection of the airway	
		change in texture	patient's swallow may initiate at different times for different textures	
		three-second prep	thinking about swallowing is part of the neural preparation	
		change in bolus size (increase or decrease)	may not see delay with larger bolus; may be able to hold smaller bolus in recesses during delay	

* Need to treat delay if greater than two seconds or if patient aspirates during the delay.

Appendix A: Cue Sheets for Choosing Compensatory Strategies During a Modified Barium Swallow. *continued*

If You See This	What Might Be Causing It?	Techniques To Try During the Study	Why?	Additional Therapy Techniques
aspiration during the swallow	reduced closure of true vocal cords	chin-down posture	to widen the valleculae and provide better airway protection by positioning larynx under tongue	breath hold/modified Valsalva
		change in texture	sometimes patients don't aspirate during the swallow on thicker textures	laryngeal closure exercises
		change in bolus size	may not aspirate on smaller bolus sizes	
		supraglottic swallow	achieves closure of true folds	
		super-supraglottic swallow	achieves closure not only at the true and false cords but above	
		head rotation*	to close off half of the larynx and help stronger cord (if there is one) move toward the weaker cord	

* At this point, you may want to put the patient in A-P view to see if the residue is asymmetrical or if contrast material moves down one side or the other. The residue will be in the weaker side of the pharynx and you would want to try turning the patient's head toward that side.

Chapter 6
The Source for Dysphagia

163

Copyright © 2000 LinguiSystems, Inc.

Appendix A: Cue Sheets for Choosing Compensatory Strategies During a Modified Barium Swallow, *continued*

If You See This	What Might Be Causing It?	Techniques To Try During the Study	Why?	Additional Therapy Techniques
aspiration during the swallow OR penetration into the upper laryngeal vestibule but the residue remains and is aspirated after the swallow or appears to be a significant risk for aspiration	not a true delay, but what appears to be a mistiming of laryngeal elevation/timing of closure	controlling bolus size	patients may be able to coordinate timing of the swallow better with a smaller amount	
		chin-down posture	to widen the valleculae and provide better airway protection	
		try different utensils (e.g., cup, cut-out cup, spoon, straw)	some patients are more coordinated when drinking from one or the other	
		super-supraglottic swallow	improves speed of onset of laryngeal elevation	
		Mendelsohn maneuver	normalizes overall timing of pharyngeal swallow events	
		change in texture	thicker liquids move more slowly to allow time for closure	
residue in pyriform sinuses	reduced laryngeal elevation	not necessarily anything if patient doesn't aspirate from this residue		falsetto/laryngeal elevation exercises Mendelsohn maneuver super-supraglottic swallow

If You See This	What Might Be Causing It?	Techniques To Try During the Study	Why?	Additional Therapy Techniques
residue in pyriform sinuses and patient either aspirates after the swallow or appears to be at significant risk for aspiration after the swallow	reduced laryngeal elevation	reduce bolus size	choose a bolus size that doesn't overload the pyriform sinuses	falsetto
		Mendelsohn maneuver	to maintain laryngeal elevation and allow pyriforms to empty	SEMG biofeedback
		multiple swallow	the second swallow may clear the residue	
		liquid or thickened liquid wash	this wash may clear out the residue (however, you also have to be careful because the liquid may wash directly into the airway)	
		super-supraglottic	speeds onset of laryngeal elevation and the cough may clear any aspirated material	
		head rotation	facilitates UES opening, closes pyriform on one side, thus reducing amount of residue which may be aspirated	
	reduced anterior movement of hyolaryngeal complex	Mendelsohn maneuver	to maintain laryngeal elevation and allow pyriforms to empty	head lift
		multiple swallows	the second swallow may clear the residue	
		reduce bolus size	choose a bolus size that doesn't overload the pyriform sinuses	
		head rotation	facilitates UES opening; closes pyriform sinuses on one side, thus reducing amount of residue that remains and may be aspirated	

Appendix A: Cue Sheets for Choosing Compensatory Strategies During a Modified Barium Swallow. *continued*

If You See This	What Might Be Causing It?	Techniques To Try During the Study	Why?	Additional Therapy Techniques
penetration into the upper laryngeal vestibule, but the residue remains and is aspirated after the swallow or appears to be a significant risk for aspiration (Note: If the penetrated material is expelled and swallowed with the rest of the bolus, you don't have to try anything as the patient is not aspirating. However, if the amount of penetration appears to place patient at risk, try these techniques.)	reduced laryngeal elevation	chin-down posture	to widen the valleculae and provide better airway protection	falsetto/laryngeal elevation exercises
		super-supraglottic swallow	improves speed of onset of laryngeal elevation and thus may eliminate penetration	SEMG biofeedback
		change of texture	patients sometimes don't penetrate thicker textures	
		controlling bolus size	patients may only penetrate large bolus sizes	
		Mendelsohn maneuver	improves overall timing of the swallow and thus may eliminate the penetration	

Appendix A: Cue Sheets for Choosing Compensatory Strategies During a Modified Barium Swallow, *continued*

If You See This	What Might Be Causing It?	Techniques To Try During the Study	Why?	Additional Therapy Techniques
penetration into the upper laryngeal vestibule, but the residue remains and is aspirated after the swallow or appears to be a significant risk for aspiration (Note: If the penetrated material is expelled and swallowed with the rest of the bolus, you don't have to try anything as the patient is not aspirating. However, if the amount of penetration appears to place patient at risk, try these techniques.)	reduced closure at entrance to airway because of reduced arytenoid tipping	chin-down posture control bolus size super-supraglottic swallow change of texture	to widen the valleculae and provide better airway protection patients may only penetrate large bolus size provides closure at entrance to airway patients sometimes don't penetrate thicker textures	falsetto/laryngeal elevation exercises

If You See This	What Might Be Causing It?	Techniques to Try During the Study	Why?	Additional Therapy Techniques
vallecular residue or residue on pharyngeal walls with aspiration after the swallow from the residue (Note: If patient is not aspirating residue, you don't have to try anything. However, if the amount of residue is significant, the risk of aspiration exists.)	reduced base of tongue pressure	effort swallow	increases the pressure placed by the base of the tongue against posterior pharyngeal wall	pretend to gargle* pretend to yawn*
		super-supraglottic swallow	in addition to increasing the effort of laryngeal closure, it increases tongue base movement and may push the bolus through	
		reduce bolus size	so as not to overload the valleculae	
		multiple swallow	second swallow may clear the residue	
		liquid or thickened liquid wash (Note: May pair with chin-down; widens valleculae in some patients and allows residue to be washed out.)	this wash may clear out the residue (however, you also have to be careful because the liquid may wash directly into the airway)	
		head rotation	moves epiglottis into a protective position, improves laryngeal closure and closes vallecula on one side (usually doesn't work as well for vallecular residue as for pyriform residue)	

* Have the patient try these techniques under fluoro to see if either/both improve movement of tongue base.

If You See This	What Might Be Causing It?	Techniques To Try During the Study	Why?	Additional Therapy Techniques
vallecular residue or residue on pharyngeal walls with aspiration after the swallow (Note: If patient is not aspirating residue, you don't have to try anything. However, if the amount of residue is significant, the risk of aspiration exists.)	reduced posterior pharyngeal wall movement	effort swallow	increases the pressure placed by the base of the tongue against posterior pharyngeal wall	tongue hold
		liquid or thickened liquid wash	this wash may clear out the residue (however, you also have to be careful because the liquid may wash directly into the airway)	pretend to gargle*
		multiple swallow	second swallow may clear the residue	pretend to yawn*
		head rotation	to close vallecula on one side (usually doesn't work as well for vallecular residue as for pyriform residue)	
vallecular residue with aspiration after the swallow	reduced laryngeal elevation	multiple swallow	second swallow may clear the residue	laryngeal elevation exercises/falsetto
		liquid wash	this wash may clear out the residue (however, you also have to be careful because the liquid may wash directly into the airway)	SEMG biofeedback
		control bolus size	so as not to overload valleculae	
		Mendelsohn maneuver	achieves better elevation and may help push the material out of the valleculae	
		head rotation	moves epiglottis into a protective position, improves laryngeal closure and closes vallecula on one side (usually doesn't work as well for vallecular residue as for pyriform residue)	

* Have the patient try these techniques under fluoro to see if either/both improve movement of tongue base.

Appendix B: FEES® Examination Protocol _____

Anatomic-Physiologic Assessment

A. **Velopharyngeal Closure**
At juncture of velum and nasopharynx, view sphincteric closure as the patient swallows and phonates oral and nasal sounds and sentences. Administer liquid while scope is in nose if nasal reflux is to be assessed.

B. **Appearance of Hypopharynx and Larynx at Rest**
Scan around entire HP to note appearance, symmetry, and abnormalities that warrant an ENT referral for suspected pathology.

C. **Handling of Secretions and Swallow Frequency**
Observe amount and location of secretions in lateral channels, laryngeal vestibule, and/or subglottally. Note this over a two- to five-minute segment as you proceed with the exam. Also note frequency of dry swallows over a period of at least two minutes. Optional: Drop green food coloring on tongue to mix with saliva if you need a better view.

D. **Base of Tongue**
Task: Say "kuh-kuh-kuh" several times.
Observe extent of movement and symmetry.

E. **Respiration**
Observe laryngeal structures for rest breathing. Note extent, symmetry, and rate of movement.
Task: Sniff or deep inhalation (note abduction).

F. **Airway Protection**
Task: Cough.
Task: Hold your breath at the level of the throat.
Task: Hold your breath very tightly.
Task: Hold your breath to the count of 7.

G. **Phonation**
Task: Hold "ee."
Task: Repeat "hee-hee-hee" 5 to 7 times.
Task: Count from 1 to 10.
Task: Glide upward in pitch.

H. **Pharyngeal Musculature**
Task: Hold your breath and blow out cheeks forcefully.
Observe the depth and symmetry of pyriform sinuses.
Task: Strain your voice and grunt or say "ee" in a very loud, high voice.
Observe middle and inferior constrictors. Note extent and symmetry of contraction.

Swallowing Food and Liquid

All foods/liquids are dyed green with food coloring.

Guidelines

- Increase amount with each presentation unless aspiration occurs.
- Repeat any amount that results in aspiration unless severe aspiration.
- Discontinue that amount if aspiration occurs twice.
- Try less than 5cc *only* if patient at very high risk for aspirating.
- Give measured amounts if exact bolus size needs to be known; otherwise give functional amounts such as teaspoons, tablespoons, and/or drinks from cup or straw.
- Give instructions to swallow on command only to sort out the specific nature of an observed problem with spillage; otherwise let patient swallow at his or her own rate.
- Give material that is light in color so that it will be visible.

Order of Consistencies will vary, depending on patient needs and the problems observed. Suggested consistencies to try to include the following:

Ice chips (½ tsp. of ice chips dyed green)
Begin with this consistency if patient is NPO at present and/or appears to be at high risk for aspiration (e.g., has standing secretions in hypopharynx).

Repeat this several times. Note the effect on clearance of secretions, ability of patient to swallow the ice chips, and sensitivity of patient to any aspiration of ice chips.

Pureed foods (5cc, 10cc, 15cc of applesauce, pudding, etc.)

Soft solid food (e.g., cheese sandwich)
Allow the patient to take a bite-sized portion.

Hard, chewy, crunchy food
Give this consistency if regular diet is being considered.

Thin liquid (5cc, 10cc, 15cc, 20cc, 5 consecutive swallows)
Milk or other translucent thin liquid (white in color) is good for visibility.

Thick liquid (5cc, 10cc, 15cc, 20cc, 5 consecutive swallows)
Give this consistency if indicated (from performance on thin liquids or pureed).
Give nectar and honey consistencies for more precise information.

Therapeutic Positions, Maneuvers, and Other Alterations in Bolus Delivery

Apply these at all appropriate points in the exam — generally as soon as the problem is observed. Use the strategy appropriate for the observed problem, including head turn; chin tuck; effortful swallow; supraglottic swallow or modification of this; Mendelsohn maneuver; dry swallows; and delivery by spoon, straw, or cup.

Hypopharyngeal/Laryngeal Sensory Testing

Can be directly tested by lightly touching the pharyngeal mucosal wall with the tip of the scope, then the base of the tongue, and, if no response, the tip of the epiglottis. If quantitative measure of sensory threshold can be obtained, this is preferable.

Karnell, M. P. and S. Langmore. *FEES® Examination Protocol.* In *Medical Speech-Language Pathology: A Practitioner's Guide.* NYC: Thieme Medical Publishers, Inc., 1998, p. 576.

Appendix C: Observation Rating Scales ⸻

Duke University Rating of Radiologic Swallowing Abnormalities[1]

Oral Preparatory Phase

0   Profound dysfunction: oral stasis, no material is propelled into the pharynx

1   Severe dysfunction: effortful oral preparation, dispersion of the bolus along the tongue and into the buccal cavities, significant oral residue after the swallow that is not cleared, extreme slowness and inefficiency in propelling the bolus into the pharynx, no masticatory ability, drooling usually occurs

2   Moderate dysfunction: slow oral preparation and motility of boluses, mastication very slow but thorough, some residue along the tongue, inefficiency and effort in propelling the bolus into the pharynx, drooling may occur

3   Mild dysfunction: mildly slow bolus preparation, but adequate bolus cohesion and motility; mastication slower than normal but thorough; mild lip incompetency with drooling may be present

4   Normal control and bolus transit, no oral residue, mastication is brisk and thorough

Reflex Initiation Phase

0   Profound: absent reflex

1   Severe: reflex initiated in the lower pharynx (pyriform sinuses) after prolonged pooling

2   Moderate: reflex initiated in the lower pharynx after brief hesitation

3   Mild: reflex initiated in the midpharynx (vallecular spaces) after brief hesitation

4   Normal: reflex initiated at the back or base of the tongue (above the epiglottis), no hesitation in bolus motility from posterior tongue into pharynx

Pharyngeal Phase

0   Profound residue: reflex is minimal or absent and the bolus fills the mid- and lower pharynx, suctioning or vigorous pharyngeal gag and cough are required to clear the pharynx

1   Severe residue: more than half the bolus remains in the pharynx after the swallow; much effort required to clear the residue, possibly requiring sips of liquid barium or water; poor peristalsis typically associated with: (a) weak propulsion force of tongue at reflex initiation, (b) visibly reduced laryngeal elevation and epiglottic tilting, and/or (c) incomplete midpharyngeal and laryngopharyngeal closure during the swallow

2   Moderate residue: more than 10% but less than 50% of the bolus remains in the mid- and/or lower pharynx, requires an extra swallow to clear, usually occurs in association with (a-c) above

3   Mild residue: less than 10% of a small bolus remains in the mid- and/or lower pharynx after the first swallow.

4   Normal: no residue, slight coating only may be present

Pharyngeal Appearance Observed in Anterior-Posterior Projection

0   No pharyngeal transit: profound residue in the mid- and/or lower pharynx bilaterally, usually seen only when the reflex is absent

1   Severe: bilateral pharyngeal weakness characterized by moderate or severe residue in the bilateral pharyngeal spaces (midpharynx, lower pharynx, or both), often the pharynx will appear bilaterally patulous or bilateral pulsion diverticula will be observed

2   Moderate: pharyngeal hemiplegia characterized by definite asymmetry, pharyngeal motility only on the opposite (functional) side

3a Mild: pharyngeal hemiparesis characterized by bilateral pharyngeal transit that is visibly superior on the opposite side and/or the hemiparetic side may show a pyriform sinus "droop," and/or the hemiparetic side may show hypotonia of the thyro-hyoid membrane presenting as a "pulsion diverticulum"

3b Slight: postural abnormality; pharyngeal asymmetry with no observable anatomic or physiologic basis (e.g., due to torticollis, poor sitting balance, or head deviation due to neglect, distractibility, etc.) (Note: When non-dysphagic individuals turn or tilt the head to one side, pharyngeal asymmetry is a normal finding, but pharyngeal asymmetry is considered to be abnormal when head and neck postures are involuntary.)

4   Normal: both symmetrical appearance and symmetrical bolus transit, no anatomic or physiologic abnormalities observed

Aspiration

0   Profound: more than trace aspiration (audible or silent), may include repeated instances of aspiration despite postural or other modifications to prevent aspiration. If the reflex is absent, risk for aspiration is profound and also warrants a rating of "zero." (Note: "trace" refers to less than 10% of the bolus)

1   Severe: more than trace aspiration (audible or silent), may include repeated instances of aspiration despite postural or other modifications to prevent aspiration

2   Moderate: trace silent aspiration (no laryngeal cough during aspiration through the larynx is referred to as "silent aspiration")

3   Mild: trace audible aspiration (when aspiration occasions a cough, it is referred to as "audible aspiration")

4   No aspiration (risk for aspiration may be present and should be noted relative to other observations)

Pharyngeal-Esophageal Phase Screening

0   Absent swallow reflex, no relaxation of the upper esophageal sphincter (UES), no material enters the esophagus

1   Severe pyriform sinus residue, sporadic or effortful passage of food or liquid into the upper esophagus, definite indication that the UES is failing to relax, usually associated with a severely incomplete swallowing reflex and reduced laryngeal excursion

2   Residue is present in the pyriform sinus(es) in equal or greater amount than in the vallecular space(s), suggesting UES dysfunction; potentially secondary to one or more of the following: (a) decreased pharyngeal peristalsis; (b) dyscoordination (mistiming) of pharyngeal peristalsis and cricopharyngeal relaxation (the material is eventually cleared from the pharynx, but repeated swallows are necessary); (c) incomplete relaxation of the upper esophageal sphincter - when larger boluses are administered, the caliber of the UES is diminished and manometry may be indicated; (d) hypotonia of the UES and/or dyscoordination of UES relaxation manifest as reflux from the upper esophagus into the pyriform sinuses after the swallow

3   Residue is present in the vallecular space(s) primarily; adequate relaxation of the UES, but the evaluation is limited to small boluses only (larger boluses were precluded by the presence of, or risk for, aspiration)

4   Normal relaxation of the UES, evaluated using a gulp or large naturalistic swallow(s)

8-Point Penetration-Aspiration Scale[2]

1   Material does not enter the airway.
2   Material enters the airway, remains above the vocal folds, and is ejected from the airway.
3   Material enters the airway, remains above the vocal folds, and is not ejected from the airway.
4   Material enters the airway, contacts the vocal folds, and is ejected from the airway.
5   Material enters the airway, contacts the vocal folds, and is not ejected from the airway.
6   Material enters the airway, passes below the vocal folds, and is ejected into the larynx or out of the airway.
7   Material enters the airway, passes below the vocal folds, and is not ejected from the trachea despite effort.
8   Material enters the airway, passes below the vocal folds, and no effort is made to eject.

[1] Horner, J. et al. "Swallowing in Torticollis Before and After Rhizotomy." *Dysphagia*, Vol. 7, No. 3, 1992, pp. 123-125. (Duke Rating Scale)

[2] Rosenbek, J. et al. "A Penetration-Aspiration Scale." *Dysphagia*, Vol. 11, 1996, p. 94.

Chapter 7

Planning Dysphagia Treatment

A complete evaluation of dysphagia does not stop at the diagnosis of the presence of a disorder in the oral or pharyngeal phase. The evaluation must provide information for treatment planning. The first decision in treatment planning is to choose a long-term goal, which must be based on the prognosis for the patient. Based on the results of the evaluation(s), what is the expectation for the patient? Long-term goals must be written in functional terms so that someone other than an SLP (e.g., a reviewer) can understand them. With most dysphagia patients, the long-term goals could be something such as "Patient will achieve safe and efficient swallowing to sustain adequate nutrition and hydration orally" or "Patient will be able to eat normal texture diet." The issue of safety is an important one, particularly when treating Medicare patients. Use the words "increased safety of eating" in your long-term goals whenever possible.

If your long-term goal for a Medicare patient is to have the patient take some pleasure feedings by mouth, Medicare is not inclined to pay for services. You have to expect that the services you provide are going to make a significant improvement in a reasonable amount of time. Therefore, if you start therapy thinking that the patient who is on total tube feeding will eventually end up still needing tube feeding and be able take about 10% of his nutrition by mouth, it is probably not an appropriate long-term goal.

Nor is an evaluation complete if the report simply lists the symptoms observed. The evaluation must include information about the physiological cause of the symptoms. This information allows for selection of appropriate short-term goals and treatment objectives to help the patient achieve a functional outcome.

Symptoms are those characteristics observed during a clinical/bedside evaluation or during an instrumental assessment. A symptom is a description of what is seen. Symptoms may be categorized according to the phase of the swallow.

- In the oral preparatory phase, symptoms might include loss of food out the front of the mouth or inability to form a cohesive bolus.

- In the oral (voluntary) phase, a symptom could be an inability to move the bolus of food toward the back of the mouth.

- In the pharyngeal phase, symptoms observed at bedside during a clinical evaluation might include coughing or swallowing multiple times.

- During a videofluoroscopic evaluation, symptoms could include food entering the airway before, during, or after the swallow or food remaining in the valleculae or pyriform sinuses.

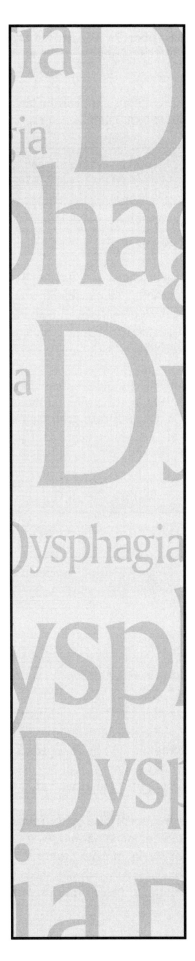

A treatment plan can be developed based on the symptoms observed. The following table describes possible **short-term goals** based on observed symptoms.

Symptom	Short-Term Goal
Patient can't move food back in the mouth.	Patient will improve ability to move food back in the mouth.
Patient has food left in the valleculae.	Patient will reduce food left in the valleculae.
Patient loses food out the front of the mouth.	Patient will decrease anterior loss of food.

The problem with writing short-term goals based on a symptom is that one symptom may have more than one physiological cause. For example, food left in the valleculae is most often due to reduced base of tongue to posterior pharyngeal wall pressure (Kahrilas et al., 1992), but may also be related to reduced laryngeal elevation (Logemann, 1998). Depending on the reason for the vallecular residue, very different short-term goals would be selected.

Another problem with writing short-term goals from the symptom observed is that these goals are not written in functional terms. **Functional short-term goals** are those that are written in terms payers, consumers, and other health-care professionals can understand. They tie the physiological cause of the symptom to the functional outcome desired. The difference between short-term goals and functional short-term goals are reflected in the following table.

Short-Term Goal	Physiological Cause	Functional Short-Term Goal
Patient will reduce anterior loss.	reduced lip closure	Patient will keep lips closed to prevent food from falling out the front of the mouth.
Patient will reduce aspiration after the swallow.	reduced laryngeal elevation	Patient will increase laryngeal elevation to reduce amount of food remaining in the pyriform sinuses that may fall into the airway after the swallow.
	reduced closure at entrance to airway	Patient will increase closure at entrance to airway to keep food from entering the top of the larynx and falling into the airway after the swallow.

Functional short-term goals list the physiology that needs to improve (e.g., increase laryngeal elevation), which symptom will be changed as a result (e.g., to reduce the amount of food remaining in the pyriform sinuses), and what the impact will be on function, particularly related to the safety of the swallow (e.g., to keep the food from falling into the airway after the swallow).

A treatment plan with functional short-term goals provides information that is understandable to a number of audiences. What it does not provide is a way to document progress toward those goals. A patient may work for weeks or even months to achieve a short-term goal, and you need a way to demonstrate the progress being made on a day-to-day basis. Functional short-term goals can be broken into more measurable steps called treatment objectives (Swigert, 1999).

Treatment objectives are smaller, more well-defined steps that often describe a treatment technique. These treatment objectives must be based on the physiological symptom. Treatment objectives may be categorized as compensatory (compensation), facilitation/therapeutic, or diet (Swigert, 1996).

1. **Compensatory techniques** are those designed to compensate for lost function. Logemann (1998) states that compensatory treatment procedures are those that control the flow of food and eliminate the patient's symptoms without necessarily changing the physiology of the swallow. These are techniques that are most often used by the patient during meals. They might include changes in posture, increased sensory input, use of prosthetics, changes in food placement, or changes in food presentation. Logemann includes changing food consistency as a type of compensatory treatment procedure.

2. **Facilitation/therapeutic techniques** are designed to improve function, or as Logemann indicates, to change swallow physiology. They are used during treatment and may or may not be used during meals. Facilitation techniques might include oral-motor exercises, laryngeal elevation, and exercises for increasing laryngeal closure.

3. Swigert (1996) lists **diet changes** as a separate category of treatment objective.

Some techniques are both a compensation and a facilitation. That is, the technique can be used to compensate for lost function and can also improve function. For example, the super-supraglottic swallow can be used during eating to increase purposeful closure of the airway to keep food from entering the laryngeal vestibule (Martin et al., 1993) thus compensating for lost function. This same technique, when practiced repetitively, may actually restore function so the laryngeal vestibule closes more effectively even when the technique is no longer used.

Type of Treatment Objectives Used to Treat Dysphagia	
Treatment Objective (Technique) Type	Designed to:
Compensation (c)	Compensate for lost function. Includes changes in posture, increasing sensory input before or during the swallow, food placement, and food presentation. Often used during feeding.
Facilitation (f)	Improve function. Used most often during therapy and not necessarily at therapeutic feedings.
Diet (d)	Compensate for lost function. Includes changes in diet texture and temperature.
Compensation and facilitation (c,f)	Compensate for lost function and improves function. The super-supraglottic swallow may compensate for reduced laryngeal closure, but may also improve laryngeal closure and the rate of laryngeal elevation.

Treatment objectives must be specific to the physiological cause of the symptoms. For instance, the symptom of aspiration after the swallow could occur because there is residue in the pyriform sinuses after the swallow. This residue is due to reduced anterior and superior movement of the larynx (Logemann, 1998). Therefore, one might select treatment techniques which will help increase laryngeal elevation. These techniques might be compensatory, facilitation, and/or diet techniques written as treatment objectives. For example, a technique such as the Mendelsohn maneuver could be both a compensation and a facilitation. As a compensation, the Mendelsohn increases the extent and duration of laryngeal elevation (Robbins and Levine, 1993; Bartolome and Neumann, 1993). This keeps the cricopharyngeus open longer and allows more of the bolus to pass into the esophagus. Subsequently, less remains in the pyriform sinuses to be aspirated later. The maneuver should also have some carryover so that excursion of the larynx improves over time (Bryant, 1991), thus serving a facilitation role. A change in diet, such as eliminating sticky foods that pool more easily in the pyriform sinuses, might be another treatment objective chosen.

However, the physiological cause of the symptom of aspiration after the swallow could also be reduced closure at the entrance to the airway which allows material to penetrate into the laryngeal vestibule during the swallow and be aspirated after. If that were the case, the compensation technique chosen would be the super-supraglottic swallow. This technique can also serve as a facilitation. Another compensation chosen might be the postural change of chin-down posture to provide more airway protection during the swallow. The diet change selected might be to present slightly thicker materials which might not penetrate into the upper laryngeal vestibule so quickly and easily.

Relationship of Functional Short-Term Goals, Treatment Objectives, and Type of Treatment Objective to Symptom of Aspiration After the Swallow

Possible Physiological Cause of Aspiration After Swallow	Functional Short-Term Goal	Treatment Objective	Type of Treatment Objective
reduced laryngeal elevation	Patient will increase elevation of the larynx to reduce the amount of food remaining in the pyriform sinuses that falls into the airway after the swallow.	Patient will complete the Mendelsohn maneuver. Patient will perform falsetto. Patient will avoid sticky foods.	Compensation Facilitation Facilitation Diet
reduced closure at entrance to airway	Patient will increase closure at entrance to the airway to keep food from entering the top of the larynx and falling into the airway after the swallow.	Patient will perform super-supraglottic swallow Patient will use chin-down posture. Patient will take only liquids thickened to syrup.	Compensation Facilitation Compensation Diet

If only compensation and diet change treatment objectives are appropriate for a patient (e.g., no potential for improved physiology or inability to participate in treatment) then the functional short-term goal should be reworded. As written, the short-term goals presume working toward improved function. Examples are provided in the table on page 179.

Comparison of Short-Term Goals Which Do/Do Not Use Facilitation Techniques	
Functional short-term goals when facilitation treatment objectives are included:	Reworded functional short-term goals if only compensation and diet treatment objectives are appropriate:
Patient will increase elevation of the larynx to reduce the amount of food remaining in the pyriform sinuses that falls into the airway after the swallow.	Patient will compensate for decreased laryngeal elevation to reduce the amount of food remaining in the pyriform sinuses that falls into the airway after the swallow.
Patient will increase closure at entrance to the airway to keep food from entering the top of the larynx and falling into the airway after the swallow.	Patient will compensate for decreased closure at the entrance to the airway to keep food from entering the top of the larynx and falling into the airway after the swallow.

The only remaining refinement needed is to write the treatment objectives in a more measurable way. Each treatment objective can be described in terms of when and how often the patient is to use the technique and with how much cueing. For instance, if the Mendelsohn maneuver as described in the example above is to be used as a compensation during meals, the objective might read: "Patient will use Mendelsohn maneuver during liquid swallows 100% of the time with consistent verbal cues given by clinician." Including target percentages, description of intensity, frequency of cueing, and situations in which the technique is to be used provide you with precise measurement capabilities. This allows you to document accomplishment of small steps toward achieving the functional short-term goal.

In summary, treatment planning for dysphagia requires that you observe symptoms carefully; use appropriate diagnostic techniques to determine the physiological cause of the symptom; write short-term goals in functional language; and select appropriate, measurable treatment objectives.

The chart on pages 180-181 provides a list of the symptoms you will observe and the different physiological causes for those symptoms. Using this chart will allow you to select the appropriate short-term goal(s) to treat your patient. On the pages following the chart, you will find 24 short-term goals based on the symptom and its physiological cause. Each short-term goal has numerous treatment objectives (techniques) which are written so that you can fill in percentages. Each treatment objective is also described as compensatory, facilitation, diet, or combination of compensation/facilitation. When choosing a technique that is both a compensation and a facilitation, indicate on your treatment plan in which way or ways it is intended to be used. For example, Short-Term Goal 13 is to be used if the patient is aspirating during the swallow because of reduced closure of the vocal cords. Treatment Objective AD/lc-6 is use of the supraglottic swallow. You might select that for this patient to use during meals as a compensation. You might not want the patient to use it during meals because he is unable to remember to follow the directions, or may become fatigued. In that case, you might choose AD/lc-6 as a facilitation. Or you might have the patient use the technique during meals and therapeutically as both compensation and facilitation.

Short-Term Goals 11 through 24 relate to aspiration before, during, or after the swallow. Sometimes the patient does not aspirate but appears to be at high risk to aspirate. In that case, these short-term goals would be appropriate. For example, the patient may not be observed to aspirate, but has such significant residue in the pyriforms due to reduced laryngeal elevation that the risk is high that he will aspirate. In that case, Short-Term Goal 15 would be appropriate. In some instances the goal will need to be reworded slightly. For example, Short-Term Goal 11 states "Patient will improve back of tongue control to keep food from falling over the back of the tongue into the airway." If the patient is not actually aspirating, you might reword the goal to say "Patient will improve back of tongue control to reduce risk of food falling over the back of the tongue into the airway."

179

Symptom/Physiological Cause/Safety or Function Issue

Symptom	Physiology	Safety/Function	Short-Term Goal	Code
anterior loss	decreased jaw closure	food falls out front of mouth	Anterior Loss/jaw closure	AL/jc
	decreased lip closure	food falls out front of mouth	Anterior Loss/lip closure	AL/lc
	decreased oral sensation	food falls out front of mouth	Anterior Loss/oral sensation	AL/os
decreased bolus formation	decreased oral sensation	food remaining in mouth food falling into airway	Bolus Formation/oral sensation	BF/os
	decreased tongue movement (includes tongue shaping)	food remaining in mouth food falling into airway	Bolus Formation/tongue movement	BF/tm
	decreased tone in cheeks	food remaining in mouth food falling into airway	Bolus Formation/tone in cheeks	BF/tc
decreased bolus propulsion	decreased tongue movement	food remaining in mouth food falling into airway	Bolus Propulsion/tongue movement	BP/tm
	decreased oral coordination	food remaining in mouth food falling into airway	Bolus Propulsion/oral coordination	BP/oc
	decreased oral sensation	food remaining in mouth food falling into airway	Bolus Propulsion/oral sensation	BP/os
	agnosia	food remaining in mouth not able to eat enough food falling into airway	Bolus Propulsion/agnosia	BP/ag
aspiration before the swallow	decreased back of tongue control	food in airway	Aspiration Before/tongue control	AB/tc
	delayed pharyngeal swallow with food in valleculae before swallow, falling directly into airway or food in pyriforms before the swallow	food in airway	Aspiration Before/delayed reflex	AB/dr

Symptom	Physiology	Safety/Function	Short-Term Goal	Code
aspiration during the swallow	decreased closure of larynx	food in airway	Aspiration During/laryngeal closure	AD/lc
	mistiming of laryngeal elevation and closure	food in airway	Aspiration During/ mistiming of laryngeal closure	AD/mc
aspiration after from pyriform sinus residue	decreased laryngeal elevation	food falling into airway	Aspiration After/pyriform/ laryngeal elevation	AA/p/le
	decreases anterior movement of hyolaryngeal complex	food falling into airway	Aspiration After/pyriform/ hyolaryngeal movement	AA/p/hm
aspiration after from penetration into laryngeal vestibule	decreased laryngeal elevation	food falling into airway	Aspiration After/laryngeal vestibule/ laryngeal elevation	AA/lv/le
	decreased arytenoid tipping	food falling into airway	Aspiration After/laryngeal vestibule/ arytenoid tipping	AA/lv/at
	slow or mistimed closure of larynx	food falling into airway	Aspiration After/laryngeal vestibule/mistiming of closure	AA/lv/mc
aspiration after from vallecular residue (unilateral or bilateral)	decreased base of tongue movement	food falling into airway	Aspiration After/valleculae/ tongue base	AA/v/tb
	decreased anterior movement of posterior pharyngeal wall	food falling into airway	Aspiration After/valleculae/ posterior pharyngeal wall	AA/v/ppw
	decreased elevation of larynx	food falling into airway	Aspiration After/valleculae/ laryngeal elevation	AA/v/le
residue in pyriform sinus(es) lateral pharyngeal wall(s) with aspiration	decreased pharyngeal wall contraction	food falling into airway	Aspiration After/walls/ pharyngeal wall movement	AA/w/pw
	decreased base of tongue movement	food falling into airway	Aspiration After/walls/ tongue base	AA/w/tb

181

Long-Term/Functional Goals _____

1. Patient will safely consume _____ diet with _____ liquids without complications such as aspiration pneumonia.
2. Patient will be able to eat foods and liquids with more normal consistency.
3. Patient will be able to complete a meal in less than _____ minutes.
4. Patient will maintain nutrition/hydration via alternative means.
5. Patient's quality of life will be enhanced through eating and drinking small amounts of food and liquid.

Master List of Short-Term Goals _____

Short-Term Goal 1	Anterior Loss/jaw closure	(AL/jc)
Short-Term Goal 2	Anterior Loss/lip closure	(AL/lc)
Short-Term Goal 3	Anterior Loss/oral sensation	(AL/os)
Short-Term Goal 4	Bolus Formation/oral sensation	(BF/os)
Short-Term Goal 5	Bolus Formation/tongue movement	(BF/tm)
Short-Term Goal 6	Bolus Formation/tone in cheeks	(BF/tc)
Short-Term Goal 7	Bolus Propulsion/tongue movement	(BP/tm)
Short-Term Goal 8	Bolus Propulsion/oral coordination	(BP/oc)
Short-Term Goal 9	Bolus Propulsion/oral sensation	(BP/os)
Short-Term Goal 10	Bolus Propulsion/agnosia	(BP/ag)
Short-Term Goal 11	Aspiration Before/tongue control	(AB/tc)
Short-Term Goal 12	Aspiration Before/delayed reflex	(AB/dr)
Short-Term Goal 13	Aspiration During/laryngeal closure	(AD/lc)
Short-Term Goal 14	Aspiration During/mistiming of closure	(AD/mc)
Short-Term Goal 15	Aspiration After/pyriform/laryngeal elevation	(AA/p/le)
Short-Term Goal 16	Aspiration After/pyriform/hyolaryngeal complex movement	(AA/p/hm)
Short-Term Goal 17	Aspiration After/laryngeal vestibule/laryngeal elevation	(AA/lv/le)
Short-Term Goal 18	Aspiration After/laryngeal vestibule/arytenoid tipping	(AA/lv/at)
Short-Term Goal 19	Aspiration After/laryngeal vestibule/mistiming of closure	(AA/lv/mc)
Short-Term Goal 20	Aspiration After/valleculae/tongue base	(AA/v/tb)
Short-Term Goal 21	Aspiration After/valleculae/posterior pharyngeal wall	(AA/v/ppw)
Short-Term Goal 22	Aspiration After/valleculae/laryngeal elevation	(AA/v/le)
Short-Term Goal 23	Aspiration After/walls/pharyngeal wall	(AA/w/pw)
Short-Term Goal 24	Aspiration After/walls/tongue base	(AA/w/tb)

Treatment Objectives to Achieve Short-Term Goals ─────

```
c    =  compensatory techniques compensate for a deficit
f    =  facilitation techniques to improve function
c, f =  compensatory techniques that facilitate return of function
d    =  diet texture changes
```

Short-Term Goal 1 – Anterior Loss/jaw closure (AL/jc)

Patient will improve jaw closure to reduce anterior loss to keep food and liquid in the mouth while eating.

Treatment Objectives

AL/jc-1   Patient will eliminate loss of food/liquid out the front of mouth when clinician provides jaw support on _____ of _____ trials. (c)

AL/jc-2   Patient will open jaw against resistance provided by clinician on _____ of _____ trials. (f)

AL/jc-3   Patient will close jaw against resistance provided by clinician on _____ of _____ trials. (f)

AL/jc-4   Patient will take only _____ liquids with/without cues on _____ of _____ trials. (d)

AL/jc-5   Patient will avoid foods in liquid base with/without cues. (d)

Short-Term Goal 2 – Anterior Loss/lip closure (AL/lc)

Patient will improve lip closure to reduce anterior loss to keep food and liquid in the mouth while eating.

Treatment Objectives

AL/lc-1   Patient will eliminate loss of food/liquid from front of mouth when clinician provides support to upper/lower lip(s) on _____ of _____ trials. (c)

AL/lc-2   Patient will achieve lip closure around object (Lifesaver on string, Popsicle, ice cube) for _____ seconds on _____ of _____ trials. (f)

AL/lc-3   Patient will achieve lip closure against resistance provided by clinician placing fingers on upper and lower lips on _____ of _____ trials. (f)

AL/lc-4   Patient will pucker lips (as if to blow a kiss) on _____ of _____ trials. (f)

AL/lc-5   Patient will achieve lip closure while keeping jaw open on _____ of _____ trials. (f)

AL/lc-6   Patient will puff cheeks and keep lips tightly sealed on _____ of _____ trials. (f)

AL/lc-7   Patient will hold tongue depressor between closed lips (not teeth) for count of 10 on _____ of _____ trials. (f)

AL/lc-8   Patient will grin (retracting corners of lips) as wide as possible without showing teeth on _____ of _____ trials. (f)

Treatment Objectives to Achieve Short-Term Goals, *continued*

AL/lc-9   Patient will take only _____ liquids with/without cues on _____ of _____ trials. (d)

AL/lc-10   Patient will avoid foods in liquid base with/without cues. (d)

Short-Term Goal 3 – Anterior Loss/oral sensation (AL/os)

Patient's oral sensation will improve to reduce anterior loss to keep food in the mouth while eating.

Treatment Objectives

AL/os-1   Patient will report increased sensitivity to cold when clinician rubs lips with cold spoon on _____ of _____ trials. (f)

AL/os-2   Patient will take only _____ liquids with/without cues on _____ of _____ trials. (d)

AL/os-3   Patient will avoid foods in liquid base with/without cues. (d)

Short-Term Goal 4 – Bolus Formation/oral sensation (BF/os)

Patient's oral sensation will increase to improve the ability to put food/liquid into a cohesive bolus to reduce the risk of food residue falling into the airway.

BF/os-1   Patient will use external pressure with fingers on cheek to decrease pocketing with/without cues on _____ of _____ trials. (c)

BF/os-2   Patient will place bolus of food on stronger side with/without cues on _____ of _____ trials. (c)

BF/os-3   Patient will clean buccal cavity with fingers/tongue during/after meal with/without cues on _____ of _____ trials. (c)

BF/os-4   Patient will "rinse and spit" at end of each meal with/without cues on _____ of _____ trials. (c)

BF/os-5   Patient will alternate thin/_____-thickened liquid wash every _____ bite(s) with/without cues on _____ of _____ trials. (c)

BF/os-6   Oral sensitivity input will be heightened by providing pressure with the spoon when boluses are presented. (c)

BF/os-7   Patient will eat only foods that form a cohesive bolus with/without cues. (d)

BF/os-8   Patient will only eat pureed foods with/without cues. (d)

BF/os-9   Oral sensitivity will be heightened by patient taking foods that require some mastication. (d)

BF/os-10   Oral sensitivity will be heightened by presenting boluses of a distinct flavor/temperature/texture (specify: _____). (d)

Short-Term Goal 5 – Bolus Formation/tongue movement (BF/tm)

Patient will increase tongue movement to improve the ability to put food and liquid into a cohesive bolus to reduce the risk of food falling into the airway.

Treatment Objectives

BF/tm-1   Patient will place bolus on stronger side with/without cues on _____ of _____ trials. (c)

BF/tm-2   Patient will tilt head to stronger side with/without cues on _____ of _____ trials. (c)

BF/tm-3   Patient will "rinse and spit" at end of each meal with/without cues on _____ of _____ trials. (c)

BF/tm-4   Patient will use multiple swallows for _____ consistencies with/without cues on _____ of _____ trials. (c)

BF/tm-5   Patient will alternate thin/_____-thickened liquid wash every _____ bite(s) with/without cues on _____ of _____ trials. (c)

BF/tm-6   Patient will move tongue in clockwise motion between teeth and closed lips on _____ of _____ trials. (f)

BF/tm-7   Patient will protrude tongue to try to touch the chin and nose with tongue tip on _____ of _____ trials. (f)

BF/tm-8   Patient will push up with back of tongue against tongue depressor on _____ of _____ trials. (A helpful cue is to ask the patient to make a /k/.) (f)

BF/tm-9   Patient will click tongue against roof of mouth on _____ of _____ trials. (f)

BF/tm-10   Patient will push tongue tip out against tongue depressor on _____ of _____ trials. (f)

BF/tm-11   Patient will push blade of tongue upward against tongue depressor on _____ of _____ trials. (f)

BF/tm-12   Patient will push R/L lateral border of tongue against tongue depressor on _____ of _____ trials. (f)

BF/tm-13   Patient will protrude tongue into R/L cheek on _____ of _____ trials. (f)

BF/tm-14   Patient will protrude tongue tip into R/L cheek against resistance provided by clinician through external pressure on _____ of _____ trials. (f)

BF/tm-15   Patient will eat only foods that form a cohesive bolus with/without cues. (d)

BF/tm-16   Patient will only eat pureed foods with/without cues. (d)

Short-Term Goal 6 — Bolus Formation/tone in cheeks (BF/tc)

The tone in patient's cheek(s) will increase to improve the ability to put food and liquid into a cohesive bolus to reduce the risk of food residue falling into the airway.

Treatment Objectives

BF/tc-1   Patient will use external pressure with fingers to cheek to decrease pocketing with/without cues on _____ of _____ trials. (c)

BF/tc-2   Patient will clean buccal cavity with fingers/tongue during/after meal with/without cues on _____ of _____ trials. (c)

BF/tc-3   Patient will place bolus of food on stronger side with/without cues on _____ of _____ trials. (c)

BF/tc-4   Patient will rinse and spit at end of each meal with/without cues on _____ of _____ trials. (c)

BF/tc-5   Patient will alternate thin/_____-thickened liquid wash every _____ bite(s) with/without cues on _____ of _____ trials. (c)

BF/tc-6   Patient will produce "oo" and then "ee" with exaggerated lip movement on _____ of _____ trials. (f)

BF/tc-7   Patient will pucker lips, then move lips from side to side on _____ of _____ trials. (f)

BF/tc-8   Patient will only eat foods that form a cohesive bolus with/without cues. (d)

BF/tc-9   Patient will only eat pureed foods with/without cues. (d)

Short-Term Goal 7 — Bolus Propulsion/tongue movement (BP/tm)

Patient will increase tongue movement to improve the ability to move a bolus to the back of the mouth in a coordinated fashion to reduce the risk of it falling into the airway.

Treatment Objectives

BP/tm-1   Patient will place bolus of food/liquid on midline of tongue with/without cues on _____ of _____ trials. (c)

BP/tm-2   Patient will place bolus of food/liquid on stronger side of mouth with/without cues on _____ of _____ trials. (c)

BP/tm-3   Patient will tip chin up slightly to help bolus move back in the mouth on _____ of _____ trials. (c) (Caution: This can be done only if the patient is not at risk for any aspiration as confirmed through a modified barium swallow.)

BP/tm-4   Patient will take small sip of liquid/_____-thickened liquid with bolus to help move the food backward with/without cues on _____ of _____ trials. (c)

BP/tm-5 Patient will take small sip of liquid/_____-thickened liquid after swallowing food to help clear residue from mouth with/without cues on _____ of _____ trials. (c)

BP/tm-6 Patient will move lemon swab placed between tongue and hard palate from front to back on _____ of _____ trials. (f)

BP/tm-7 Patient will sweep tongue from alveolar ridge to junction of hard and soft palate on _____ of _____ trials. (f)

BP/tm-8 Patient will pop tongue against hard palate on _____ of _____ trials. (f)

BP/tm-9 Patient will eat only foods that form a cohesive bolus with/without cues on _____ of _____ trials. (d)

BP/tm-10 Patient will avoid very sticky foods with/without cues on _____ of _____ trials. (d)

BP/tm-11 Patient will eat only pureed foods with/without cues. (d)

Short-Term Goal 8 — Bolus Propulsion/oral coordination (BP/oc)

Patient will increase oral coordination to improve the ability to move a bolus to the back of the mouth in a coordinated fashion to reduce the risk of it falling into the airway.

Treatment Objectives

BP/oc-1 Awareness of bolus will be increased through downward pressure of the spoon on the tongue on _____ of _____ trials. (c)

BP/oc-2 Patient will be allowed to self-feed liquids/solids from spoon/cup/straw/fingers on _____ of _____ trials. (c)

BP/oc-3 Awareness of bolus will be increased through temperature/taste/size of bolus on _____ of _____ trials. (d)

BP/oc-4 Awareness of bolus will be increased through presentation of foods that require mastication on _____ of _____ trials. (d)

Short-Term Goal 9 — Bolus Propulsion/oral sensation (BP/os)

Patient's oral sensation will increase to improve the ability to move a bolus to the back of the mouth in a coordinated fashion to reduce the risk of it falling into the airway.

Treatment Objectives

BP/os-1 Awareness of bolus will be increased through downward pressure of the spoon on the tongue on _____ of _____ trials. (c)

Chapter 7
The Source for Dysphagia   187

BP/os-2   Patient will be allowed to self-feed liquids/solids from spoon/cup/straw/fingers on _____ of _____ trials. (c)

BP/os-3   Patient will use effort swallow with/without cues on _____ of _____ trials. (c)

BP/os-4   Patient will move lemon swab placed between tongue and hard palate from front to back on _____ of _____ trials. (f)

BP/os-5   Awareness of bolus will be increased through temperature/taste/size of bolus on _____ of _____ trials. (d)

BP/os-6   Awareness of bolus will be increased through presentation of foods that require mastication on _____ of _____ trials. (d)

Short-Term Goal 10 – Bolus Propulsion/agnosia (BP/ag)

Patient will increase awareness of food/liquid and utensils in the mouth to improve the ability to move a bolus to the back of the mouth in a coordinated fashion to reduce the risk of it falling into the airway.

Treatment Objectives

BP/ag-1   Awareness of bolus will be increased through downward pressure of the spoon on the tongue on _____ of _____ trials. (c)

BP/ag-2   Empty cup or spoon will be presented when patient is holding bolus in oral cavity on _____ of _____ trials. (c)

BP/ag-3   Awareness of bolus will be increased through temperature/taste/size of bolus on _____ of _____ trials. (d)

BP/ag-4   Awareness of bolus will be increased through presentation of foods that require mastication on _____ of _____ trials. (d)

Short-Term Goal 11 – Aspiration Before/tongue control (AB/tc)

Patient will improve back of tongue control to keep food from falling over the back of the tongue and into the airway.

Treatment Objectives

AB/tc-1   Patient will use chin-down posture for _____ consistencies with/without cues on _____ of _____ trials. (c)

AB/tc-2   Patient will control bolus size to _____ with/without cues on _____ of _____ trials. (c)

AB/tc-3   Patient will use a cut-out cup/cup/straw/spoon for all liquid intake with/without cues on _____ of _____ trials. (c)

AB/tc-4   Patient will exert pressure with back of tongue up against tongue depressor on _____ of _____ trials. (A helpful cue is to ask the patient to try to say a /k/.) (f)

AB/tc-5   Patient will produce forceful /k/ at the end of words on _____ of _____ trials. (f)

AB/tc-6   Patient will take only liquids of _____ consistency with/without cues on _____ of _____ trials. (d)

AB/tc-7   Patient will avoid foods in liquid base with/without cues on _____ of _____ trials. (d)

Short-Term Goal 12 — Aspiration Before/delayed reflex (AB/dr)

Patient will decrease delay in initiation of pharyngeal swallow to reduce food falling into the airway during the delay before the swallow.

Treatment Objectives

AB/dr-1   Patient will control bolus size to _____ with/without cues on _____ of _____ trials. (c)

AB/dr-2   Patient will use chin-down posture for _____ consistencies with/without cues on _____ of _____ trials. (c) (Note: May not be helpful if bolus reaches pyriforms during the delay.)

AB/dr-3   Patient will use a cut-out cup/cup/straw/spoon for all liquid intake with/without cues on _____ of _____ trials. (c)

AB/dr-4   Patient will empty mouth before next bite with/without cues on _____ of _____ trials. (c)

AB/dr-5   Patient will decrease length of time from command to swallow to onset of swallow from _____ to _____ seconds following thermal-tactile application/neurosensory stimulation/cold bolus/sour bolus/three second prep/suck-swallow on _____ of _____ trials. (c,f) (Note: When choosing more than one technique, separate treatment objectives can be written by using letters (a), (b), etc.)

AB/dr-6   Patient will decrease length of time from command to swallow to onset of swallow from _____ to _____ seconds after thermal application/neurosensory stimulation/cold bolus/sour bolus/three second prep/suck swallow on carryover swallows at end of session on _____ of _____ trials. (c,f) (Note: When choosing more than one technique, separate treatment objectives can be written by using letters (a), (b), etc.)

AB/dr-7   Patient will initiate swallow within 1-2 seconds of command to swallow without any stimulation on _____ of _____ trials. (c,f)

AB/dr-8   Patient will avoid foods in liquid base with/without cues on _____ of _____ trials. (d)

AB/dr-9   Patient will take only liquids of _____ consistency with/without cues on _____ of _____ trials. (d)

Short-Term Goal 13 – Aspiration During/laryngeal closure (AD/lc)

Patient will increase closure of the true folds to keep food from falling into the airway during the swallow.

Treatment Objectives

AD/lc-1   Patient will control bolus size to _____ with/without cues on _____ of _____ trials. (c)

AD/lc-2   Patient will empty mouth before next bite with/without cues on _____ of _____ trials. (c)

AD/lc-3   Patient will use cut-out cup/cup/straw/spoon for liquid presentations with/without cues on _____ of _____ trials. (c)

AD/lc-4   Patient will use head rotation to R/L with/without cues on _____ of _____ trials. (c)

AD/lc-5   Patient will use chin-down for _____ consistencies with/without cues on _____ of _____ trials. (c)

AD/lc-6   Patient will use supraglottic swallow for _____ consistencies with/without cues on _____ of _____ trials. (c,f)

AD/lc-7   Patient will demonstrate Valsalva maneuver (breath hold) on _____ of _____ trials. (f)

AD/lc-8   Patient will take only liquids of _____ consistency with/without cues on _____ of _____ trials. (d)

AD/lc-9   Patient will avoid foods in liquid base with/without cues on _____ of _____ trials. (d)

Short-Term Goal 14 – Aspiration During/mistiming of closure (AD/mc)

Patient will improve rate of laryngeal elevation/timing of closure to keep food from falling into the airway during the swallow.

Treatment Objectives

AD/mc-1   Patient will control bolus size to _____ with/without cues on _____ of _____ trials. (c)

AD/mc-2   Patient will empty mouth before next bite with/without cues on _____ of _____ trials. (c)

AD/mc-3   Patient will use cut-out cup/cup/straw/spoon for liquid presentations with/without cues on _____ of _____ trials. (c)

AD/mc-4   Patient will use chin-down for _____ consistencies with/without cues on _____ of _____ trials. (c)

AD/mc-5   Patient will use super-supraglottic swallow for _____ consistencies with/without cues on _____ of _____ trials. (c,f) (Note: Improves speed of onset of laryngeal elevation.)

AD/mc-6   Patient will use Mendelsohn maneuver for _____ consistencies with/without cues on _____ of _____ trials. (c,f) (Note: Normalizes timing of pharyngeal swallow events.)

AD/mc-7   Patient will take only liquids of _____ consistency with/without cues on _____ of _____ trials. (d)

AD/mc-8   Patient will avoid foods in liquid base with/without cues on _____ of _____ trials. (d)

Short-Term Goal 15 – Aspiration After/pyriform/laryngeal elevation (AA/p/le)

Patient will increase laryngeal elevation to reduce residue in the pyriform sinus(es) and reduce risk of the residue falling into the airway after the swallow.

Treatment Objectives

AA/p/le-1   Patient will alternate thin/_____ consistency liquid wash every _____ bite(s) with/without cues on _____ of _____ trials. (c)

AA/p/le-2   Patient will use multiple swallows for each bite with/without cues on _____ of _____ trials. (c)

AA/p/le-3   Patient will control bolus size to _____ with/without cues on _____ of _____ trials. (c)

AA/p/le-4   Patient will use head rotation to R/L with/without cues on _____ of _____ trials. (c)

AA/p/le-5   Patient will remain seated upright at 90° with/without cues for 30 minutes after any PO intake. (c)

AA/p/le-6   Patient will use Mendelsohn maneuver for _____ consistencies with/without cues on _____ of _____ trials. (c,f)

AA/p/le-7   Patient will use super-supraglottic swallow for _____ consistencies with/without cues on _____ of _____ trials. (c,f)

AA/p/le-8   Patient will produce /i/ in continuous fashion, including falsetto, on _____ of _____ trials. (f)

AA/p/le-9   Patient will increase laryngeal elevation via SEMG biofeedback on _____ of _____ trials. (f)

AA/p/le-10   Patient will avoid sticky foods with/without cues. (d)

AA/p/le-11   Patient will take only liquids of _____consistency with/without cues. (d)

AA/p/le-12   Patient will avoid foods in liquid base with/without cues on _____ of _____ trials. (d)

Short-Term Goal 16 – Aspiration After/pyriform/hyolaryngeal complex movement (AA/p/hm)

Patient will increase anterior movement of the hyolaryngeal complex to reduce residue in the pyriform sinuses and reduce the risk of the residue falling into the airway after the swallow.

Treatment Objectives

AA/p/hm-1   Patient will alternate thin/_____ consistency liquid wash every _____ bite(s) with/without cues on _____ of _____ trials. (c)

AA/p/hm-2   Patient will use multiple swallows for each bite with/without cues on _____ of _____ trials. (c)

AA/p/hm-3   Patient will control bolus size to _____ with/without cues on _____ of _____ trials. (c)

AA/p/hm-4   Patient will use head rotation to R/L with/without cues on _____ of _____ trials. (c)

AA/p/hm-5   Patient will remain seated upright at 90° with/without cues for 30 minutes after any PO intake. (c)

AA/p/hm-6   Patient will use Mendelsohn maneuver for _____ consistencies with/without cues on _____ of _____ trials. (c,f)

AA/p/hm-7   Patient will perform head lift maneuver for _____ seconds on _____ of _____ trials. (f)

AA/p/hm-8   Patient will perform _____ repetitive head lift maneuvers. (f)

AA/p/hm-9   Patient will avoid sticky foods with/without cues. (d)

AA/p/hm-10 Patient will take only liquids of _____ consistency with/without cues. (d)

AA/p/hm-11 Patient will avoid foods in liquid base with/without cues on _____ of _____ trials. (d)

Short-Term Goal 17 – Aspiration After/laryngeal vestibule/laryngeal elevation (AA/lv/le)

Patient will improve laryngeal elevation to reduce penetration into the upper laryngeal vestibule to reduce the risk of the penetrated material being aspirated after the swallow.

Treatment Objectives

AA//lv/le-1 Patient will control bolus size to _____ with/without cues on _____ of _____ trials. (c)

AA/lv/le-2 Patient will use chin-down posture for _____ consistencies with/without cues on _____ of _____ trials. (c)

AA/lv/le-3 Patient will use supraglottic swallow for _____ consistencies with/without cues on _____ of _____ trials. (c) (Note: Compensatory as patient will expectorate residual material left above larynx.)

AA/lv/le-4 Patient will use Mendelsohn maneuver for _____ consistencies with/without cues on _____ of _____ trials. (c,f)

AA/lv/le-5   Patient will use super-supraglottic swallow for _____ consistencies with/without cues on _____ of _____ trials. (c,f) (Note: Improves speed of onset of laryngeal elevation.)

AA/lv/le-6   Patient will produce /i/ in continuous fashion, including falsetto on _____ of _____ trials. (f)

AA/lv/le-7   Patient will increase laryngeal elevation via SEMG biofeedback on _____ of _____ trials. (f)

AA/lv/le-8   Patient will take only liquids of _____ consistency with/without cues. (d)

AA/lv/le-9   Patient will avoid foods in liquid base with/without cues on _____ of _____ trials. (d)

Short-Term Goal 18 – Aspiration After/laryngeal vestibule/arytenoid tipping (AA/lv/at)

Patient will improve arytenoid tipping/closure at entrance to airway to reduce penetration into the upper laryngeal vestibule to reduce the risk of the penetrated material being aspirated after the swallow.

Treatment Objectives

AA/lv/at-1   Patient will control bolus size to _____ with/without cues on _____ of _____ trials. (c)

AA/lv/at-2   Patient will use chin-down posture for _____ consistencies with/without cues on _____ of _____ trials. (c)

AA/lv/at-3   Patient will produce /i/ in continuous fashion, including falsetto, on _____ of _____ trials. (f)

AA/lv/at-4   Patient will use super-supraglottic swallow for _____ consistencies with/without cues on _____ of _____ trials. (c,f)

AA/lv/at-5   Patient will take only liquids of _____ consistency with/without cues. (d)

AA/lv/at-6   Patient will avoid foods in liquid base with/without cues on _____ of _____ trials. (d)

Short-Term Goal 19 – Aspiration After/laryngeal vestibule/mistiming of closure (AA/lv/mc)

Patient will improve the rate of laryngeal elevation/timing of closure to reduce penetration into the upper laryngeal vestibule to reduce the risk of the penetrated material being aspirated after the swallow.

Treatment Objectives

AA/lv/mc-1   Patient will control bolus size to _____ with/without cues on _____ of _____ trials. (c)

AA/lv/mc-2   Patient will use chin-down posture for _____ consistencies on _____ of _____ trials. (c)

AA/lv/mc-3   Patient will use supraglottic swallow for _____ consistencies with/without cues on _____ of _____ trials. (c) (Note: Compensatory as patient will expectorate residual material in the larynx.)

Treatment Objectives to Achieve Short-Term Goals, *continued*

AA/lv/mc-4   Patient will use Mendelsohn maneuver for _____ consistencies with/without cues on _____ of _____ trials. (c,f) (Note: Normalizes timing of pharyngeal swallow events.)

AA/lv/mc-5   Patient will use super-supraglottic swallow for _____ consistencies with/without cues on _____ of _____ trials. (c,f) (Note: Improves speed of onset of laryngeal elevation.)

AA/lv/mc-6   Patient will produce /i/ in continuous fashion, including falsetto on _____ of _____ trials. (f)

AA/lv/mc-7   Patient will only take liquids of _____ consistencies with/without cues. (d)

AA/lv/mc-8   Patient will avoid foods in liquid base with/without cues on _____ of _____ trials. (d)

Short-Term Goal 20 – Aspiration After/valleculae/tongue base (AA/v/tb)

Patient will increase base of the tongue movement to reduce vallecular residue (unilateral or bilateral) to reduce the risk of the residue being aspirated after the swallow.

Treatment Objectives

AA/v/tb-1   Patient will take no larger than _____ bolus size with/without cues on _____ of _____ trials. (c)

AA/v/tb-2   Patient will empty mouth before next bite with/without cues on _____ of _____ trials. (c)

AA/v/tb-3   Patient will stay seated upright at 90° for 30 minutes after any PO with/without cues. (c)

AA/v/tb-4   Patient will use multiple swallows with/without cues on _____ of _____ trials. (c)

AA/v/tb-5   Patient will use thin/_____ consistency liquid wash with/without chin-down to widen valleculae every _____ bite(s) with/without cues on _____ of _____ trials. (c)

AA/v/tb-6   Patient will use head rotation to R/L with/without cues on _____ of _____ trials. (c)

AA/v/tb-7   Patient will use effort swallow with/without cues on _____ of _____ trials. (c,f)

AA/v/tb-8   Patient will use super-supraglottic swallow with _____ consistencies on _____ of _____ trials. (c,f) (Note: Improves tongue base retraction.)

AA/v/tb-9   Patient will demonstrate tongue base retraction on _____ of _____ trials. (f)

AA/v/tb-10   Patient will pretend to gargle on _____ of _____ trials. (f)

AA/v/tb-11   Patient will pretend to yawn on _____ of _____ trials. (f)

AA/v/tb-12   Patient will avoid sticky foods with/without cues on _____ of _____ trials. (d)

AA/v/tb-13   Patient will avoid foods in liquid base with/without cues on _____ of _____ trials. (d)

Short-Term Goal 21 — Aspiration After/valleculae/posterior pharyngeal wall (AA/v/ppw)

Patient will increase movement of the posterior pharyngeal wall to reduce vallecular residue to reduce the risk of the residue being aspirated after the swallow.

Treatment Objectives

AA/v/ppw-1   Patient will take no larger than _____ bolus size with/without cues on _____ of _____ trials. (c)

AA/v/ppw-2   Patient will empty mouth before next bite with/without cues on _____ of _____ trials. (c)

AA/v/ppw-3   Patient will stay seated upright at 90° for 30 minutes after any PO with/without cues. (c)

AA/v/ppw-4   Patient will use multiple swallows with/without cues on _____ of _____ trials. (c)

AA/v/ppw-5   Patient will use thin/_____ consistency liquid wash with/without chin-down to widen valleculae every _____ bite(s) with/without cues on _____ of _____ trials. (c)

AA/v/ppw-6   Patient will use head rotation to R/L with/without cues on _____ of _____ trials. (c)

AA/v/ppw-7   Patient will use effort swallow with/without cues on _____ of _____ trials. (f)

AA/v/ppw-8   Patient will swallow saliva using tongue hold on _____ of _____ trials. (f)

AA/v/ppw-9   Patient will pretend to gargle on _____ of _____ trials. (f)

AA/v/ppw-10   Patient will pretend to yawn on _____ of _____ trials. (f)

AA/v/ppw-11   Patient will avoid sticky foods with/without cues on _____ of _____ trials. (d)

AA/v/ppw-12   Patient will avoid foods in liquid base with/without cues on _____ of _____ trials. (d)

Short-Term Goal 22 — Aspiration After/valleculae/laryngeal elevation (AA/v/le)

Patient will increase laryngeal elevation to reduce vallecular residue to reduce the risk of the residue being aspirated after the swallow.

Treatment Objectives

AA/v/le-1   Patient will alternate thin/_____ consistency liquid wash with/without chin-down to widen valleculae every _____ bite(s) with/without cues on _____ of _____ trials. (c)

AA/v/le-2   Patient will use multiple swallows for each bite with/without cues on _____ of _____ trials. (c)

AA/v/le-3   Patient will control bolus size to _____ with/without cues on _____ of _____ trials. (c)

AA/v/le-4   Patient will remain seated upright at 90° with/without cues for 30 minutes after any PO intake. (c)

AA/v/le-5   Patient will use head rotation to R/L with/without cues on _____ of _____ trials. (c)

AA/v/le-6   Patient will use Mendelsohn maneuver for _____ consistencies with/without cues on _____ of _____ trials. (c,f)

AA/v/le-7   Patient will increase laryngeal elevation via SEMG biofeedback on _____ of _____ trials. (f)

AA/v/le-8   Patient will produce /i/ in continuous fashion, including falsetto, on _____ of _____ trials. (f)

AA/v/le-9   Patient will avoid sticky foods with/without cues. (d)

AA/v/le-10   Patient will take only liquids of _____ consistency with/without cues. (d)

AA/v/le-11   Patient will avoid foods in liquid base with/without cues on _____ of _____ trials. (d)

Short-Term Goal 23 – Aspiration After/walls/pharyngeal wall (AA/w/pw)

Patient will increase movement of pharyngeal wall(s) to reduce residue on pharyngeal wall(s) (unilateral or bilateral) to reduce the risk of the residue being aspirated after the swallow.

Treatment Objectives

AA/w/pw-1   Patient will alternate thin/_____ consistency liquid wash with/without chin-down to widen valleculae every _____ bite(s) with/without cues on _____ of _____ trials. (c)

AA/w/pw-2   Patient will use multiple swallows for each bite with/without cues on _____ of _____ trials. (c)

AA/w/pw-3   Patient will control bolus size to _____ with/without cues on _____ of _____ trials. (c)

AA/w/pw-4   Patient will use head rotation to R/L with/without cues on _____ of _____ trials. (c)

AA/w/pw-5   Patient will remain seated upright at 90° with/without cues on _____ of _____ trials. (c)

AA/w/pw-6   Patient will use effort swallow with/without cues on _____ of _____ trials. (c,f)

AA/w/pw-7   Patient will swallow saliva using tongue hold on _____ of _____ trials. (f)

AA/w/pw-8   Patient will avoid sticky foods with/without cues on _____ of _____ trials. (d)

AA/w/pw-9   Patient will avoid foods in liquid base with/without cues on _____ of _____ trials. (d)

Short-Term Goal 24 — Aspiration After/walls/tongue base (AA/w/tb)

Patient will increase movement of the tongue base to reduce bilateral residue on pharyngeal walls to reduce the risk of the residue being aspirated after the swallow.

Treatment Objectives

AA/w/tb-1   Patient will alternate thin/_____ consistency liquid wash with/without chin-down to widen valleculae every _____ bite(s) with/without cues on _____ of _____ trials. (c)

AA/w/tb-2   Patient will use multiple swallows for each bite with/without cues on _____ of _____ trials. (c)

AA/w/tb-3   Patient will control bolus size to _____ with/without cues on _____ of _____ trials. (c)

AA/w/tb-4   Patient will use head rotation to R/L with/without cues on _____ of _____ trials. (c)

AA/w/tb-5   Patient will remain seated upright at 90° with/without cues on _____ of _____ trials. (c)

AA/w/tb-6   Patient will use tongue base retraction on _____ of _____ trials. (f)

AA/w/tb-7   Patient will pretend to gargle on _____ of _____ trials. (f)

AA/w/tb-8   Patient will pretend to yawn on _____ of _____ trials. (f)

AA/w/tb-9   Patient will avoid sticky foods with/without cues on _____ of _____ trials. (d)

AA/w/tb-10   Patient will avoid foods in liquid base with/without cues on _____ of _____ trials. (d)

The goals are worded as compensatory techniques (i.e., being used with food during a meal). Therefore, if you choose to use the goal as a facilitory technique without food, you may have to reword the treatment objective. For example, Treatment Objective AA/lv/le-4 "Patient will use Mendelsohn maneuver for pudding consistencies with/without cues on 7 of 10 trials" would be worded that way if you use it in a compensatory fashion during meals. If, however, you see the patient only for facilitation without the presentation of food, you might reword it to say "Patient will use Mendelsohn maneuver for saliva swallows with/without cues on 7 of 10 trials."

Treatment Techniques

The following treatment techniques can help the patient achieve his treatment objectives and short-term goals. They are grouped into compensatory (c), facilitation (f), and diet (d). Some techniques can be both compensatory and facilitation (designed to improve function) if used during therapeutic feeding to compensate for a deficit.

Information is also provided from the research literature on the efficacy of certain techniques. Those techniques are marked with an asterisk (*). (See Appendix D, pages 215-219). The references may be helpful when you need to talk with a physician, nurse, family member, etc. about what you are doing with a patient.

Most of these techniques are also described on a patient handout in Chapter 4, pages 85-91.

Compensatory Treatment Techniques

These compensate for deficits and are most often used with therapeutic feedings.

1. **Appropriate Seating**

   During the oral intake of medicines, foods, and/or liquids, it is optimal for a patient to be seated at a 90° angle, whether in a bed or in a chair.

   At bedside, a draw sheet can be used to assist in positioning. A draw sheet is a sheet placed under the patient's torso. To use the draw sheet, put the bed in a flat position and have someone stand on either side of the patient holding onto the draw sheet. Using the sheet, pull the patient toward the head of the bed. Raise the head of the bed to its highest point and lower the foot of the bed to its lowest point. The patient should then be sitting at a 90° angle. Pillows may need to be placed behind the patient's back and/or head to achieve the correct position. A towel roll can further assist with keeping the head upright.

   Similarly, for the patient seated in a chair, the 90° angle is necessary prior to and during feeding. If the chair in which the patient is seated has a soft or slanted back, pillows can help attain the desired angle.

   The 90° position allows the patient to control material in the oral cavity with a minimal impact of gravity. This position must be maintained during and following the meal. Repositioning is frequently required during the meal.

2. **Chin-Down***

   The chin-down position assists patients who have decreased back of tongue control. For patients who exhibit materials falling over the back of their tongues, a chin-down position will help them gain oral and pharyngeal control of the bolus. Orally, the patient gains volitional control for propulsion of the bolus. Pharyngeally, the chin-down position widens the valleculae in many patients to allow for collection of material without spill to the pyriform sinuses or into the trachea.

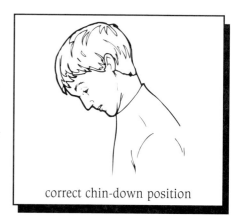

correct chin-down position

The chin-down or chin tuck also protects the trachea opening from aspiration by tucking the airway beneath the tongue base and epiglottis. The degree of chin tuck required to provide optimal protection and control varies from patient to patient based on the degree of compromised functioning.

It should be noted that the chin tuck or down positioning is not the same as a leaning forward posture. The patient's back should remain in the 90° position with the chin tucking toward the chest.

incorrect chin-down position

3. **Head Rotation***

Head rotation assists patients who have unilateral pharyngeal paresis or paralysis by decreasing the pharyngeal space by 50 percent.

On the videofluoroscopic evaluation, unilateral paralysis can be observed in the anterior/posterior view by looking for the variation in pooling within the pyriform sinuses. If the pooling is significantly asymmetrical, pharyngeal weakness or paralysis may be present.

For the patient with pharyngeal paralysis, the patient should rotate his head ALL THE WAY toward the damaged side. This closes the pyriform sinus on that side, increases vocal fold closure, and reduces resting tone in the cricopharyngeal muscle. The amount of pyriform sinus pooling will be decreased by directing the flow of the bolus down the stronger, more intact side.

Under videofluoroscopy, you can also try rotating the patient's head to the "good" side, as Logemann has found some improvement with this technique.

4. **Head Tilt***

A posterior head tilt is rarely recommended, but it may be helpful with patients who exhibit decreased ability to propel the bolus posteriorly to initiate a swallow. Typically, this involves patients who have undergone partial or total glossectomies, laryngectomies, and those with tongue scarring.

Tipping the head back allows gravity to propel the bolus posteriorly to initiate the swallow reflex. This technique should only be used with patients who are intact neurologically and present an efficient and strong response to penetration into the airway.

For patients who exhibit hemiparesis of the tongue and pharynx, a lateral head tilt to the patient's intact side may help. The bolus would be directed to the side of the oral cavity with greater muscle tone which assists in oral preparatory control.

5. **Oral Sensitivity Training**

Patients who aren't eating by mouth may show reduced sensitivity to material in the oral cavity. If a patient's oral cavity is very dry from mouth breathing and having no liquids, it is inappropriate to initially present food to the patient without first completing some oral sensitivity training. Be sure the patient is positioned upright and then use a toothette or a swab to moisten the oral cavity. Adequate saliva is essential for a patient to be able to form a good bolus. If the patient is able to complete such a maneuver, you may even have him swish and spit some liquid from his mouth.

6. Sour Bolus*

    Some patients may benefit from presentation of a sour bolus, like 50% real lemon juice and 50% water. This can significantly improve the onset of the oral and/or pharyngeal stages of the swallow. You can also utilize Italian lemon ice in small amounts. For the patient who is NPO, lemon glycerine swabs provide a source of sour stimulation.

7. Food Placement

    Patients usually do best if the food is placed at midline on their tongues. Some patients may do better if the food is placed on their stronger sides, especially if it's food that needs to be chewed.

8. External Pressure to the Cheek*

    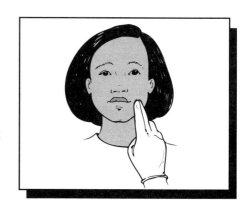

    Placing pressure on the affected cheek may also assist a patient with oral cavity weakness. By doing so, the patient receives several benefits. The pressure decreases the amount of material falling into the weaker lateral sulcus and helps the tongue action in the formation of a cohesive bolus. This tactile cue also reminds the patient to check the buccal pocket or lateral sulcus for material which could have fallen there. This technique compensates for decreased muscle tone.

9. Labial and Chin Support

    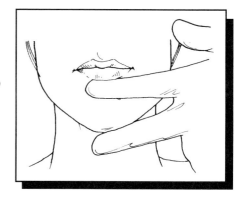

    Similar to external pressure to the cheek, you can provide the patient with assistive support at the lip and chin. Place your finger under the chin or lower lip to help maintain closure of the mouth. For the patient with a labial droop, fingertip support may be sufficient to provide closure of the lips to keep the material in the oral cavity. This is particularly helpful for thin liquid maintenance.

    For more severely-involved patients, support can be provided to compensate for both labial and jaw weakness. Position the thumb along the mandible with your index finger beneath the lower lip and your middle finger beneath the patient's chin.

10. Food Presentation*

    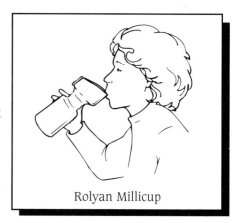

    Rolyan Millicup

    You may recommend different ways for food to be presented depending upon your goal. For example, if you want bolus size control, you may recommend that all presentations be made from a spoon. Or you can put a small amount of liquid into a cup before giving the cup to the patient. Remember that a cup tends to cause a patient to tip his head back when taking a drink. A cut-out cup can help reduce this tendency.

    A new product, the Rolyan Millicup is designed to measure out specific sip sizes (2.5 ml, 5 ml, 10 ml, 15 ml, and 20 ml). The patient or the clinician squeezes the cup, forcing the liquid into the measured reservoir. The patient then has only that amount accessible when he picks up the cup to take a drink. The cup provides nose clearance to encourage chin tuck.

A straw may help some patients maintain a chin-down posture while taking liquids. However, many patients have more difficulty when sucking from a straw as they tend to suck the material right into the airway.

Controlling the size of the bolus is important not only related to how much a person can hold in the oral cavity, but also how much the valleculae and pyriform sinuses can hold. As long as the bolus size is controlled to a small amount (5 to 8cc), the bolus can rest in the valleculae and pyriforms without aspiration while the patient waits to elicit the reflex.**

One other consideration about food presentation is whether you want the patient to mix liquids with solids. Some patients need to make sure they've swallowed several times to clear the oral cavity before any liquid is presented. Others do better if allowed to have a liquid to wash down the material.

**5cc is about a teaspoonful. 8-10cc is a comfortable mouthful.

11. **Multiple Swallow***

Some patients may need to be cued to quickly use a second dry swallow to clear residue from the pyriform sinuses and valleculae.

Facilitation Techniques

These techniques are designed to improve function.

1. **Laryngeal Adduction***

Vocal fold adduction exercises are helpful as facilitation techniques. These are the same techniques used in voice therapy to achieve better laryngeal closure. They include pushing, pulling, and hard glottal attack. Pushing and pulling cause the patient to bear down and tighten closure at the level of the vocal folds. Have the patient pull against a bed rail, your hand, or even try to pull up under the seat of the chair in which he is sitting. Ambulatory patients can lean against the wall to push. While the patient is pushing or pulling, have him phonate a vowel sound. Hard glottal attack involves having the patient hold his breath and then forcefully repeat vowels or words beginning with vowels.

2. **Breath Hold (Valsalva maneuver)**

Another technique which is helpful in achieving better closure of the larynx is the Valsalva maneuver or breath-hold technique. Ask the patient to take a breath and hold it tight for several seconds. Watch carefully, as many patients think they are holding their breath but they continue to breathe. If you watch their upper chest you can usually tell when they are really holding their breath. Some patients try to hold their breath by squeezing their lips shut. Discourage this by showing them how you can hold your breath with your mouth open.

3. **Falsetto/Pitch**

    Falsetto exercises are designed to improve elevation of the larynx. Better elevation means there will be better airway closure and less residue in the pyriform sinuses.

    Ask the patient to produce /i/ in a continuous note as he increases his pitch until he reaches the falsetto and to hold it there. Some patients may have more success with simple pitch change activities when asked to sing up the scale.

4. **Tongue Hold***

    This technique is designed to increase the forward movement of the posterior pharyngeal wall as it moves forward to meet the base of the tongue. Ask the patient to protrude his tongue and hold it between his teeth while he swallows. This is done with saliva swallows as it is difficult to control a food bolus while performing this technique.

5. **Tongue Base Retraction**

    Ask the patient to pull the base of his tongue towards the back wall of the throat (posterior pharyngeal wall) with lots of effort and to hold it there for several seconds. This is good to develop strength in the base of the tongue to reduce vallecular residue.

6. **Head Lift***

    This technique, described by Shaker et al. (1997) is designed to increase forward movement of the hyoid bone, which actually helps the entire hyolaryngeal complex move forward. This results in the cricopharyngeus opening more widely and staying open longer which should allow more residue to drain from the pyriform sinuses.

    The exercise has two parts: sustained and repetitive. For each, the patient lies flat on a bed or on the floor with no pillow under his head. For the sustained part of the exercise, have the patient lift his head (keeping his shoulders on the surface) and look at his toes. Have him hold the position for 60 seconds. For the repetitive part, keep the patient in the same position. Have him raise and lower his head 30 times in a row.

7. **Neurosensory Stimulation**

    This technique is a nice alternative when a patient won't open his mouth to allow you to perform thermal/tactile application. This technique helps to improve the triggering of the swallow.

    Fill a finger of a glove with water, tie it off, and freeze it. If you forget to plan ahead, you can also fill the finger of the glove with crushed ice and tie it off. Have the patient suck on the cold finger of the glove and then swallow. This technique combines the thermal aspect of thermal/tactile application with suck-swallow.

8. **Suck-Swallow**

    The suck-swallow has been shown to increase the speed of initiation of the pharyngeal swallow. Ask the patient to pretend he is sucking something very thick up through a very narrow straw for 2-3 seconds. Then have the patient swallow.

Chapter 7
The Source for Dysphagia   202

9. **Three-Second Prep**

This technique is based in neuropsychological research, which indicates that getting into a mental "set" to perform an action helps you initiate the action. Ask the patient to think about getting ready to swallow while you count to three. When you get to three, the patient should swallow.

10. **Surface Electromyographic Stimulation (SEMG)***

Crary (1997), Huckabee (1999), and others describe the use of SEMG as a means of biofeedback when teaching patients the Mendelsohn maneuver. Surface electrodes are placed below the chin. This allows you to see the amount and the duration of the elevation of the larynx on an LCD display or on a computer screen. Both Crary and Huckabee report success in improving the swallow of patients with chronic dysphagia often secondary to brain stem stroke when using an intensive treatment regimen of biofeedback.

11. **Pretend to Gargle**

This technique increases the movement of the posterior pharyngeal wall and the base of the tongue (Logemann, personal communication, 1998).

12. **Pretend to Yawn**

This technique also increases the movement of the posterior pharyngeal wall and the base of the tongue (Logemann, personal communication, 1998).

13. **Oral-Motor Exercises***

The exercises described below may be helpful for:

- bolus maintenance (keeping the bolus from falling over the base of the tongue, out the front of the mouth, or into the sulci)

- bolus preparation/manipulation (moving the bolus around in the mouth)

- bolus propulsion (moving the bolus posteriorly)

This list is not meant to be all-inclusive, but provides examples of exercises which may be helpful. Remember to wear gloves when performing any oral-motor exercises in or near the patient's mouth.

Bolus Maintenance

Therapist initiated:

1. Place your thumb and index finger on the patient's upper lip just below the nostrils, and give a quick stretch outward toward the corners of the mouth. Release pressure suddenly. Repeat with the lower lip.

2. Using your index finger and thumb on the corners of the patient's mouth, stretch out toward the cheeks. Release suddenly.

3. Briefly tap directly on the bone under the patient's chin to create a reflex action to assist in jaw closure.

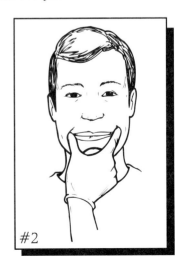

#2

4. Place your hand below the patient's chin to provide resistance to the jaw opening, and then place your hand in front of the chin to resist protrusion.

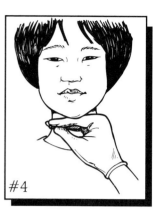

#4

Patient initiated:

1. Suck on a straw, Lifesaver on a string, Popsicle, juice bar, or ice cube to increase muscle tension and stimulate contraction for closure and seal.

2. Pucker your lips as if to kiss. Kiss the back of your hand or throw a kiss.

3. Open your mouth and then try to close your lips while keeping your jaw open.

4. Blow with your lips closed, puffing up cheeks. Try to move the air from side to side. Then have the therapist push on one cheek at a time to move the air.

5. Close your lips and press hard.

6. Move your tongue in a clockwise motion between your teeth and the inside of your closed lips. Repeat in a counter-clockwise direction.

7. Try to touch your chin and then your nose with your tongue.

Bolus Formation

Therapist initiated:

1. Press downward on the back of the patient's tongue with a spoon or tongue depressor. Release suddenly while the patient articulates /k/ or words beginning and/or ending with /k/ such as *car, key, cool, bake, book, cake, cook,* or *kick.*

2. Place a tongue depressor against the tip of the patient's tongue, and have the patient push his tongue tip out against it.

3. Press down on the patient's tongue with the tongue depressor, and have the patient push his tongue upward against it.

4. Place a tongue depressor along the lateral margin of the patient's tongue on the stronger side, and have the patient push against it with his tongue.

Patient initiated:

1. Blow with your lips closed, puffing up your cheeks. Try to move the air from side to side.

2. Click your tongue as if to make a galloping horse sound.

3. Chew on gauze flavored with lemon juice or sugar water. Attempt to move it between the left and right molar areas keeping one end firmly held outside of the mouth.

4. Move a lemon swab placed between your tongue and palate from side to side and then backward and forward using your tongue.

Bolus Propulsion

Patient initiated:

1. Stick your tongue out of your mouth as far as possible making sure that it comes straight out and does not deviate to the side.

2. Move your tongue from one corner of your mouth to the other taking care to touch each corner completely.

3. Move your tongue in a clockwise direction around both your upper and lower lips. Take care to make a complete excursion and not to miss any areas. Repeat in a counter-clockwise direction.

4. Move your tongue tip from the front of your mouth to the back, beginning with the tip on the alveolar ridge.

Compensatory and Facilitation Techniques

These compensatory techniques can also help facilitate the return of function.

1. **Thermal/Tactile Application***

   Thermal/tactile application, which is sometimes called thermal stimulation, is typically used with patients who show a delay of greater than two seconds in initiating the swallow reflex or who aspirate during the delay. The stimulation does not cause the reflex to happen, but heightens the awareness of that region in the mouth to increase the likelihood that a swallow will occur.

   Be sure to take quantitative data during this maneuver. Before you begin this technique, count how long it takes the patient to achieve a baseline swallow. Count again after completing the thermal stimulation to see if there is improvement. After the session has ended, take another measurement of how long it takes the patient to elicit a swallow to determine if there has been any carryover.

   Generally a double 00 laryngeal mirror is used. Hold the mirror like a pencil so you can easily rotate it in your hand. Dip it in ice and rub it up and down five times on one of the patient's anterior faucial arches. Then dip it back into the ice quickly, rotate it so the flat head of the mirror is facing in the other direction, and rub it on the other faucial arch. Instruct the patient to swallow so that the voluntary component of the swallow is invoked.

   You can pair thermal/tactile application with small amounts of liquid if the patient is allowed to have anything to drink. This may help elicit a swallow reflex. If you find a patient who wants to close his mouth around the mirror, apply downward pressure to the jaw and give verbal cues to keep the mouth open. When the swallow reflex is triggered, several simultaneous motor acts occur:

   - closure of the velopharyngeal port
   - closure of larynx (true and false vocal cords)
   - laryngeal elevation
   - closure at top of larynx by epiglottis
   - hyoid elevation

- anterior movement of the larynx
- anterior movement of the hyoid

These actions serve to close the airway and also to open the upper esophageal sphincter.

2. Supraglottic Swallow*

The supraglottic swallow is indicated for patients who cannot attain laryngeal closure or airway closure prior to, during, and after a swallow. The supraglottic swallow works to provide five areas of approximating laryngeal valving sufficient to achieve strong laryngeal closure prior to and during the swallow. Following a swallow, the patient coughs to clear any residual material, and then swallows again. This technique brings airway closure under a patient's voluntary control.

Step 1: Patient takes in a breath and lets out a little air.

Step 2: Patient holds his breath.

Step 3: Food is placed within the oral cavity.

Step 4: Patient swallows, maintaining breath holding until swallow is completed.

Step 5: Patient coughs.

Step 6: Patient swallows again to clear material expelled.

This technique can be completed during direct and/or indirect therapy to increase the patient's ability to achieve laryngeal closure. If done indirectly, eliminate Step 3.

It may be difficult to tell if the patient is really using the technique. One means for assessing if the patient is able to coordinate the steps is to watch for lack of chest wall movement during periods of breath holding.

3. Super-Supraglottic Swallow*

The super-supraglottic swallow follows the identical sequence to the supraglottic swallow, but the patient is instructed to use additional force during the sequence to provide greater muscular tension. Recent studies show the super-supraglottic swallow improves rate of laryngeal elevation and improves movement of the tongue base.

4. Effort Closure*

This technique gets the patient's tongue base moving. Pooling in the valleculae typically means the tongue base isn't making contact with the posterior pharyngeal wall and the epiglottis never gets squeezed all the way down.

Instruct the patient to "swallow real hard and squeeze with the tongue all the way along." Increasing tongue base retraction is like telling the patient to "swallow his tongue" or to "swallow hard enough to push a Ping-Pong ball down."

5. Mendelsohn maneuver*

This technique is designed to maintain elevation of the larynx at its highest point which decreases pooling in the pyriform sinuses. It maintains the opening of the cricopharyngeus for a longer period of time. It may also improve coordination of the whole swallow sequence.

This technique is typically prescribed when the patient is demonstrating aspiration after the swallow from the pooled material in the pyriform sinuses. This is a difficult procedure for patients to learn to use. The Mendelsohn is basically accomplished by voluntarily continuing tongue contraction to prolong the rise of the larynx.

Patients may have problems trying to hold the larynx up too early or catching it late. Let the patient feel the laryngeal elevation with his hand, but make sure he understands that he is not holding the larynx with his hand. If he can't follow your directions, ask, "Can you feel the point where your throat all comes together? When that happens, squeeze really hard with the back muscles of your tongue to hold that feeling." Cue the patient to push the tongue hard up against the roof of his mouth.

Diet Modification Techniques

1. Consistency of Liquids

For most dysphagic patients who have difficulties in the oral preparatory and oral voluntary phases, some kind of diet modifications will be necessary. The biggest change is typically made in the consistency of liquids. It's important to remember that liquids are not only things in a cup, but other things such as soups and broth on vegetables. Also, things that melt to a liquid in the mouth before being swallowed must be considered a liquid like ice cream and Jell-O.

If a patient has extremely poor tongue control and particularly, poor control of the back of the tongue, liquids will roll over the base of the tongue before the patient has control of the bolus and is ready to begin a swallow.

Liquids can be thickened with commercial products such as NutraThik, Thick-It or Classic Instant Food Thickener. Foods other than commercial thickeners can also be used to change the consistency of liquids, but they may change the food flavor or texture. These foods include rice, tapioca, instant or mashed potatoes, unflavored gelatin, or baby cereal.

Using different amounts of a food thickener can result in liquids changing from thin liquid to syrup consistency, honey consistency, or even a pudding consistency. These thickeners work best if shaken rather than stirred. A clean specimen cup is ideal for mixing at bedside.

One of the most difficult challenges when working with dysphagic patients is getting them to take enough thickened liquids to meet their fluid needs. The dietitian can help you incorporate high-fluid content foods like pureed fruits, custard, gelatins, and frozen juice into the patient's diet. Work closely with the dietitian regarding the patient's nutritional needs and calorie counts.

2. Temperatures of Food

You will need to experiment with each patient to determine if he responds better to room temperature, cold, or hot foods. This is very individualized.

3. Textures of Foods*

A pureed diet will vary a great deal from one institution to another. Many institutions have developed diets specifically for their dysphagia patients. For patients with mechanical problems in the oral phase, liquids, thickened liquids, and pureed foods are often the easiest to swallow.

Patients with pharyngeal problems who are at risk for aspiration sometimes have more difficulty with thinned, runny purees because the disordered mechanism cannot respond in time with sufficient control to protect the airway. In those instances, foods like baked potatoes or macaroni and cheese maintain a cohesive texture and do not easily break up in the mouth. They can typically be swallowed as a single bolus and are probably better tolerated than runny purees. There is some evidence that these kinds of foods may trigger a weak reflex better than a runny pureed food.

As the patient progresses, food items that require more manipulation are added and the consistency of the liquids is thinned. Generally foods that fall or break apart in the mouth like dried muffins, pound cake, plain rice, coconut, and foods with more than one consistency like fruit cocktail or soup with pieces should be avoided. This precaution helps avoid small pieces of food entering the airway.

One other thing to consider when dysphagia patients are receiving a pureed diet is the fact that it is not generally very palatable nor is it visually appealing. A creative clinical nutrition specialist can be a big help in changing the way foods look. Molds are available to change the shape of pureed fruits and vegetables. For example, a mold can be used to change a bowl of pureed peas into what appears to be a pile of little round peas. Pureed meats can be molded in a loaf pan and then sliced. In addition, a mixture called *slurry* can be poured over bread and cake products. The bread retains its shape, but turns into a pureed texture. Slurry is made by mixing milk and a food thickener.

Five levels of dysphagia diets are described on pages 209-213. They consider many factors for patients at different levels.

Dysphagia Diet Level I

Rationale: This diet is for patients with severely impaired swallowing who have significant pooling in the hypopharynx with sticky foods. Foods that are sticky (like peanut butter) or non-cohesive (like rice) are omitted.

Description: The diet is a modified pureed diet with runny smooth textures. All foods should have a honey consistency and homogeneous textures with no nuts, seeds, or lumps. All liquids including water, broth, and strained soups should be thickened to honey consistency.

Nutritional Adequacy: This diet does not provide adequate fluid or nutrients to meet the Recommended Dietary Allowances. Consider tube feedings to meet requirements. This diet is not intended for long-term use.

Food Group	Foods Allowed
beverages/milk	All liquids must be thickened to a honey consistency, including water.
meats and meat substitutes (4-6 servings/day)	pureed meat with gravy or broth added to achieve a honey consistency, custard-style blended yogurt
starches, breads, and cereals (6-11 servings/day)	mashed potatoes with gravy, Cream of Wheat, rice cereal
fruits (2-4 servings/day)	pureed fruits without skins or seeds, thickened juices
vegetables (3-5 servings/day)	pureed vegetables without skins or seeds, thickened juices
soups	pureed, strained soups thickened to a runny honey consistency
desserts	sherbet, ice cream
condiments	margarine, butter, artificial sweetener, sugar, gravy, sour cream, ketchup, mustard, steak sauce, mayonnaise, herbs, spices

Dysphagia Diet Level II

Rationale: This diet is for patients with severely impaired swallowing who are receiving swallowing re-training. Foods that are sticky (like peanut butter) or non-cohesive (like rice) are omitted. This diet may be appropriate for persons with severely reduced oral preparatory phase abilities and reduced laryngeal closure.

Description: The diet is a modified pureed diet with thick, smooth textures. All foods should have a pudding consistency. All liquids including water, broth, and strained soups should be thickened to pudding consistency.

Nutritional Adequacy: This diet does not provide adequate fluid or nutrients to meet the Recommended Dietary Allowances. Consider tube feedings to meet requirements. This diet is not intended for long-term use.

Food Group	Foods Allowed
beverages/milk	All liquids must be thickened to a pudding consistency, including water.
meats and meat substitutes (4-6 servings/day)	pureed meat, pureed cottage cheese, custard-style blended yogurt
starches, breads, and cereals (6-11 servings/ day)	mashed potatoes with gravy, whipped sweet potatoes, Cream of Wheat, rice cereal, oatmeal
fruits (2-4 servings/day)	pureed fruits without skins or seeds, thickened juices
vegetables (3-5 servings/day)	pureed vegetables without skins or seeds, thickened juices
soups	pureed, strained soups thickened to a pudding consistency
desserts	pudding
condiments	margarine, butter, artificial sweetener, sugar, gravy, sour cream, ketchup, mustard, steak sauce, mayonnaise, herbs, spices

Dysphagia Diet Level III

Rationale: This diet is for patients with impaired swallowing who can chew some very soft foods, but cannot swallow thin liquids safely. This diet may be appropriate for persons with moderately impaired oral preparatory phase abilities and/or pharyngeal disorders.

Description: Most foods are still pureed with the addition of some textures which form a cohesive bolus. Foods that are sticky, non-cohesive, or a mixed consistency are omitted. All liquids, including water, are thickened to honey, syrup, or pudding consistency.

Nutritional Adequacy: This diet provides nutritional adequacy as indicated by the Recommended Dietary Allowances, depending upon amount consumed. More frequent feedings may be necessary. Monitor fluid intake.

Food Group	Foods Allowed
beverages/milk	All liquid including water must be thickened to a honey, syrup, or pudding consistency. Milk shakes, buttermilk, eggnog, fruit nectars, tomato, and V8 juice are acceptable if liquids are required to be only syrup thick.
meats and meat substitutes (4-6 servings/day)	pureed meat, plain baked fish without bones, macaroni and cheese, cottage cheese, pimento cheese, custard-style blended yogurt, pureed soup beans
starches, breads, and cereals (6-11 servings/ day)	oatmeal, Cream of Wheat, rice cereal, grits, pancakes, mashed potatoes with gravy, whipped sweet potatoes, baked potato without skin, canned yams
fruits (2-4 servings/day)	applesauce, soft baked apples without peel, banana, pureed fruit
vegetables (3-5 servings/day)	pureed vegetables, plain vegetable soufflé
soups	strained soups thickened to proper consistency
desserts	pudding, cheesecake without crust
condiments	margarine, butter, artificial sweetener, sugar, honey, syrup, gravy, sour cream, cream cheese, cheese sauce, ketchup, mustard, steak sauce, mayonnaise, herbs, spices

Dysphagia Diet Level IV

Rationale: This diet is for patients whose oral skills have improved to the point that they can chew and form a bolus with many foods. It is based on a mechanical soft diet and the foods should maintain a cohesive texture. These patients would still be at risk with thin liquids and mixed consistency foods.

Description: Textures are soft with no tough or stringy foods. In addition, no nuts, seeds, or raw foods are allowed. Meats should be ground. All liquids should be thickened.

Nutritional Adequacy: This diet provides nutritional adequacy as indicated by the Recommended Dietary Allowances, depending upon amount consumed.

Food Group	Foods Allowed	Foods to Avoid
beverages/milk	as advised	as advised
meats and meat substitutes (4-6 servings/day)	ground meats, scrambled eggs, fried eggs, poached eggs, hard-boiled eggs, plain baked fish, breaded baked fish, tuna fish, tuna fish salad, salmon loaf, chicken salad, macaroni and cheese, cottage cheese, pimiento cheese, cheese slices, blended yogurt, casseroles made with appropriate ingredients	stringy meats and cheese, fried meats, dry meat, tough meats, sausage, bacon, hot dogs, peanut butter
starches, breads, and cereals (6-11 servings/day)	all hot cereals, pancakes, waffles, doughnuts, muffins, biscuits, corn bread, crackers, all potatoes (no skin), noodles, pasta	cold cereals containing nuts or dried pieces of fruit, bread, bagels, English muffins, French toast, dinner rolls, rice
fruits (2-4 servings/day)	canned pears, peaches, apricots, applesauce, soft baked apples (no peel), apple slices (no peel), bananas, strawberries, blueberries, cherries, stewed prunes	fresh fruit and berries not listed, dried fruits, fruit cocktail, mixed fruit salad, citrus sections, grapes, raisins
vegetables (3-5 servings/day)	soft-cooked vegetables drained well, soufflés, corn pudding, beans, winter squash, casseroles made with appropriate ingredients	salads; coleslaw; mixed vegetables; corn; tomatoes; succotash; sauerkraut; yellow squash; and raw, steamed crunchy vegetables
soups	creamed soups	all other soups, broth
desserts	pudding; ice cream; sherbet; frozen yogurt; cream pies; cheesecake; pies or cobblers made with allowed fruits; soft cookies; chocolate, butterscotch, and caramel sauces	cakes, hard cookies, Jell-O, hard candy, chewing gum, chewy desserts
condiments	margarine, butter, sugar, artificial sweetener, honey, syrup, jelly, jam, sour cream, cream cheese, cheese sauce, gravy, mustard, ketchup, mayonnaise, steak sauce, barbecue sauce, herbs, spices	nuts, coconut, seeds, olives, pickles, relishes, stringy cheese sauce, any foods not listed

Dysphagia Diet Level V

Rationale: This diet is very similar to Level IV, but is designed for patients who are safe with thin liquids.

Description: Textures are soft with no tough or stringy foods. In addition, no nuts; seeds; raw, crisp, or deep-fried foods are allowed.

Nutritional Adequacy: This diet is designed to provide an adequate quantity of nutrients as indicated by the Recommended Dietary Allowances, depending upon amount consumed.

Food Group	Foods Allowed	Foods to Avoid
beverages/milk	all allowed	none
meats and meat substitutes (4-6 servings/day)	ground meat, eggs, macaroni and cheese, meat loaf, baked fish, salmon loaf, tuna fish, tuna fish salad, cheese slices, cottage cheese, pimiento cheese, grilled cheese, yogurt, chicken salad, casseroles made with appropriate ingredients	fried, dry, tough, stringy meats; peanut butter; melted stringy cheese; sandwiches not listed
starches, breads, and cereals (6-11 servings/day)	all hot cereals, dry cereals not containing nuts or dried fruit pieces, pancakes, waffles, muffins, biscuits, corn bread, doughnuts, crackers, noodles, pasta, rice, stuffing, dumplings, potatoes (no skin), bread, toast, dinner rolls	dry cereals containing nuts or dried fruit, granola, bagels, English muffins, muffins containing nuts, bread sticks, French bread
fruits (2-4 servings/day)	canned fruits, soft baked apples (no peel), citrus sections, cherries, congealed fruit salads, apple wedges (no peel), bananas, strawberries, blueberries, stewed prunes, melons, flaked coconut	fresh fruits and berries not listed, raisins, dried fruits
vegetables (3-5 servings/day)	soft-cooked vegetables, soufflés, beans, corn, summer squash, winter squash, chopped spinach and greens, mixed vegetables, tomatoes, sauerkraut, casseroles made with appropriate ingredients	raw, crisp, crunchy vegetables; salads; cole slaw
soups	all allowed	none
desserts	soft cookies; pudding; ice cream; sherbet; Jell-O; cake; cheesecake; cream pies; fruit pies or cobblers made with allowed fruits; chocolate, caramel, or butterscotch sauces	hard cookies, hard candy, chewing gum, chewy desserts
condiments	margarine, butter, sugar, artificial sweetener, honey, syrup, jelly, sour cream, cream cheese, cheese sauce, gravy, mustard, ketchup, mayonnaise, steak sauce, barbecue sauce, relishes, herbs, spices	nuts, olives, pickles, stringy cheese sauce, seeds, jams, popcorn, chips

Descriptions of Food Consistencies

Mixed Consistency

cereal with milk
congealed salads
fruit cocktail
fruits in juice or syrup
green beans
lettuce, salads
peas, corn
stewed tomatoes
vegetables not drained
melons
citrus fruits

Thin Liquids

broth
coffee
fruit juices
hot chocolate
ice cream
Italian ice
Jell-O
milk
nutritional supplements (e.g., Ensure Plus)
Popsicles
sherbet
sodas
strained soups (all types)
tea
thin gravy or cheese sauce
thin milk shakes
water

Fruits with High Water Content

any citrus
melons
pineapple
tomatoes

Vegetables with High Water Content

carrots
greens
squash
zucchini

Non-Cohesive Consistency

biscuits
cereal with milk
citrus fruit
corn
corn bread
crackers (including graham)
fruit cocktail
green beans
greens (all varieties)
hard-boiled eggs
lettuce
noodles
pasta
plain, chopped, raw vegetables and fruit
plain ground meats without gravy
rice
salads
scrambled eggs
stewed tomatoes
tomatoes
yellow squash

Sticky Consistency

bananas
jelly
mashed potatoes without gravy
oatmeal
peanut butter
pie filling
white bread

Appendix D: Efficacy References for Treatment Techniques

Chin Down

Rasley, A., J. Logemann, P. Kahrilas, A. Rademaker, B. Pauloski, and W. Dodds. "Prevention of Barium Aspiration During Videofluoroscopic Swallowing Studies: Value of Change in Posture." *American Journal of Roentgenology*, Vol. 160, May 1993, pp. 1005-1009.

Singh, V., M. J. Brockbank, R. A. Frost, and S. Tyler. "Multi-Disciplinary Management of Dysphagia: The First 100 Cases." *The Journal of Laryngology and Otology*, Vol. 109, 1995, pp. 419-424.

Welch, M. V., J. A. Logemann, A. W. Rademaker, and P. J. Kahrilas. "Changes in Pharyngeal Dimensions Effected By Chin Tuck." *Archives of Physical Medicine and Rehabilitation*, Vol. 74, 1993, pp. 178-181.

Head Rotation

Logemann, J., P. Kahrilas, M. Kobara, and N. Vakil. "The Benefit of Head Rotation on Pharyngoesophageal Dysphagia." *Archives of Physical Medicine and Rehabilitation*, Vol. 70, 1989, pp. 767-771.

Logemann, J. and P. Kahrilas. "Relearning to Swallow After Stroke — Application of Maneuvers and Indirect Biofeedback: A Case Study." *Neurology*, Vol. 40, 1990, pp. 1136-1138.

Rasley, A., J. Logemann, P. Kahrilas, A. Rademaker, B. Pauloski, and W. Dodds. "Prevention of Barium Aspiration During Videofluoroscopic Swallowing Studies: Value of Change in Posture." *American Journal of Roentgenology*, Vol. 160, May 1993, pp. 1005-1009.

Silbergleit, A., W. Waring, M. Sullivan, and F. Maynard. "Evaluation, Treatment, and Follow-Up Results of Post-Polio Patients With Dysphagia." *Otolaryngology-Head and Neck Surgery*, Vol. 104, No. 3, 1991, pp. 333-338.

Welch, M. V., J. A. Logemann, A. W. Rademaker, and P. J. Kahrilas. "Changes in Pharyngeal Dimensions Effected By Chin Tuck." *Archives of Physical Medicine and Rehabilitation*, Vol. 74, 1993, pp. 178-181.

Head Tilt

Singh, V., M. J. Brockbank, R. A. Frost, and S. Tyler. "Multi-Disciplinary Management of Dysphagia: The First 100 Cases." *The Journal of Laryngology and Otology*, Vol. 109, 1995, pp. 419-424.

Sour Bolus

Logemann, J. A., B. R. Pauloski, L. Colangelo, C. Lazarus, M. Fujiu, and P. J. Kahrilas. "Effects of a Sour Bolus on Oropharyngeal Swallowing Measures in Patients With Neurogenic Dysphagia." *Journal of Speech and Hearing Research*, Vol. 38, No. 3, 1995, pp. 556-563.

External Pressure to the Cheek

Singh, V., M. J. Brockbank, R. A. Frost, and S. Tyler. "Multi-Disciplinary Management of Dysphagia: The First 100 Cases." *The Journal of Laryngology and Otology*, Vol. 109, 1995, pp. 419-424.

Food Presentation

Lazarus, C. L., J. A. Logemann, A. W. Rademaker, P. J. Kahrilas, T. Pajak, R. Lazar, and A. Halper. "Effects of Bolus Volume, Viscosity and Repeated Swallows in Nonstroke Subjects and Stroke Patients." *Archives of Physical Medicine and Rehabilitation*, Vol. 74, 1993, pp. 1066-1070.

Perlman, A. "The Successful Treatment of Challenging Cases." *Clinics in Communication Disorders*, Vol. 3, No. 4, 1993, pp. 37-44.

Silbergleit, A., W. Waring, M. Sullivan, and F. Maynard. "Evaluation, Treatment, and Follow-Up Results of Post-Polio Patients With Dysphagia." *Otolaryngology-Head and Neck Surgery*, Vol. 104, No. 3, 1991, pp. 333-338.

Singh, V., M. J. Brockbank, R. A. Frost, and S. Tyler. "Multi-Disciplinary Management of Dysphagia: The First 100 Cases." *The Journal of Laryngology and Otology*, Vol. 109, 1995, pp. 419-424.

Multiple Swallow

Silbergleit, A., W. Waring, M. Sullivan, and F. Maynard. "Evaluation, Treatment, and Follow-Up Results of Post-Polio Patients With Dysphagia." *Otolaryngology-Head and Neck Surgery*, Vol. 104, No. 3, 1991, pp. 333-338.

Singh, V., M. J. Brockbank, R. A. Frost, and S. Tyler. "Multi-Disciplinary Management of Dysphagia: The First 100 Cases." *The Journal of Laryngology and Otology*, Vol. 109, 1995, pp. 419-424.

Laryngeal Adduction

Kasprisin, A. T., H. Clumeck, and M. Nino-Murcia. "The Efficacy of Rehabilitative Management of Dysphagia." *Dysphagia*, Vol. 4, 1989, pp. 48-52.

Singh, V., M. J. Brockbank, R. A. Frost, and S. Tyler. "Multi-Disciplinary Management of Dysphagia: The First 100 Cases." *The Journal of Laryngology and Otology*, Vol. 109, 1995, pp. 419-424.

Tongue Hold

Fujiu, M. and J. A. Logemann. "Effect of a Tongue-Holding maneuver on Posterior Pharyngeal Wall Movement During Deglutition." *American Journal of Speech-Language Pathology*, Vol. 5, 1996, pp. 23-30.

Fujiu, M., J. A. Logemann, and B. R. Pauloski. "Increased Postoperative Posterior Pharyngeal Wall Movement in Patients with Anterior Oral Cancer: Preliminary Findings and Possible Implications for Treatment." *American Journal of Speech-Language Pathology*, Vol. 4, 1995, pp. 24-30.

Head Lift (Shaker) Maneuver

Easterling, C., C. Kern, T. Nitschke, B. Grande, G. M. Cullen, and R. Shaker. "A Novel Rehabilitative Exercise for Dysphagic Patients: The Effect on Swallow Function and Biomechanics." In Press.

Easterling, C., M. Kern, T. Nitschke, B. Grande, S. Daniels, G. M. Cullen, B. T. Massey, and R. Shaker. "Effect of a Novel Exercise on Swallow Function and Biomechanics in Tube Fed Cervical Dysphagia Patients: A Preliminary Report." *Dysphagia*, Vol. 14, 1999.

Easterling, C., M. Kern, T. Nitschke, B. Grande, M. Kazandjian, K. Dikeman, B. T. Massey, and R. Shaker. "Restoration of Oral Feeding in 17 Tube Fed Patients by the Shaker Exercise." In Press.

Shaker, R., M. Kern, E. Bardan, A. Taylor, E. T. Stewart, R. G. Hoffman, R. Arndorfer, C. Hofman, and J. Bonnevier. "Augmentation of Deglutitive Upper Esophageal Sphincter Opening in the Elderly by Exercise." *The American Journal of Physiology*, Vol. 272, 1997, pp. 1518-1522.

SEMG

Bryant, M. "Biofeedback in the Treatment of a Selected Dysphagic Patient." *Dysphagia*, Vol. 6, 1991, pp. 140-144.

Crary, M. A. "A Direct Intervention Program for Chronic Neurogenic Dysphagia Secondary to Brainstem Stroke." *Dysphagia*, Vol. 10, 1995, pp. 6-18.

Crary, M. A. "Surface Electromyographic Characteristics of Swallowing in Dysphagia Swallowing Secondary to Brainstem Stroke." *Dysphagia*, Vol. 12, No. 4, 1997, pp. 180-188.

Gutpa, V., N. P. Reddy, and E. P. Canilang. "Surface EMG Measurements at the Throat During Dry and Wet Swallowing." *Dysphagia*, Vol. 11, No. 3, 1996, pp. 180-185.

Huckabee, M. L. and M. P. Cannito. "Outcomes of Swallowing Rehabilitation in Chronic Brainstem Dysphagia: A Retrospective Evaluation." *Dysphagia*, Vol. 14, 1999, pp. 93-109.

Perlman, A. L. and J. P. Grayhack. "Use of the Electroglottograph for Measurement of Temporal Aspects of the Swallow: Preliminary Observations." *Dysphagia*, Vol. 6, 1991, pp. 88-93.

Oral-Motor Exercises

Helfrich-Miller, K., K. Rector, and J. Straka. "Dysphagia: Its Treatment in the Profoundly Retarded Patient with Cerebral Palsy." *Archives of Physical Medicine and Rehabilitation*, Vol. 67, 1986, pp. 520-525.

Kasprisin, A. T., H. Clumeck, and M. Nino-Murcia. "The Efficacy of Rehabilitative Management of Dysphagia," *Dysphagia*, Vol. 4, 1989, pp. 48-52.

Logemann, J. A., B. R. Pauloski, A. W. Rademaker, and L. Colangelo. "Speech and Swallowing Rehabilitation in Head and Neck Cancer Patients." *Oncology*, Vol. 11, No. 5, 1997, pp. 651-659.

Singh, V., M. J. Brockbank, R. A. Frost, and S. Tyler. "Multi-Disciplinary Management of Dysphagia: The First 100 Cases." *The Journal of Laryngology and Otology*, Vol. 109, 1995, pp. 419-424.

Thermal/Tactile Application

Cook I. J., W. J. Dodds, R. O. Dantas, et al. "Opening Mechanism of the Human Upper Esophageal Sphincter." *American Journal of Physiology*, Vol. 257, 1989, pp. 748-759.

Helfrich-Miller, K., K. Rector, and J. Straka. "Dysphagia: Its Treatment in the Profoundly Retarded Patient with Cerebral Palsy." *Archives of Physical Medicine and Rehabilitation*, Vol. 67, 1986, pp. 520-525.

Kaatzke-McDonald, M. N., M. App, E. Post, and P. J. Davis. "The Effects of Cold, Touch, and Chemical Stimulation of the Anterior Faucial Pillar on Human Swallowing." *Dysphagia*, Vol. 11, 1996, pp. 198-206.

Kasprisin, A. T., H. Clumeck, and M. Nino-Murcia. "The Efficacy of Rehabilitative Management of Dysphagia." *Dysphagia*, Vol. 4, 1989, pp. 48-52.

Lazzara, G., C. Lazarus, and J. Logemann. "Impact of Thermal Stimulation on the Triggering of the Swallowing Reflex." *Dysphagia*, Vol. 1, 1986, pp. 73-77.

Linden, P., D. Tippet, J. Johnston, A. Siebens, and J. French. "Bolus Position at Swallow Onset in Normal Adults: Preliminary Observations." *Dysphagia*, Vol. 4, 1989, pp. 146-150.

Rosenbek, J., J. Robbins, B. Fishback, and R. Levine. "Effects of Thermal Application on Dysphagia After Stroke." *Journal of Speech and Hearing Research*, Vol. 34, December 1991, pp. 1257-1268.

Rosenbek, J. C., J. Robbins, W. O. Willford, G. Kirk, A. Schiltz, T. W. Sowell, S. E. Deutsch, F. J. Milanti, J. Ashford, G. D. Gramigna, A. Fogarty, K. Dong, M. T. Rau, T. E. Prescott, A. M. Lloyd, M. T. Sterkel, and J. E. Hansen. "Comparing Treatment Intensities of Tactile-Thermal Application." *Dysphagia*, Vol. 13, No. 1, 1998, pp. 1-10.

Rosenbek, J. C., E. B. Roecker, M. L. Wood, and J. A. Robbins. "Thermal Application Reduces the Duration of Stage Transition in Dysphagia After Stroke." *Dysphagia*, Vol. 11, 1996, pp. 225-233.

Singh, V., M. J. Brockbank, R. A. Frost, and S. Tyler. "Multi-Disciplinary Management of Dysphagia: The First 100 Cases." *The Journal of Laryngology and Otology*, Vol. 109, 1995, pp. 419-424.

Supraglottic Swallow

Kahrilas, P. J., J. Logemann, and M. Gibbens. "Food Intake by Maneuver: An Extreme Compensation for Impaired Swallowing." *Dysphagia*, Vol. 7, 1992, pp. 155-159.

Kasprisin, A. T., H. Clumeck, and M. Nino-Murcia. "The Efficacy of Rehabilitative Management of Dysphagia." *Dysphagia*, Vol. 4, 1989, pp. 48-52.

Logemann, J. and P. Kahrilas. "Relearning to Swallow After Stroke — Application of Maneuvers and Indirect Biofeedback: A Case Study." *Neurology*, Vol. 40, 1990, pp. 1136-1138.

Logemann, J. A., P. Gibbons, A. W. Rademaker, B. R. Pauloski, P. J. Kahrilas, M. Bacon, J. Bowman, and E. McCracken. "Mechanisms of Recovery of Swallow After Supraglottic Laryngectomy." *Journal of Speech and Hearing Research*, Vol. 37, 1994, pp. 965-974.

Silbergleit, A., W. Waring, M. Sullivan, and F. Maynard. "Evaluation, Treatment, and Follow-Up Results of Post-Polio Patients With Dysphagia." *Otolaryngology-Head and Neck Surgery*, Vol. 104, No. 3, 1991, pp. 333-338.

Singh, V., M. J. Brockbank, R. A. Frost, and S. Tyler. "Multi-Disciplinary Management of Dysphagia: The First 100 Cases." *The Journal of Laryngology and Otology*, Vol. 109, 1995, pp. 419-424.

Super-Supraglottic Swallow

Kahrilas, P. J., J. Logemann, and M. Gibbens. "Food Intake by Maneuver: An Extreme Compensation for Impaired Swallowing." *Dysphagia*, Vol. 7, 1992, pp. 155-159.

Logemann, J. A., B. R. Pauloski, A. W. Rademaker, and L. Colangelo. "Super-supraglottic Swallow in Irradiated Head and Neck Cancer Patients." *Head & Neck*, Vol. 19, 1997, pp. 535-540.

Martin B. J. W., J. Logemann, R. Shaker, and W. Dodds. "Normal Laryngeal Valving Patterns During Three Breathhold Maneuvers: A Pilot Investigation." *Dysphagia*, Vol. 8, 1993, pp. 11-20.

Effortful Swallow

Kahrilas, P. J., S. Lin, J. A. Logemann, G. A. Ergun, and F. Facchini. "Deglutitive Tongue Action: Volume Accommodation and Bolus Propulsion." *Gastroenterology*, Vol. 104, 1991, pp. 152-162.

Kahrilas, P. J., J. Logemann, and M. Gibbens. "Food Intake by Maneuver: An Extreme Compensation for Impaired Swallowing." *Dysphagia*, Vol. 7, 1992, pp. 155-159.

Kahrilas P. J., J. Logemann, S. Lin, and G. A. Ergun. "Pharyngeal Clearance During Swallow: A Combined Manometric and Videofluoroscopic Study." *Gastroenterology*, Vol. 103, 1992, pp. 128-136.

Pounderoux, P. and P. J. Kahrilas. "Deglutitive Tongue Force Modulation by Volition, Volume, and Viscosity in Humans." *Gastroenterology*, Vol. 108, 1995, pp. 1418-1426.

Mendelsohn maneuver

Bartolome, G. and D. Neuman. "Swallowing Therapy in Patients with Neurological Disorders Causing Crichopharyngeal Dysfunction." *Dysphagia*, Vol. 8, 1993, pp. 146-149.

Bryant, M. "Biofeedback in the Treatment of a Selected Dysphagic Patient." *Dysphagia*, Vol. 6, 1991, pp. 140-144.

Kahrilas, P. J., J. Logemann, C. Kruglar, and E. Flanagan. "Volitional Augmentation of Upper Esophageal Sphincter Opening During Swallowing." *American Journal of Physiology*, Vol. 260, 1991, pp. 450-456.

Lazarus, C., J. A. Logemann, and P. Gibbons. "Effects of Maneuvers on Swallowing Function in a Dysphagic Oral Cancer Patient." *Head & Neck*, Vol. 15, 1996, pp. 419-424.

Logemann, J. and P. Kahrilas. "Relearning to Swallow After Stroke — Application of Maneuvers and Indirect Biofeedback: A Case Study." *Neurology*, Vol. 40, 1990, pp. 1136-1138.

Logemann, J., P. Kahrilas, J. Chang, B. R. Pauloski, P. Gibbons, A. Rademaker, and S. Lin. "Closure Mechanisms of the Laryngeal Vestibule During Swallowing." *American Journal of Physiology*, Vol. 262, 1992, pp. 338-344.

Perlman, A. "The Successful Treatment of Challenging Cases." *Clinics in Communication Disorders*, Vol. 3, No. 4, 1993, pp. 37-44.

Textures of Foods

Perlman, A. "The Successful Treatment of Challenging Cases." *Clinics in Communication Disorders*, Vol. 3, No. 4, 1993, pp. 37-44.

Chapter 8

Documentation of Treatment

Sometimes it seems we spend more time documenting what we do than doing what we do. Each treatment setting has different demands for documentation and different formats that must be learned. Regardless of the setting, being able to accurately and quickly capture on paper what the patient has done in treatment is essential. This written record is one of the most important ways in which we communicate with physicians, other health care providers, case managers, and payers. The written record begins with an evaluation report and includes the treatment plan, progress notes, monthly summaries and recertifications, and discharge summaries.

Documenting Baseline Behaviors

It is essential to document baseline behaviors so you have a comparison factor when writing progress notes and monthly reports. It's important to obtain baseline information on both short-term goals and treatment objectives. Examples of baseline statements related to the short-term goals and treatment objectives follow:

Short-Term Goals	Baseline Behaviors for Short-Term Goals
Patient will improve lip closure to reduce anterior loss to keep food and liquid in the mouth while eating.	Patient currently loses all liquids out the front of the mouth from cup or straw.
Patient will increase closure of the true vocal folds to keep food from falling into the airway during the swallow.	Patient currently aspirates 20% of every thin liquid bolus during the swallow.
Patient will increase base of tongue movement to reduce vallecular residue to reduce the risk of the residue being aspirated after the swallow.	Patient currently shows residue in the valleculae with any consistency thicker than thin liquids.

Treatment Objectives	Baseline Behaviors for Treatment Objectives
Patient will pucker lips as if to blow a kiss on 9 of 10 trials.	Patient unable to achieve a pucker.
Patient will use supraglottic swallow for thin consistencies with cues on 9 of 10 trials.	Patient is able to perform the supra-glottic swallow (with saliva) on 2 of 10 trials.
Patient will use multiple swallows without cues on 10 of 10 trials.	Patient currently uses multiple swallows only 50% with maximum cues.

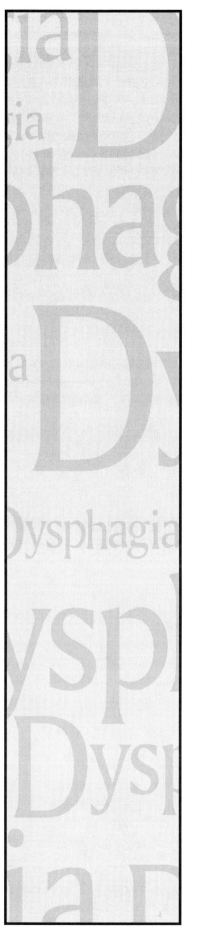

Obtaining baseline information can help you:

1. establish initial status and expectation

2. provide supportive information for documenting progress on treatment objectives

3. document change in functional status

4. document appropriate treatment recommendations

5. provide information for any quality improvement activities you are completing

Progress Notes, Monthly Reports, and Discharge Summaries

Progress notes can be completed on a daily, weekly, or monthly basis. Medicare makes no specific determination as to the frequency of documentation for these notes. However, if Medicare conducts an audit, they will expect that your documentation supports the progress you have claimed. In addition, Medicare can deny payment based on one specific session or an entire group of sessions. Therefore, if you are writing a progress note for a week and your documentation is not sufficient to show significant improvement, the entire week's worth of sessions may be denied.

Increasing demand for productivity in many settings has forced clinicians to reassess the time they spend in documentation. For example, in long-term care under the prospective payment system (PPS), the length of the session is recorded in minutes, not units. This has made clinicians even more aware of the time they spend in documentation. Notes are now written at the bedside while discussing the patient's performance during the session with the patient. This is the only way to capture note writing as productive time. Although forced into this practice by the payment system, taking time at the end of each session to make sure you and the patient agree on what progress is being made is a good idea. Writing notes with the patient present is also a good idea in home health, rather than saving the notes to be written at the end of the day.

Your progress note documentation can take a variety of formats including S.O.A.P. notes, various charts or graphs, or standardized forms. If you write your notes on a weekly basis, it's important that you have a graph to document the number of visits or units completed on each date. When writing your progress notes, use words that effectively describe progress. For example:

- describe oral sensitivity training vs. oral care

  don't say: Provided oral care to patient whose mouth was very dry.

  do say: Patient initially unable to elicit swallow and this may have been related to dry oral mucosa. Provided oral sensitivity training with lemon swab to increase saliva production.

- training and instruction vs. exercises or drill

  don't say: Completed lingual lateralization exercises with patient or practiced lip closure drills with patient.

  do say: Provided training and instruction in lingual lateralization. Patient needs model but then is able to lateralize tongue tip to right corner 70% and to left corner 65%.

- analysis and feedback vs. monitoring and observation

  don't say: Monitored patient's use of chin-down during observation at lunch.

  do say: Therapeutic feeding completed during lunch. Patient cued to use chin-down posture to reduce risk of food falling over base of tongue. Analysis revealed patient used chin-down with cues 90% (required physical assist 10%). Provided feedback to patient about accuracy of use of this technique.

- choking vs. coughing

  don't say: Patient coughed twice during presentation of thin liquids via straw.

  do say: When thin liquids presented via straw, patient choked 2/10 trials. Analysis reveals this is when patient takes large sips.

More key words are listed on page 225.

S.O.A.P. Notes

The well-recognized S.O.A.P. note format is not required, but it can be helpful because it forces you to analyze a patient's performance. S.O.A.P. stands for S = Subjective, O = Objective, A = Analysis, P = Plan.

S = Subjective: Include initial observations of the patient as you enter the room or anything the family has said about how the patient is doing. You might include statements like "Mrs. P. was choking on her coffee when I arrived," or "The patient reports nurse gave pills without crushing them and she had difficulty swallowing them."

O = Objective: Include any objective data you took in the session on your treatment objectives, like percentages and patient's response to your analysis and feedback.

A = Analysis: Summarize and put in functional terms exactly what happened during each session. Instead of concentrating directly on the treatment objectives, talk about how progress on the treatment objectives moved the patient closer toward achieving the functional goals. Use comparative statements like "better than the session yesterday" or "increased performance on percent of ability to perform exercises."

P = Plan: Explain what you intend to do in the next session. It can be as simple as "Continue per treatment plan" or can have specific suggestions. You may have noted in the session that the patient does better with a new compensatory technique than you had initially determined. In this case, your plan might be to include this compensatory technique in future sessions.

Keep in mind the requirements Medicare has for documentation and how they can fit into your progress notes. Some important points to include in your notes are:

1. number of treatments completed or the dates of treatment

2. the statement of positive expectation

3. techniques to achieve short-term goals

4. statement regarding short-term goal achievement or progress

5. any expected changes within the course of the next term of treatment

Monthly Reports

In most settings, you'll need to write monthly summaries to document progress and ask for more treatment. Monthly reports should indicate changes in functional behavior from the time of the initial evaluation or from the most recent monthly summary.

Summary reports for Medicare patients may also be called *recertifications*. A recertification means that the physician is asked to state more services are needed. Recertifications should be completed on a 30-day basis in skilled nursing facilities and in outpatient facilities, and on a 60-day basis in home health. Each recertification should be signed by the physician.

The functional behaviors to document are changes which have improved the patient's ability to function within her environment. In the area of dysphagia, a functional swallow is a swallow which sustains nutrition orally. How you achieve this goal is not the issue. The desired outcome for Medicare reimbursement is that the functional goal is achieved. Examples of functional behavior statements are:

- Patient is able to eat soft foods without any choking behavior.

- Patient is able to maintain food in her mouth without losing any out the front.

- Patient is able to eat a meal in significantly less time than at evaluation.

Significant Progress

Medicare states that significant progress should be made for intervention services to continue. By definition, significant progress means a generally measurable and substantial increase in the patient's present level of communication, independence, and competence compared to her levels when treatment was begun. Progress must be substantial and efficient in relation to how long the progress took.

Insufficient Statement: "The patient's oral stage swallowing skills have significantly improved."

Better Statement: "Because of improved oral muscle control, the patient is able to swallow liquids thickened to nectar consistency."

Even Better Statement: "Improved tongue control has resulted in improved oral stage swallow. Previously, liquids needed to be thickened to a pudding consistency to be swallowed safely, but now less thickener is needed and the patient can swallow liquids of nectar consistency. Treatments to improve tongue strength and coordination will continue to allow the patient to swallow thin liquids (water, juice, coffee) without a thickener."

When treatment techniques are of an indirect nature (e.g., not working with food), the significance of progress may be questioned. For example, if you have a patient who is using thermal application to decrease swallow reflex response time, does a change from a 20-second delay to a consistent change of a 10-second delay signify significant progress? Would a Medicare reviewer who sees that the patient is still unable to consume PO intake understand that this is significant progress? You must document why the 10-second change in delay is a significant factor and why you think further progress can be made. Also discuss how continued progress will help the patient reach her functional goal.

"The patient was initially able to swallow after a 20-second delay. Following thermal application, the patient is now consistently swallowing after a 10-second delay. With continued decrease in this delay, the patient should be able to begin to eat food safely."

Positive Expectation

Your monthly report must show a positive expectation for continued treatments that require your skilled services. What abilities has the patient shown to make you think your intervention is going to be of continued help?

For example, you might report baseline information that the patient was initially able to perform the supraglottic swallow on 20% of trials, but that the patient has shown excellent response to learning the supraglottic swallow and can now perform it 100% of the time. Further, you might state that it's expected with continued intervention that she will be able to use this technique to safely swallow thin liquid boluses of any size without standby assistance.

This information uses a comparative statement to show the progress and expectation for continued improvement. You're also using the client's previously learned skills to show what the patient may be able to accomplish. Be careful that you don't make it sound so positive that your services are no longer needed. You might say "The patient is able to maintain adequate airway closure during swallow within structured therapeutic settings." This indicates that the expectation is to move the patient to the point where she can do so independently.

Skilled Services Must Be Documented

Your monthly report should include descriptions to show that the patient was provided with skilled intervention and not something that anyone can do. The following examples could be used to show skilled service:

- training and instruction provided to increase strength and coordination of facial and oral muscles

- training and instruction of appropriate compensatory positioning strategies provided to the patient and nursing staff to insure safe and efficient swallowing behavior

- training and instruction provided to increase laryngeal elevation during the swallow

Discharge or Re-evaluation

We are often faced with the decision of when to end therapy, when to re-evaluate, and whether to discharge a patient from a functional maintenance program. Guidelines for termination of direct skilled intervention services can include the following:

1. The physician orders the service discontinued.

2. The patient reaches a plateau in progress.

3. The patient achieves her treatment goals.

4. The patient no longer needs skilled therapy services.

5. The patient is discharged from the facility/clinic.

If any of these conditions exist, then skilled intervention is no longer appropriate. However, alternative intervention might be indicated under certain conditions, such as a continuation under functional maintenance or as part of continued patient/family training.

Unfortunately, services are also sometimes discontinued because the patient's payer will no longer pay for the service and the patient is unable to pay. For example, in long-term care, the patient may no longer qualify for one of the rehabilitation categories under Part A - PPS. The patient may also have reached the cap on the limit of dollars that can be spent for that service. You must then make sure other caregivers know the techniques needed to keep the patient eating safely.

Discharge summaries should use the baseline information which you obtained in your initial functional goals and then give statements to show the progress the patient has made toward achieving those functional goals.

Other Documentation Demands

In addition to documentation of the speech-language pathology services provided, you may be called upon to complete other scales and ratings for a facility or agency. In long-term care, SLPs are often involved in scoring the Minimum Data Set (MDS). It is important to participate as much as possible to assure a more accurate rating of the patient. In home health, you may also be asked to complete the Outcomes and Assessment Information Set (OASIS). Both the MDS and the OASIS have scales which attempt to rate the patient's ability to eat/swallow. You should be aware of the drawbacks to instruments such as these. They are often written so broadly (to attempt to capture self-feeding and eating) that they offer no meaningful information, and certainly will not accurately be able to reflect any progress.

Key Words and Phrases for Progress Notes _____

These words and phrases can help provide proper documentation and should be used in progress notes.

safety   likelihood of change
danger of reoccurrence   medical complications
high risk factor   reasonable probability
choking   prevent deterioration
potential for complication   observation and assessment
promote recovery and insure medical safety   medical needs
safe and effective delivery   special medical complications
prior level of function   reasonable and necessary
skilled level of care   requires the skills of a therapist
on a daily basis

Words and Phrases to Avoid _____

These words and phrases are occasionally used in progress notes and re-certifications. They should always be avoided in proper Medicare documentation. If any of the following words or phrases accurately describes what is happening with your patient, the patient is most likely not a good candidate for treatment.

custodial care   maintenance therapy
intermittent care/service   poor rehab potential
inability to follow directions   chronic/long-term condition
refuses to participate   drill
monitoring

Sample Speech-Language Pathology Treatment Plan ___

Patient's Name _Fred_____ Birthdate _____ Age _68_

Date therapy begun _____ Date therapy ended _____

Frequency and duration of treatment sessions _daily therapy for 8 weeks_____ Total units _____

Therapy conducted at _Happy Hills SNF_

Diagnosis _Moderately impaired oral preparatory phase_

_____ _Mild pharyngeal dysphagia_

_____

Prognosis and estimated length of treatment _Excellent for return to PO; 6-8 weeks_____

Follow-up _____

Long-Term Goal:

Patient will safely consume a regular diet to maintain adequate nutrition and hydration.

Short-Term Goal 2 — Anterior Loss/lip closure (AL/lc):

Patient will improve lip closure to reduce anterior loss to keep foods and liquid in the mouth while eating.

Treatment Objectives

AL/lc-1   Patient will eliminate loss of liquid from front of mouth when clinician provides support to lower lip on 10 of 10 trials. (c)

AL/lc-3   Patient will achieve lip closure against resistance provided by clinician placing fingers on upper and lower lip on 10 of 10 trials. (f)

AL/lc-4   Patient will pucker lips as if to blow a kiss on 10 of 10 trials. (f)

Short-Term Goal 5 — Bolus Formation/tongue movement (BF/tm):

Patient will increase tongue movement to improve the ability to put food and liquid into a cohesive bolus to reduce the risk of food falling into the airway.

Treatment Objectives

BF/tm-1   Patient will place bolus of food on stronger side without cues on 10 of 10 trials. (c)

BF/tm-4   Patient will use multiple swallows for masticated consistencies with cues on 10 of 10 trials. (c)

BF/tm-5   Patient will alternate mildly thickened liquid wash every several bites with cues on 10 of 10 trials. (c)

Short-Term Goal 6 — Bolus Propulsion/tone in cheeks (BP/tc)

The tone in patient's cheek(s) will increase to improve the ability to put food and liquid into a cohesive bolus to reduce the risk of food residue falling into the airway.

Treatment Objectives

BF/tc-1   Patient will use external pressure with fingers on cheek to decrease pocketing without cues on 10 of 10 trials. (c)

BF/tc-2   Patient will clean buccal cavity with tongue after meal without cues on 10 of 10 trials. (c)

Short-Term Goal 7 – Bolus Propulsion/tongue movement (BP/tm)

Patient will increase tongue movement to improve the ability to move a bolus to the back of the mouth in a coordinated fashion to reduce the risk of it falling into the airway.

Treatment Objectives

BP/tm-6   Patient will move lemon swab placed between tongue and hard palate between front to back on 8 of 10 trials. (f)

BP/tm-7   Patient will sweep tongue from alveolar ridge to junction of hard and soft palate on 9 of 10 trials. (f)

Short-Term Goal 11 – Aspiration Before/tongue control (AB/tc)

Patient will improve back of tongue control to keep food from falling over the back of tongue and into the airway.

Treatment Objectives

AB/tc-1   Patient will use chin-down posture for thin liquids without cues on 10 of 10 trials. (c)

AB/tc-2   Patient will control bolus size to teaspoon without cues on 10 of 10 trials. (c)

AB/tc-3   Patient will use cut-out cup for all liquid intake without cues on 10 of 10 trials. (c)

AB/tc-4   Patient will exert pressure with back of tongue up against tongue depressor on 9 of 10 trials. (f)

AB/tc-5   Patient will produce forceful /k/ at the end of words on 10 of 10 trials. (f)

Short-Term Goal 20 – Aspiration After/valleculae/tongue base (AA/v/tb)

Patient will increase base of tongue movement to reduce vallecular residue (unilateral or bilateral) to reduce the risk of the residue being aspirated after the swallow.

Treatment Objective

AA/v/tb-7   Patient will use effort swallow without cues on 10 of 10 trials. (c,f)

Examples of Progress Notes

Daily

S: Patient states he tried his effort swallow last night when his daughter brought him some pudding from home and thinks he did well.

O: Patient seen for training and instruction in facilitation techniques designed to improve lip closure, strength of back of tongue, and coordinated movement of tongue from front to back of mouth. (AL/lc-3) Patient able to achieve lip closure when SLP provided resistance on 5 of 10 trials. Instructed patient to look in mirror and concentrate on using both sides of his lips. (AB/tc-4) Patient able to exert pressure with back of tongue up against tongue blade on 7 of 10 trials. (AB/tc-5) Patient able to produce forceful /k/ at end of words on 7 of 10 trials.

A: Patient responding well to treatment. Very cooperative. Back of tongue strength is improving as evidenced by ability to produce more words with forceful /k/ (up to 70% from 50%). Lip closure still a problem due to reduced strength. Patient will need to continue with compensatory techniques at meals.

P: Continue per plan with emphasis on lip closure activities.

Weekly

Patient: Fred

Dates and units (15-minute sessions):
Monday	9/8	3 units
Tuesday	9/9	3 units
Wednesday	9/10	2 units
Thursday	9/11	3 units
Friday	9/12	3 units

S: Patient seen at meals for therapeutic feeding intervention this week. On Wednesday, his daughter was present, and after training and instruction, finished the meal with the patient.

O: Patient presented with pureed textures and one soft vegetable. (AL/lc-1) Provided support to lower lip when patient took sips of liquid from cup in 5cc amounts. This is essential since patient is using chin-down posture (AB/tc-1) for all thin liquid swallows and without the lip support, he would lose everything anteriorly. With lip support, the patient has loss on only 2 of 10 trials. (BF/tc-1) At beginning of the week, training and instruction were provided in use of external pressure with fingers to cheek to reduce the amount of food that gets pocketed there. By Friday, patient was remembering to put his own fingers on his cheek on 6 of 10 trials without cues. (BF/tm-4) Patient responded well to analysis and feedback about his use of multiple swallows. He is using a second swallow consistently without cues for the masticated food. (AB/tc-3) Patient uses chin-down posture with the cut-out cup when it is provided on his tray. Several times this week his liquids were sent in a regular cup.

A: Patient doing well with compensatory techniques to prevent aspiration. No choking observed this week at meals except when liquids were sent in regular cup which made it difficult for patient to maintain a chin-down posture.

P: Continue with therapeutic intervention at meals. Shift more responsibility to patient for use of the compensatory techniques without cues.

Weekly with Percentages Only

Dates seen and (units)

9/8	(3 units, 1 unit)
9/9	(3 units, 2 units)
9/10	(2 units, 1 unit)
9/11	(3 units, 1 unit)
9/12	(3 units, 1 unit)

S: Patient states he thinks it is taking less time for him to eat his meals. States liquids have been in cut-out cups at every meal.

O: Patient seen for therapeutic feeding at breakfast each day. Provided training and instruction in use of compensatory techniques needed to prevent aspiration. Also saw patient for treatment with facilitation techniques at times other than meals. Gave patient feedback and analysis concerning his performance on treatment objectives. His performance scores are:

AL/lc-1	90%	BF/tm-5	90%	AB/tc-2	100%
AL/lc-3	50%	BF/tc-1	70%; 100% with cues	AB/tc-3	100%
AL/lc-4	60%	BF/tc-2	90%	AB/tc-4	85%
BF/tm-1	60%	BP/tm-6	70%	AB/tc-5	70%
BF/tm-4	80%	AB/tc-1	90%	AA/v/tb-1	75%

A: Patient doing well with use of compensatory techniques during therapeutic feeding sessions. Responding well to analysis provided by increasing his use of techniques without cues. Lip strength is still a problem (AL/lc-3&4) but looking in mirror seems to help.

P: Continue per plan with emphasis on lip closure activities. Continue with training of patient and staff.

Monthly

During the past month of therapy, training and instruction were provided to increase the strength and coordination of back of tongue movements, tone in cheeks, lip closure, base of tongue to posterior pharyngeal wall pressure, and A-P tongue movement. During those sessions, the patient's responses to treatment were analyzed and the patient demonstrated appropriate response to therapy. Feedback was given to the patient regarding perceived strength of back of tongue, adequacy of lip closure, and ability to move tongue from front to back to manipulate a bolus.

In addition, the patient was provided with training and instruction on effort swallow to clear vallecular residue. The patient has been provided instruction on using small sips of honey-thick liquid to help clear the oral cavity of residue to reduce the risk of food falling into his airway after the swallow.

The patient has made significant progress on the treatment objectives listed. He demonstrates the ability to safely and efficiently swallow. The patient has also demonstrated ability to produce words ending with /k/ very forcefully indicating that the back of tongue strength has increased significantly, helping to reduce residue in valleculae, and to reduce the risk of aspiration.

The patient has been able to swallow thin liquids in small sips using the chin-down posture without the presumed risk of aspiration. The patient also has had no temperature spikes and lung sounds are clear.

At the beginning of treatment, the patient was choking on thin liquids and was unable to adequately form a bolus with any masticated foods. He is now eating a diet comprised mostly of soft foods, although he still needs pureed meats. The oral-motor training techniques have allowed him to form an adequate bolus and clear the residue from his cheeks.

Patient will need continued treatment to be able to take larger amounts of thin liquid without compensatory techniques. He also needs continued training to improve his ability to manipulate soft foods in the oral cavity and to further reduce anterior loss with thin liquids.

Sample Discharge Summaries

Active Treatment

Patient Name _Fred_   Patient # _____

Date _11-2_

Over the last eight weeks, Fred has been seen for individual therapy. Initially therapy took place on a daily basis, but it has been reduced to three times a week. Fred is being discharged from active treatment at this time and will continue to be followed in the Rehab Dining Room.

At the beginning of treatment, Fred was choking on thin liquids and was unable to adequately form a bolus with any masticated foods. Now he is eating a mechanical soft diet but still needs to have meats pureed. He is able to take thin liquids in uncontrolled amounts without any compensatory techniques. He is also able to successfully clear his oral cavity of residue using his tongue and a rinse after each meal.

Fred has some mild anterior loss from the lips which he compensates for by using a finger to support his lower lip. He no longer appears to be at risk for aspiration and is able to feed himself with only standby verbal cues to remember his techniques.

Functional Maintenance

Patient Name _Ethel_   Patient # _____

Date _12-31_

Staff has been trained in techniques necessary to help this patient eat an adequate amount of food to maintain nutrition and hydration without choking. Ethel is consistently eating a pureed diet and thin liquids in small boluses from a spoon and a cup when staff is consistently able to apply added pressure to the tongue with the spoon or tap the lips with an empty spoon. The patient now initiates posterior movement of the bolus within five seconds on a consistent basis.

Ethel's last calorie count was adequate as long as she is given two supplemental shakes a day. She should do fine with this regimen, but if deterioration in skills is observed, she will need a reassessment.

Sample Progress Report/Re-certification

Patient __Fred__
Physician _____
Facility __Happy Hills SNF__
Date of evaluation __09-02__   Date of report __10-02__
Date of last recertification __n/a__
Medical Diagnosis __S/P CVA__
Communicative Disorder Diagnosis __Oral and pharyngeal dysphagia__

Treatment Objectives

Progress

AL/lc-1   Patient will eliminate loss of liquid from front of mouth when clinician provides support to lower lip on 10 of 10 trials. (c)

from 60% to 90%

AL/lc-3   Patient will achieve lip closure against resistance provided by clinician placing fingers on upper and lower lip on 10 of 10 trials. (f)

from 10% to 50%

AL/lc-4   Patient will pucker lips as if to blow a kiss on 10 of 10 trials. (f)

from 50% to 100%

BF/tm-1   Patient will place bolus of food on stronger side without cues on 10 of 10 trials. (c)

_100%_

BF/tm-4   Patient will use multiple swallows for masticated consistencies with cues on 10 of 10 trials. (c)

80% with cues

BF/tm-5   Patient will alternate mildly thickened liquid wash every several bites with cues on 10 of 10 trials. (c)

_90%_

BF/tc-1   Patient will use external pressure with fingers on cheek to decrease pocketing without cues on 10 of 10 trials. (c)

_100%_

BF/tc-2   Patient will clean buccal cavity with tongue during and after meal with cues on 9 of 10 trials. (c)

_100%_

Treatment Objectives, *continued*

Progress

BP/tm-6   Patient will move lemon swab placed between tongue and hard palate between front to back on 8 of 10 trials. (f)

from 60% to 90%

BP/tm-7   Patient will sweep tongue from alveolar ridge to junction of hard and soft palate on 9 of 10 trials. (f)

from 70% to 80%

AB/tc-1   Patient will use chin-down posture for thin liquids without cues on 9 of 10 trials. (c)

100% except when liquids come in regular cup

AB-tc-2   Patient will control bolus size to teaspoon without cues on 10 of 10 trials. (c)

still requires cues about 1/2 time

AB/tc-3   Patient will use cut-out cup for all liquid intake without cues on 10 of 10 trials. (c)

100% when kitchen sends cup

AB/tc-4   Patient will exert pressure with back of tongue up against tongue depressor on 9 of 10 trials. (f)

from 70% to 80%

AB/tc-5   Patient will produce words ending in /k/ with forceful production of /k/ on 10 of 10 trials. (f)

from 60% to 80%

AB/v/tb-7   Patient will use effort swallow without cues on 10 of 10 trials. (c, f)

70% without cues; 100% with cues

Narrative Interpretation (relationship to long-term and short-term goals)   *During the past month of therapy, training and instruction were provided to increase the strength and coordination of back of tongue movements, lip closure, and A-P tongue movement. The patient has made significant progress on the treatment objectives listed. He now demonstrates the ability to safely and efficiently swallow. He is eating a diet comprised mostly of soft foods although he still needs pureed meats. The oral-motor training techniques have allowed him to form an adequate bolus and clear the residue from his cheeks. In addition, the patient has had no temperature spikes and lung sounds are clear.*

Sample Progress Report/Re-certification, *continued*

Positive Expectation to Continue   _Patient continues to work hard and be cooperative during therapy. He will need continued treatment to be able to take larger amounts of thick liquid and hopefully not have to use compensatory techniques. He also needs continued training to improve his ability to manipulate masticated foods in the oral cavity._

Need for Continued Skilled Service   _Without continued skilled intervention, patient will always have to use a compensatory technique and take only small amounts of thin liquids._

Changes in Treatment Plan (Goals/Frequency)   _Reduce frequency to 3 times a week._

_____   _____   _____
        Speech-Language Pathologist   License #   Date

I certify the above patient requires therapy services, is under a plan of care established or reviewed every 30 days by me, and requires the above treatment specified on a continuing basis with the following changes:

Physician Notice: (Circle one)   I do / do not find it necessary to see this patient within the next 30 days.

_____   _____
            Physician   Date

Sample Discharge Report _____

Patient _Fred_____	Physician _R. U. Eting_____
Date of Discharge _11-02_____ Birthdate_____	Date of Initial Evaluation _09-02____
Facility _Happy Hills SNF_____	Duration of Therapy _8 weeks_____

Progress in Therapy/Goals Met: _Patient has met all goals established. He can take thin liquids in_
uncontrolled amounts without compensatory techniques. Initially he had to use several techniques to prevent
_choking. He is now on a mechanical soft diet with pureed meats._____

Goals Not Met: _____
_____
_____
_____

Reason for Discharge/Patient's Current Status: _Patient no longer appears to be at risk for_
_aspiration and is able to feed himself with only standby verbal cues to remember his techniques._____

Follow-Up Recommendations: _If patient's condition should change, he will require a re-evaluation by_
_speech-language pathology, but it is not suspected at this point._____

_____   _____   _____
Speech-Language Pathologist   License #   Date

_____   _____
Physician   Date

Chapter 9

Special Considerations in Intensive Care

What's so different about evaluating and treating patients with dysphagia while they are in intensive care? The obvious answer is that they are critically ill compared to patients on a medical floor, at home, or in a skilled nursing facility. The fact that they are critically ill has implications for how we evaluate and treat. Patients who are critically ill may experience much more significant responses to changes in their environment. For instance, just moving a patient in bed to achieve a good position for feeding may result in a significant change in his respiratory rate and/or blood pressure. These patients' conditions may fluctuate widely from day to day or within a day. Therefore, recommendations made one day may be inappropriate the next if the patient's status has changed. This requires frequent monitoring to assure that recommendations thought to maintain safety of swallowing aren't now putting the patient at risk of aspiration. If the patient is a post-surgical patient, he may experience rapid improvement in his condition. This also requires careful monitoring so that changes in your recommendations can be made as soon as it is appropriate.

Working in the intensive care requires that you have knowledge of a variety of instruments, devices, and monitors. You must be able to read the monitors and understand when a change is significant enough to require the attention of the nurse or respiratory therapist. It is also important to gather other history pertaining to the patient's critically ill status and make adjustments in the bedside/clinical screening of swallowing, as other techniques (e.g., suctioning) are possible with patients who have tracheostomies.

Why Are SLPs Called Into the Intensive Care?

As little as a decade ago, it was rather unusual for an SLP to be consulted while a patient was still in intensive care. It was thought that the patient was too sick for any rehabilitation while in critical condition. In many hospitals nowadays, it is not unusual for an SLP (and other rehab professionals) to be consulted within 24 hours of admit, particularly for patients who have suffered a cerebrovascular accident (CVA).

With the advent of managed care, the minute the patient arrives at the hospital, the emphasis is on discharge. In order for patients to be discharged sooner to another level of care, rehabilitation services must begin as soon as possible. In addition, there is recognition that early initiation of dysphagia services can prevent costly complications such as aspiration pneumonia.

Many hospitals use critical pathways. These pathways are an attempt to standardize the timing of care provided to patients with a particular diagnosis. Standardizing care reduces variations in care, and variations in care are costly.

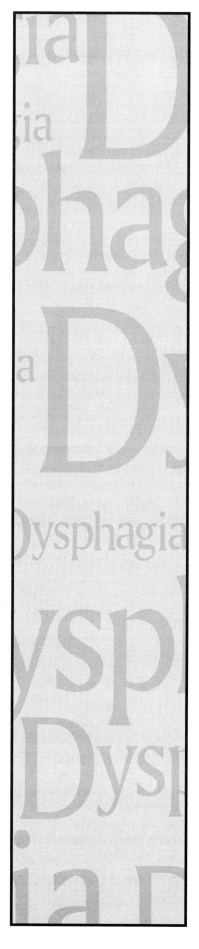

For example, if a critical pathway for patients who need a total hip replacement calls for the same type of hip joint to be used with each patient, then the hospital can negotiate a better rate on the joint because they will be buying more of that product. Along those same lines, if the pathway calls for rehabilitation of CVA patients to begin on day one, then all patients receive timely evaluations and begin rehabilitation programs geared to their deficits. This can reduce costs because complications are avoided.

Instruments and Devices

One of the biggest differences seen when providing services in intensive care is the amount of instrumentation in use. Instruments and devices may simply monitor a body function or may actually perform that function for the patient.

Ventilators

A ventilator is a medical device that ventilates a patient. Ventilation is the process of moving gases into and out of the lungs. Respiration is the actual exchange of gases between the air breathed in and the cells of the body. Therefore, the machine provides the ventilation, or movement of air. Respiration takes place in the lungs after the air has been placed there by the ventilator.

Patients are placed on mechanical ventilation for several reasons.

- They are experiencing periods of apnea.

- They are in acute ventilatory failure.

- They are in impending ventilatory failure.

- They need hyperventilation for intracranial pressure control.

Respiratory or ventilatory failure means that the exchange of oxygen and/or carbon dioxide between the alveoli and the pulmonary capillaries is inadequate. The goal of mechanical ventilation is to push enough volume of air into the lungs to allow the exchange of gases in the alveoli to maintain metabolic requirements of the patient. The ventilator provides temporary (or sometimes permanent) support to any patient who cannot breathe well enough on his own to maintain adequate oxygenation. Mechanical ventilation allows the patient to rest and not have to expend so much energy on breathing.

Ventilators seen in critical care units are called *positive pressure ventilators*. These work by pushing air into the airway to inflate the alveoli in the lungs. The desired pressure you want to achieve is set on the ventilator. The volume needed to achieve that pressure varies. In order to use a positive pressure ventilator, the patient has to have an endotracheal tube or a tracheostomy tube. (See page 241 for pictures.)

Talk to the respiratory therapist at your facility to learn more about ventilators. In addition, a text by Mason (1994) provides detailed information about ventilators and tracheostomies. You should be familiar with the modes of ventilation as well as with some of the alarms on the ventilator.

Modes of Ventilation

When respiratory therapists describe the mode of ventilation, they mean the type of breath support the ventilator is providing to the patient. This includes how often the breath is given, what triggers the machine to give the breath, the size of the breath given, and the pressure to be maintained. Some of the more common settings are:

1. *Assist Control* — In this mode, the patient starts to take a breath on his own, and whenever he does, the machine gives a little help to achieve an adequate breath. The ventilator is set so that if the patient doesn't try to take a breath on his own often enough, the machine will take over and give a breath. Patients are usually fairly stable before they are placed on this mode.

2. *Mandatory Control* — This mode does not rely on the patient trying to take a breath on his own. It is usually used with acute cases of respiratory failure or when a patient is sedated or paralyzed.

3. *Intermittent Mandatory (IMV)* — This setting allows the patient to breathe spontaneously, but also gives a set number of mandatory breaths. This setting can be confusing for a patient who is trying to breathe on his own, because the machine's breaths are not timed between his attempts to breathe. IMV is rarely used.

4. *Synchronized Intermittent Mandatory (SIMV)* — This is a much better option than IMV. The machine allows the patient to breathe spontaneously as deeply and as quickly as he wants to. The ventilator is set to wait for the next inspiratory effort, and then gives a mandatory breath along with the patient's inspiratory effort. This setting is used to help wean the patient from the ventilator. The settings are gradually changed to give fewer and fewer mandatory breaths.

Two modes are considered augmentative. That is, they are used along with other pressure support settings.

5. *Positive End Expiratory Pressure (PEEP)* — In individuals with healthy lungs and normal pulmonary function, the alveoli in the lungs maintain a certain amount of pressure so the lungs don't collapse. This makes it easier to inflate the lungs on the next breath. This setting on the ventilator gives added pressure to maintain PEEP in the patient's alveoli. The PEEP setting is used with Assist Control or SIMV.

6. *Continuous Positive Airway Pressure (CPAP)* — This is the same as PEEP in that positive pressure is always maintained to keep alveoli inflated. This setting can be used alone as part of the weaning process.

The CPAP setting is used when patients are initiating their own breaths.

Alarms

Ventilators have several alarms. There are two basic alarms for you to understand. These two alarms will help you monitor how the patient is reacting to your treatment (e.g., Is the high pressure alarm going off because the patient is coughing?).

High pressure alarm — The ventilator indicates that it is taking too much pressure to push a breath in. This can be caused by a number of things such as secretions in the tracheostomy tube or a change in lung function. Since one of the causes is secretions in the tube, it may indicate that the patient needs to be suctioned. This alarm also goes off when the patient coughs or when too much water has accumulated in the tubing to the ventilator.

Low pressure alarm — This is also called the disconnect alarm. The ventilator is expecting a certain amount of pressure in the tubing back from the patient. If the ventilator does not feel this pressure, the low pressure alarm goes off.

This usually means the patient is disconnected from the ventilator. Other things that could cause this alarm to go off are a leaking or deflated cuff, use of an endotracheal cuff, or when a one-way speaking valve is used (the cuff is deflated). The respiratory therapist will work with you to turn off the low pressure alarm during speaking valve use.

Settings

It is helpful to understand some of the settings on the ventilator and what normal ranges typically are. Ask the respiratory therapist to show you where these values are displayed on the ventilator so that you can use them to monitor patient response. Mason (1994) provides a description of these ventilator settings and the normal values.

- *Tidal Volume* — the amount of air taken in a breath; the ventilator is set to deliver 10-15 ml per kg of ideal body weight which is usually between 500 and 1000 ml

- *Respiratory Rate* — the number of breaths taken in a minute; normal for adults is 10-15 breaths/minute

- *Inspiratory Flow Rate* — how much gas is given per minute; typically set at 40-60 liters per minute

- *Inspiratory Time:Expiratory Time (I:E ratio)* — the relationship between how long it takes to breathe in and breathe out; we usually breathe out 2 to 5 times longer than we breathe in, therefore, typical ratios are 1:2 to 1:5

- *Sensitivity* — how much pressure the patient has to generate in order to trigger the ventilator to give a breath; if the setting is too sensitive, it may trigger the machine to give a breath when it is not needed or if it is not sensitive enough, the patient may have to work too hard at breathing

- *Fractional Inspired Oxygen Concentration (FIO$_2$)* — the portion or percentage of 100% oxygen given with each inspiration; usually noted as a percent (e.g., 50% or FIO$_2$ – 0.5)

Non-invasive Ventilatory Devices

You may encounter a patient using a device called BiPap. This method does not require an endotracheal tube or a tracheostomy tube, but instead delivers continuous or intermittent positive pressure through a nasal mask or a mouth-piece. Some patients with sleep apnea use a BiPap.

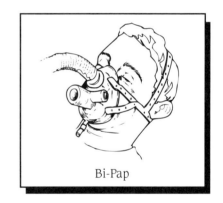

Bi-Pap

Oxygen Devices

Patients who do not need assistance in maintaining ventilation of air into the lungs may still need supplemental oxygen. This oxygen may be delivered in a variety of ways.

Rebreather — A rebreather is a mask that allows a higher percentage of oxygen to be delivered to the patient than either a nasal cannula (which allows a maximum of 44% oxygen) or an oxygen mask (which allows up to 65% oxygen). As a patient breathes in, not all of the air gets to the lungs to be exchanged. Some of it is trapped in the upper airway, called anatomical deadspace. This exhaled gas is unaltered and is still the original composition that was inhaled. The rebreather captures this exhaled gas (which was trapped in the upper airway) so that it can be inhaled on the next inspiration.

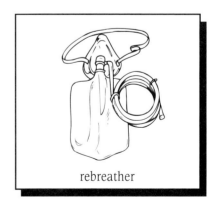

rebreather

T-piece — The T-piece attaches to the tracheostomy tube and to a source of oxygen to allow the oxygen to blow by the tracheostomy. The other end of the T is left open for the oxygen to blow out.

Trach collar — Patients may also receive the oxygen from a tracheostomy collar at the tracheotomy site.

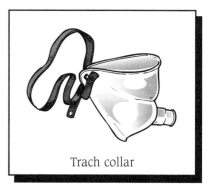

T-piece

Monitors

Patients in intensive care are usually attached to several kinds of monitors or to a monitor which measures several functions at once. There are many different types of monitors, so ask the critical care nurse to explain the specific monitors used at your facility. Two basic bodily functions typically monitored are:

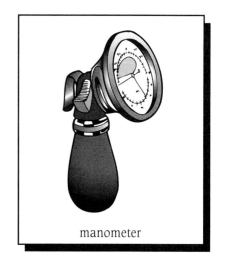

Trach collar

Heart rate: Cardiac monitors display heart rate as well as other cardiac rhythms. Normal heart rate for adults is 60-80 beats per minute. Patients may experience increased heart rate whenever they are engaged in physical activity (such as being positioned in the bed). This is to be expected. However, if they exhibit an extremely fast heart rate (100-120 bpm), it is called tachycardia. An extremely slow heart rate (40-50 bpm) is called bradycardia. The monitors are usually set to alarm if the patient's heart rate gets too fast or too slow. If the alarm isn't set, the nurse can tell you the appropriate range for the patient's heart rate.

Oxygen saturation: The amount of oxygen that saturates the blood is measured by a device called a pulse oximeter. A small, infrared sensor device is placed on a body part rich in capillaries such as a finger, toe, or ear lobe. The sensor determines arterial oxygen saturation (SaO_2). The device also measures pulse rate (heart rate). Typically the patient should be at 90% or above on saturation. The pulse oximeter has an alarm which is set to signal when the patient's saturation level drops below the desired amount.

Manometer

A tracheal cuff manometer is used to measure the amount of pressure in the trach cuff. If a cuff is over-inflated, too much pressure is exerted on the tracheal walls. This can cause erosion of the tissue, resulting in a fistula. The cuff manometer indicates the safe range for pressure. Anytime you are reinflating a cuff, a manometer should be used. You might think that you could just look at the syringe, note how much air you took out of the cuff, and return the same amount. This does not work because the amount of pressure changes when the patient moves. Also, each time the patient inhales, the trachea expands. Therefore, there are several factors that may have changed since you removed the air which necessitates remeasuring the amount of pressure needed with the manometer.

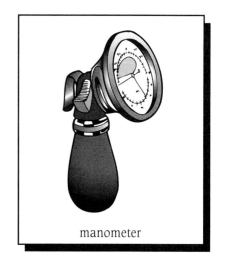

manometer

Intubation and Tracheostomy Tubes

In order for a patient to be placed on a ventilator, an artificial airway has to be established. When a patient is going to have surgery or when he initially needs to be ventilated, the first choice is typically an endotracheal or nasotracheal tube. Patients typically do not receive a tracheotomy until it is apparent that the need for ventilation is going to be long term.

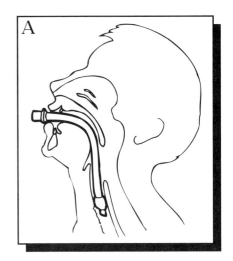

Endotracheal tube — This tube is placed with a laryngoscope so that the vocal cords can be visualized. It is also called an orotracheal tube. This method is used most frequently. (See picture A.)

Nasotracheal tube — This tube is placed in the nasopharynx and then through the pharynx and larynx into the airway. This route may be selected if there are problems in the oral cavity. Going through the nasopharynx eliminates the possibility of the patient biting on the tubing. (See picture B.)

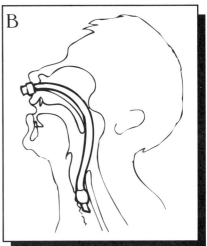

Each of these types of tubes are held in place by a cuff which is inflated with air. Patients are not able to eat with either type of tube.

Tracheostomy tube — When a patient undergoes a tracheotomy, a tracheostomy tube is placed. The tracheotomy is performed under general anesthetic. A surgical incision is made, usually between the second and third tracheal rings if the incision is made horizontally or through the second, third, and fourth tracheal rings if a vertical incision is made. The vertical incision is thought to allow for more movement of the larynx. A tracheostomy tube is then placed through the incision. This tube has a cuff on it if the patient is to be placed on a ventilator. (See picture C.)

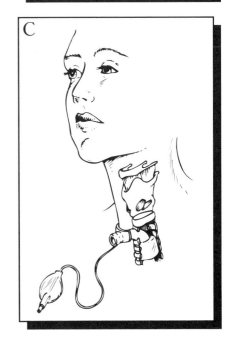

The two main types of tracheostomy tubes are plastic and metal. Plastic tubes are less expensive than metal tubes and are disposable. Plastic tubes are used if the patient is to be mechanically ventilated because the plastic tubes have a universal 15 mm hub. Metal tubes, usually made of stainless steel or sterling silver, usually do not have a cuff and do not have the universal hub. However, metal tubes are easier to clean and they lie flat against the neck.

Tubes come in different sizes, depending on the estimated size of the trachea of the individual receiving the tracheotomy. Regardless of the brand of trach tube, there are several basic parts to a tube. The flange, outer cannula, and universal hub are found on all tubes. The other parts may or may not be included.

- *outer flange* — This part rests on the patient's neck and keeps the tube from falling through the tracheostomy. The flange is tied around the patient's neck. (See picture A.)

- *outer cannula* — This is the main part of the tracheostomy tube. It goes into the airway. (See picture A.)

- *inner cannula* — This is a smaller tube which can be inserted into the outer cannula. An inner cannula makes it easier to clean the tracheostomy tube, as only this part has to be removed. (See picture B.)

- *obturator* — This fits inside the outer cannula and has a smooth, rounded tip on it that sticks out through the outer cannula. The obturator makes insertion easier, but must be taken out as soon as insertion is complete as it blocks the airway. (See picture C.)

- *universal hub* — Regardless of the size of the tracheostomy tube, a 15mm hub extends from the tube. This universally-sized hub is what attaches to the ventilator tubing or to a speaking valve. (See picture B.)

- *cuff* — The cuff surrounds the lower part of the outer cannula and is connected to a small tube which travels to the hub and beyond. It ends in a cuff pilot or pilot balloon. Air is inserted into the *cuff pilot*, typically via syringe, travels through the tubing and into the cuff to inflate it. Some tracheostomy tubes have foam cuffs, rather than balloon-type cuffs, that fill with air. Foam cuffs do not deflate, so they cannot be used with speaking valves. (See picture A.)

  Cuffs are necessary on tubes used with patients on ventilators to create a closed system. This allows all the air pushed in by the ventilator to reach the lungs. With a cuff, none of the air escapes into the upper airway through the larynx. The cuff is well below the vocal cords.

- *fenestrations* — Some tracheostomy tubes have a hole or multiple holes in the outer cannula. When the inner cannula is removed, these fenestrations allow air to travel through the vocal cords above while the cuff is still inflated. If the patient blocks the end of the tracheostomy tube, he can talk. When the inner cannula is in place, the fenestrations are blocked. (See picture A.)

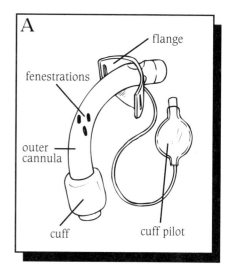

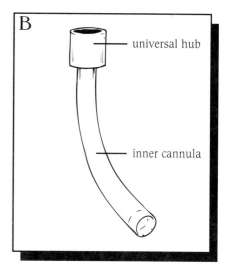

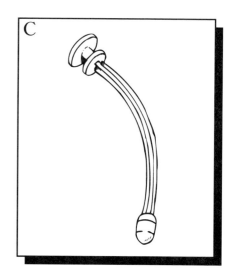

One-way Speaking Valves

Several manufacturers make one-way speaking valves which can be used on tracheostomy tubes. The valves allow the patient to continue to breathe in through the tracheostomy tube, but when he breathes out, the valve closes and the air travels up through the vocal cords. It is imperative that speaking valves be placed only after the cuff is deflated (and never used on tubes with foam cuffs, as these cuffs do not stay deflated).

Suction Kits/Catheters

Patients with tracheostomies need to be suctioned if they cannot clear the secretions in their airways by coughing. If they are on ventilators, they cannot clear their own secretions because there is no way for the secretions to be coughed out. The secretions are caught below the cuff on the trach tube.

Suctioning is a sterile process and sterile gloves must be worn when suctioning a patient. The suction catheter is attached to the tubing in the wall which is attached to the suction machine. The catheter is placed into the tracheostomy tube, and just as the catheter is pulled out of the airway, the port is covered to create suction. For more information, see pages 246-247.

Applying This Information to the Management of Patients with Dysphagia

History taking: When reviewing the chart and gathering information from the nurse, there are some things you must pay particular attention to before assessing critically-ill patients. Ask the nurse if this is a good time to evaluate the patient. Patients in intensive care require intensive nursing care, and some nursing procedures cannot wait while your assessment or treatments are done. In addition, these patients may have fluctuating periods of alertness and you want to complete the evaluation when the patient is alert. In particular, post-

surgical patients may be given pain medications that alter their level of alertness. Ask the nurse if there are any positioning restrictions for the patient (e.g., patients with temporary renal catheters in the groin may not be able to sit up).

History of oral/nasal intubation: Find out if the patient has been intubated and how long the intubation lasted. Surgery patients who experience no complications are typically extubated within hours of the surgery. Patients who have undergone a coronary artery bypass graft are typically weaned within six hours. In our experience, a short period of intubation does not necessarily seem to have a negative effect on swallowing skills. Of course there are exceptions and each case must be carefully analyzed.

Swallowing may be affected after intubation as a result of the endotracheal tube, which is placed between the vocal cords. Some edema of the cords is to be expected. In a study over 20 years ago, Burgess et al. (1979) studied short-term intubated patients after open heart surgery. A large percent of the patients demonstrated swallowing alterations immediately after extubation.

There is little information in the literature about how long an intubation has to be before you can expect problems or how long after the extubation before swallowing function recovers. One study (de Larminat, 1995) concluded that a marked impairment in the sensitivity of the swallowing response may be seen after as short a time as 24 hours of intubation.

Colice (1989, 1992) reported information about the kind of damage that can be caused by prolonged intubation (called translaryngeal intubation). In 1989, he described the typical pattern of laryngeal damage as mucosal ulcerations along the posterior-medial aspects of both vocal cords. There were also varying degrees of laryngeal edema in 94% of the patients. The author also indicated that there was no relationship found between laryngeal pathology and the development of adverse laryngeal effects. In his 1992 study, Colice reported that 9% of the patients studied who had been intubated greater than four days had a normal-appearing larynx at extubation. Seventy-eight percent had laryngeal healing by eight weeks and 7% developed a laryngeal granuloma. These studies did not assess swallowing function or safety.

Leder et al. (1998) studied 20 consecutive trauma patients who were translaryngeally intubated for at least 48 hours. He used the FEES® about 24 hours after extubation. He found aspiration in 45% of the subjects and of those, 44% were silently aspirating. Therefore, silent aspiration occurred in 20% of the study population. Eighty-nine percent of the aspirating subjects resumed an oral diet from 2-10 days following extubation. This article speaks to the importance of a dysphagia evaluation with the implied benefit of preventing complications. When you are asked to screen a patient at bedside who has just been extubated, often the best recommendation you can give is for the patient to remain NPO with NG feedings for a few days. This recommendation is especially warranted when you listen to the patient's voice and he is very breathy, indicating probable edema of the cords. This study also speaks to the importance of instrumental assessment of these patients after extubation.

Tracheostomy: Patients who have been intubated translaryngeally and cannot be successfully weaned from the ventilator have to have a tracheostomy placed. This is usually done if the weaning cannot be accomplished within 7 to 10 days after intubation. What effect can the tracheostomy tube have on swallowing function? Bonanno (1971) demonstrated that the negative effects observed in patients with a tracheostomy who exhibited dysphagia were limited laryngeal elevation and limited anterior rotation of the larynx. The tracheostomy tube appears to act as an anchor, securing the larynx to the neck and prohibiting movement. Bonanno described

this as a "direct inhibition of the hyomandibular complex. This occurs as a result of the tracheostomy tube anchoring the trachea to the strap muscles and skin of the neck . . ." so that the "usual function of the suprahyoid musculature is thereby checkreined and the laryngeal excursion is diminished."

Others report that there may also be some loss of protective reflexes and uncoordinated laryngeal closure as a result of the tracheostomy tube. Shaker et al. (1995) reported on a small study comparing six normal volunteers and six patients with tracheostomy. The authors found that although the vocal cords closed completely during swallowing, the duration of the closure was significantly shorter for those patients with tracheostomies as compared with the normal volunteers. In addition, the timing of apnea related to vocal cord closure was also altered in patients with tracheostomies.

The presence of a tracheostomy tube does not necessarily result in dysphagia. However, incidence of aspiration associated with tracheostomy tubes has been reported between 65% to 87% (Bone et al., 1974; Cameron et al., 1973). It seems logical that patients who have first had a translaryngeal intubation followed by tracheostomy are at particular risk for dysphagia.

DeVita et al. (1990) report on a study of 11 patients after prolonged translaryngeal intubation (mean duration 19.9 days), 10 of whom then received a tracheostomy. All of the patients received a modified barium swallow study. The authors found that all of the patients had at least one problem from a list of 11, and there was a mean of six defects per patient. The most common defects were delayed triggering of the swallow (seen in all patients) and pharyngeal pooling of contrast material. The patients had no evidence of neurological dysfunction. The authors' conclusions were that prolonged oral intubation with subsequent tracheostomy may cause severe dysphagia. Interestingly, five of the patients received a repeat study after the tracheostomy tube was removed and they continued to show some deficits, although the problems were mild. The authors concluded that the deficit may be due to disuse muscle atrophy with resultant weakness and discoordination of the swallow response.

Tolep et al. (1996) report that patients requiring prolonged mechanical ventilation have a high incidence of swallowing abnormalities, regardless of whether or not they had an accompanying neuromuscular disorder. Their 35 patients had first been orally intubated and then received tracheostomies. Findings on MBS studies were abnormal in 83% of patients (85% in patients with neuromuscular disorders and 80% in patients without neuromuscular disorders). The authors also examined the patients with laryngoscopy and confirmed findings of others that the abnormalities seen included decreased sensation of the vocal cords, pooled secretions above the cords, limited vocal cord movement, and edema of the arytenoids.

The findings of Elpern et al. (1994) also support that swallowing disorders were common in their group of 83 subjects who were receiving long-term mechanical ventilation. Fifty percent aspirated during modified barium swallow studies and of those, 77% were silently aspirating. The authors also found that advanced age increased the risk of aspiration.

Cuffs on Tracheostomy Tubes

Check to see if the patient has a cuffed tracheostomy tube. If so, is the cuff inflated or deflated when the patient is swallowing and do you need to reinflate the cuff after your evaluation? In general, it is preferable to complete the evaluation with the cuff deflated to allow for maximum movement of the larynx.

The cuff on a tracheostomy tube is in the trachea, well below the vocal cords. Therefore, its purpose is not to prevent aspiration, for if food or liquid reaches the cuff, it has already been aspirated

(since the definition of aspiration is food or liquid entering the airway below the cords). Elpern et al. (1987) used a blue dye procedure (See pages 247-248 for information about this technique.) to assess aspiration in patients and concluded that inflated cuffs did not prevent aspiration. In fact, the authors found that aspiration occurred with greater frequency when cuffs were inflated to occlusion than when cuff leaks were present (meaning that the cuff was not filled to tightly fit the trachea).

It is true that an inflated cuff will protect against aspiration of a large amount of vomitus, so that may be how this misunderstanding originated. (See *The Fallacy of Inflated Cuff*, page 113.) In fact, there may be negative consequences on swallowing if the cuff is inflated. It may serve as a further anchor to laryngeal elevation, and if overinflated, can impinge on the esophagus and cause food boluses to catch in the esophagus as they pass that area. Respiratory therapists and pulmonologists may insist that the cuff stay inflated if the patient is on the ventilator, since it creates a closed loop system for the ventilator. However, in a small trial with five patients, Tippett and Siebens (1991) demonstrated that a deflated cuff can be compatible with ventilation. If you want to try deflated cuffs with a patient who is on a ventilator, this article will provide more specific information.

Tracheostomy Tube Occlusion/ Use of One-way Speaking Valves

Evidence is contradictory whether patients aspirate less when the tracheostomy tube is occluded or when they are wearing a one-way speaking valve. Given the choice, it is preferable to assess swallowing while the patient is wearing the valve so that he can communicate during the evaluation, and so that you can subjectively judge vocal quality.

Patients can also phonate if the tracheostomy tube is occluded. This can be done with a gloved finger or with a plug designed to fit into the trach tube. A physician's order is generally required before the tracheostomy tube can be plugged.

Oxygen delivered at the tracheostomy will need to be switched to a nasal cannula. However, brief periods of occluding the tracheostomy with a finger are usually tolerated well by the patient, as the oxygen is only blocked temporarily. Take your finger away from the tracheostomy when the patient is not talking. Some patients can be taught to occlude their tracheostomies lightly with their own fingers. Be sure their hands are clean, or let them wear gloves, as the tracheostomy area should be kept clean.

Eibling and Gross (1996) reviewed the evidence supporting the role of subglottic pressure rise in swallowing efficiency. They explained the interdependence of subglottic air pressure and the glottic closure reflex. They stated that when subglottic air pressure builds up, stretch receptors are activated. This signals the respiratory muscles so they don't inhale during this period of swallowing. The authors hypothesized that if subglottic air pressure can't be built up because of the tracheostomy tube, then the inhibition of inspiration may also be affected. They reported on 11 patients who were known to aspirate on MBS and who were evaluated with and without the Passy-Muir Valve. The authors found significant decrease or elimination of aspiration with the Passy-Muir Valve on. They postulated that restoration of normal subglottic pressures by the Passy-Muir Valve was the key in clinical improvement.

In two separate studies (1996; 1998), Leder et al. demonstrated that occlusion of the tracheostomy tube had no effect on the prevalence of aspiration. They also found no trends related to bolus consistency, type of tube, or presence or absence of a nasogastric tube. Leder et al. (1999) also found that incidence of aspiration was not affected by the use of a one-way tracheostomy speaking valve, and concluded that the valve provided mostly nondeglutitive benefits. If you are performing an instrumental examination of swallowing, you might consider performing the assessment with and without a speaking valve (or occlusion of the tracheostomy) to see if that particular patient exhibits any differences in swallowing.

Ventilator

If the patient is on a ventilator, you may need to coordinate your assessment with the respiratory therapist if you want to make any adjustments such as deflating the cuff or placing a one-way speaking valve. The respiratory therapist can also help you take baseline information from the ventilator (e.g., respiratory rate) so you can determine if the patient's respiration changes during your evaluation.

Oxygen Saturation/Pulse Oximetry

Obtain baseline information on heart rate and oxygen saturation. Fragile patients in intensive care may react negatively to being moved in the bed and to physical exertion (e.g., eating). These cardiopulmonary adaptations should be noted. Changes in oxygen saturation levels noted on the pulse oximeter may signal a variety of things. For example, oxygen saturation levels may drop when the patient coughs. In preliminary studies, Rogers et al. (1993) and Zaidi et al. (1995) observed hypoxemic events during swallowing and hypothesized this might indicate aspiration. They thought that non-invasive monitors might yield important information about safety of swallowing at bedside. Sellars et al. (1998) performed pulse oximetry on six patients undergoing videofluoroscopic studies. The results indicated no clear-cut relationship between changes in arterial oxygenation and aspiration. The authors indicated that more research is needed to study the relationship between respiratory status and dysphagia during oral feedings.

Suctioning

Patients with tracheostomy tubes require suctioning to help them clear secretions from the airway. It is a good idea for the patient to be suctioned before you begin your assessment as this will clear the patient's airway and reduce work of breathing.

This procedure is usually performed by nurses, respiratory therapists, and in more and more facilities by the SLP. At Central Baptist Hospital in Lexington, Kentucky, the Patient Care Council granted SLPs the privilege to provide suctioning for tracheostomy patients. This improved patient care, as the SLPs are now able to suction as soon as needed rather than waiting for nursing or respiratory therapy, who may be busy with another patient.

These documents were helpful in convincing the Patient Care Council that this was within our scope:

- The scope of practice from ASHA. (You may also want to review the scope of practice in your state licensure law to see what it allows.) Although ASHA's scope does not specifically list suctioning, it states ". . . it is recognized that speech-language pathology is a dynamic and continuously developing practice area. Listing specific areas within the scope of practice does not necessarily exclude other, new, or emerging areas." Suctioning is not viewed as a new area of practice, but a tool to help us provide better patient care in areas in which we already practice (e.g., dysphagia).

- Code of Ethics of ASHA which states that "Individuals shall engage in only those aspects of the professions that are within the scope of their competence, considering their level of education, training, and experience." We used this statement to explain why we worked with the Respiratory Therapy Department to develop our education and training and to assure competence in the procedure.

- ASHA's Position Statement on Multiskilled Personnel (1996) which states that "cross-training of clinical skills is not appropriate at the professional level of practice . . ." but that "Cross-training of basic patient care skills . . . is a reasonable option." It lists suctioning as an example of a basic patient care skill.

It is advisable to work with the respiratory therapist (RT) or critical care nursing staff to learn about the procedure. You will want to practice in simulation, and then perform a number of procedures with the RT or critical care nurse. There is no prescribed number of times for you to practice. You may be ready to have your competencies checked after four or five practice runs or you may feel more comfortable after 10 or 12 practice runs. When you feel as though you have mastered the procedure, have the RT or nurse check each step to assure that you are competent to perform independently. If you do not perform the procedure frequently, you may want to have your competency rechecked periodically. A copy of the *Competency Validation Tool* we use is provided in Appendix E, page 249.

Modified Evans Blue Dye Test (MEBDT)

When evaluating patients with tracheostomies at bedside, suctioning can be used as a way to screen to see if the patient has aspirated any food or liquid. However, relying on suctioning to prove or disprove aspiration is quite risky. It is important to understand the development of this procedure and its limitations.

Use of the MEBDT to determine the occurrence of aspiration in patients with tracheostomies has been documented (Cameron et al., 1973; Spray et al., 1976; Elpern, 1987; Higgins et al., 1997). In the Cameron et al. study, when four drops of a 1% solution of blue dye were placed on patients' tongues every four hours for 48 hours, 69% were found to be aspirating. Other studies have also shown that aspiration may occur in healthy individuals, particularly during sleep (Huxley et al., 1978). That means that this procedure may have false positives.

Thompson-Henry & Braddock (1995) used a modified form of this test in which blue food coloring was mixed with 3cc to 6cc of thin liquid and semi-solid food. This test was negative for all five patients they studied; however, FEES® or MBS studies conducted 4-22 days later revealed aspiration for all five patients. The authors question the use of the MEBDT and conclude that "caution may be warranted when using this diagnostic approach as the primary indicator of a patient's swallow function."

Tippett & Siebens (1996) indicate that the Thompson-Henry & Braddock study contains several design flaws, including unspecified subject selection criteria, unspecified cuff status during FEES® and MBS, and the influence of time intervals between MEBDT and FEES® or MBS. Tippett & Siebens do reinforce Thompson-Henry & Braddock when they state that "caution may be warranted" and that false negative readings are conceivable when using the MEBDT.

Leder (1996) also points out problems with the methodology of the Thompson-Henry & Braddock study. He noted that a "prospective and randomized or consecutive study using an MBS or FEES® for an objective assessment of aspiration immediately followed by a MEBDT is needed to demonstrate the efficacy and sensitivity of the MEBDT in assessing aspiration." In 1999, Brady et al. reported on such a study in which 20 consecutive simultaneous MEBDTs and MBS studies were completed on patients with tracheostomies. Overall, the MEBDT showed a 50% false-negative error rate. The MEBDT identified aspiration in 100% of patients who aspirated more than trace amounts (greater than 10% of bolus), but did not identify aspiration of trace amounts. As Garren & Meyers (1999) pointed out in their editorial, the Brady study did not report what (if any) the relationship was between occurrences of aspiration and coughing. They also state that overall use of the MEBDT as a screening tool is "limited by its relatively low overall sensitivity."

Consequently, if the MEBDT (or, in other words, watching for food particles when the patient is suctioned) fails to demonstrate aspiration in tracheostomized patients, you cannot assume that aspiration is not occurring (i.e., a false negative result). The MEBDT cannot reliably tell you if a patient is aspirating and it certainly cannot tell you what techniques can be used to prevent aspiration. That is the value of an instrumental assessment.

Instrumental Assessments for Patients in the ICU

Patients in intensive care units, particularly those with history of intubation or tracheostomies, are at high risk for aspiration and therefore most likely will need an instrumental assessment of their swallowing. Timing of that assessment is important. If a patient has just been extubated, is nearly aphonic, and is less than optimally alert when you are consulted, the patient may be best served by encouraging continued tube feedings for several days until the patient is a better candidate for an instrumental assessment. This may be preferable to completing an instrumental assessment immediately, only to have the patient fail miserably and need another study in a few days. Of course, the instrumental assessment will provide you with information needed to plan appropriate treatment, and if the physician is insisting that the patient begin eating by mouth (perhaps they are not tolerating tube feeding), then proceeding with the instrumental assessment is warranted.

If you have access to both the MBS and the FEES®, compare the two techniques (see Chapter 6, pages 134-135) to determine which is most appropriate for the patient in the ICU. The MBS study requires transport to the Radiology department, and the patient's nurse will need to accompany the patient (and possibly the respiratory therapist if the patient is on a ventilator). It is possible to complete an MBS at bedside if the facility has an available C-arm fluoroscopy unit which can be taken to the bedside. The FEES® can be done at bedside and can be repeated more easily as the patient begins to improve so that recommendations can be modified.

Conclusion

Evaluating and treating patients with dysphagia in intensive care units is stimulating and challenging, but requires you to acquire knowledge and skills about this patient population. You must also be integrated as a member of the critical care team treating the patient in order to provide expert care.

Appendix E: Competency Validation Tool _____

Name:_____ Unit:_____ SLP:_____

Objective: To provide the patient with a clear airway before, during, and after swallowing evaluations and treatment, as well as during the use of Passy-Muir Valves.

CRITICAL BEHAVIORS	SUCCESSFULLY MET			
	YES	DATE/ INITIALS	On The Job	Simulation
1. Collect necessary equipment to perform suctioning.				
2. Explain purpose of procedure.				
3. Position the patient appropriately.				
4. Turn on suction equipment and set vacuum regulator to correct negative pressure.				
5. Wash hands.				
6. Put on non-sterile gloves.				
7. Remove yaunker from the suction unit.				
8. Open sterile catheter package on clean surface.				
9. Set up sterile solution container on sterile field and fill with sterile water.				
10. Place sterile gloves over non-sterile gloves.				
11. Connect vacuum tubing from suction unit to catheter.				
12. Lubricate catheter by dipping it into sterile water, then grasp air entrainment adapter with one hand.				
13. Hyperoxygenate patient with 100% O_2 for 1 minute. If not on vent, instruct patient to take deep breaths.				
14. Expose the airway.				
15. Hold catheter by connecting tubing, turn catheter until natural curve points in direction of bronchus to be suctioned.				
16. Insert catheter into tracheobronchial tree without application of suction until resistance met.				
17. Instruct patient to cough to allow catheter to pass into trachea.				
18. Apply suction while rotating and withdrawing catheter.				
19. Hyperoxygenate patient before repeating.				
20. Allow patient to rest.				
21. If cuff is inflated, deflate and follow procedures 14-20 again.				
22. Monitor patient's respiratory status.				
23. Perform oral-pharyngeal suctioning following lower airway suctioning.				
24. Discard gloves and suctioning supplies.				
25. Wash hands.				
26. Reassess patient's respiratory system for expected and unexpected outcomes.				
27. Document procedure in patient's record.				

Comments:_____

*Validation signature documents direct observation of criteria in accordance with hospital policy and procedure.

Initials	Signature/Title	Initials	Signature/Title

Chapter 10

Using Data in the Management of Dysphagia

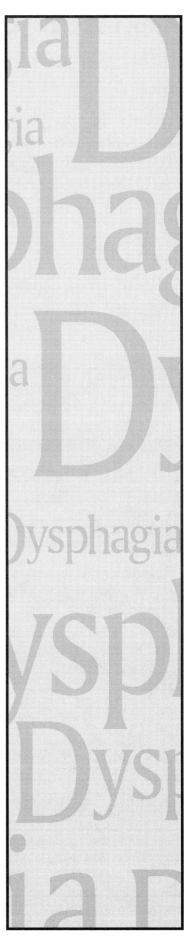

As a science-based profession, it seems a given that we would use data to manage our decisions about the treatment of patients with dysphagia. However, external demands for data have accelerated our interest in the topic. We are being asked by a variety of audiences to demonstrate the value of our treatment — to demonstrate that our involvement with patients with dysphagia is going to make a difference.

Who is making demands for data? Third-party payers want to know about the bang for their buck. If they pay for the service, what will the outcome be? Will the patient still need to be on tube feeding? Consumers and their family members want to know if the patient will be able to eat normal foods and drink regular liquids. Referring physicians may ask whether the patient's swallowing skills will improve more rapidly with treatment than without.

These demands, and many others we face, make it important that we understand the kinds of data available, as well as ways to use this data to provide better services. We must also be aware of the kinds of data we are lacking, and sorely need, to answer questions we will face in the future about our services. We can expect that not only will we receive more questions about outcomes from a variety of sources, but that those questions will become more rigorous.

What Streams of Data Do We Have Available?

As clinicians, we are all used to documenting to demonstrate change. This is done on a case-by-case basis as we develop a treatment plan, select long- and short-term goals, and establish treatment objectives to meet those goals. In this way, we are able to demonstrate the patient's progress from session to session, as well as from the beginning to the end of treatment. However, if this is the only data stream we have available, we will not be able to answer questions such as:

- How many sessions will it take before the patient no longer needs tube feeding and can eat by mouth?

- Will the patient's swallowing really improve during her short stay in acute care?

- Does more therapy yield more significant improvement?

For answers to questions such as these, outcomes data are needed. Outcomes data describe what the patient was like at the end of a period of treatment. One cannot necessarily attribute any change which took place over the course of treatment to the treatment itself (for that kind of data, see discussion of efficacy on pages 255-256). Any such interpretation of cause must be qualified, but can lend support to experimental evidence of efficacy (Frattali, 1998). Outcomes data simply state that at the end of the period of treatment, this is what the patient was like compared to what she was like at the beginning of treatment. Outcomes research is a fairly new methodology in the field of rehabilitation, and thus comes under some scrutiny as "not real science." However, as Frattali points out, "Outcomes research methodologies, because of their less stringent design characteristics, are amenable for use in real-world settings with large patient populations."

Outcomes data collection typically involves the use of a rating scale or other measurement which can be used pre- and post- to show that change has occurred.

In Which Areas of Patient Change Has Outcomes Research Focused?

Physiology

It is not surprising that, as clinicians, we are most comfortable in the realm of change in physiology. As mentioned in Chapter 7, we are used to writing deficit-based goals (e.g., patient will improve the ability to lateralize the tongue). This reflects a change in physiology, but says nothing about function (e.g., patient can clean pocketed food from cheek). In terms of outcomes, several rating scales and measures of change focus on changes in the physiological deficit.

Logemann et al. (1993), in a study examining swallow function after tonsil/base of tongue resection, used a measure called oropharyngeal swallow efficiency (OPSE) which the authors described as a "measure generated by dividing the percent of the bolus swallowed (subtracting percent aspirated and percent of oral and pharyngeal residue from 100 percent of the bolus) by oral plus pharyngeal transit times" (Logemann et al., 1989). These authors used the OPSE measurement, along with other measures of physiology such as oral transit time, laryngeal closure, pharyngeal

delay time, etc. to describe the impact of surgery on the patient's ability to swallow. This study tried to determine if the outcome (based on change in physiology of the swallow) would be different for patients having different types of surgery. They found that swallow function was equally affected in the two groups.

DeJonckere and Hordijk (1998) wanted to determine if certain factors could offer information about the prognosis for safe swallowing after surgical treatment for head and neck cancer. They used change in physiologic function as the expected outcome. They found that no single parameter of those they studied had great prognostic value to determine which patients would show improvement. Both the Dejonckere and Logemann articles are examples of trying to obtain outcomes data which could be used as basis for prognosis.

Several rating scales described in Chapter 6 measure biomechanical action during swallowing. The *Duke Rating Scale* and the *Penetration-Aspiration Scale* can be used to objectify what is observed during videofluorographic studies. The scales can also be used as pre- and post-ratings of physiological skills to demonstrate change that has taken place between the initial radiographic study and any repeat studies. Murray et al. (1996) used a rating scale from 0-3 to describe amount and location of secretions on FEES®. This rating was used to predict likelihood of aspiration, but could also be used in repeat studies to demonstrate change.

Functional Outcomes

In contrast to physiological rating scales which describe outcome as a change in some aspect of the complex physical act of swallowing (e.g., better tongue movement; increased laryngeal elevation) are rating scales which describe functional outcome. Functional outcomes describe change in a way that is meaningful to someone other than an SLP. Functional change implies a change in an applied aspect of the skill. That is, because the underlying physiology has improved, the result is a practical change. Functional outcomes in dysphagia are generally grouped into the following categories:

1. ability to eat
2. health status of the patient
3. patient/caregiver satisfaction
4. quality of life

Each of these types of functional outcomes will be discussed, with examples provided.

1. Ability to Eat

Scales designed to describe a patient's ability to eat (e.g., types of foods and liquids, amount of time it takes to eat, supervision needed) have been in use for many years. Steefel (1981) used a seven-level rating scale in 1981 which ranged from severe to normal level of functioning. The Wisconsin Speech-Language-Hearing Association recently undertook development of a seven-point scale called the *Functional Outcome Assessment of Swallowing*.

Some scales combine some functional ratings with physiological ratings. The *Dysphagia Outcome and Severity Scale* (DOSS) was described by O'Neil et al. (1999) as a scale which allows clinicians to make recommendations about diet level, independence level, and type of nutrition. Examining one of its seven levels demonstrates how physiology and function are combined on the same scale. For example, Level 3: Moderate dysphagia is described as "Total assist, supervision, or strategies; two or more diet consistencies restricted." The scale then lists symptoms which may be exhibited such as moderate retention in the pharynx or oral cavity and airway penetration. Combining severity of physiological deficits and functional skills on one scale makes the scale less meaningful to payers, although the authors state that the tool lends some objective measurement to the functional description.

Some scales are specific to a certain medical disorder. Hillel et al. (1989) developed the *Amyotrophic Lateral Sclerosis Severity Scale*, which has a swallowing scale. The swallowing scale is a 10-point scale, descending from normal swallowing at 10 through stages they describe as early eating problems (levels 8 & 7), dietary consistency changes (levels 6 & 5), needs tube feeding (levels 4 & 3), and nothing by mouth (levels 2 & 1). For the head and neck cancer population, several scales have been developed. Teichgraeber et al. (1985) developed a scale which requires the patient to answer multiple choice, yes/no, and other questions to rate their swallowing symptoms. The scale also includes ratings by an SLP and head and neck surgeon on items such as tongue mobility, weight, and status of mandible and teeth. List et al. (1990) defined points on three subscales: eating in public, understandability of speech, and normalcy of diet. The latter addresses the kind of foods that patients can eat.

Others have designed scales to measure change in functional status. These may be simple paper-and-pencil tools or more sophisticated computer software programs. Although such scales are more descriptive of a patient's progress in functional skills than progress toward achieving short-term goals, they do not allow for any comparisons to other patients or average change of other patients on a large scale basis. Comparison to a standard is called benchmarking.

National systems do allow for benchmarking. Benchmarking provides a more powerful tool in several ways. Being able to compare an individual patient's progress to a group of patients with a similar deficit provides the basis for an informed prognosis. Benchmarking meets the demands of accrediting agencies which want programs to compare themselves to a standard, and set goals to improve the program's performance. Information from a national system can form the basis for quality improvement and program management activities. In addition, national data can stimulate change in practice patterns.

Such national data may be embedded in a comprehensive assessment instrument such as the *Functional Independence Measure* (FIM) (Uniform Data System, 1995). The FIM was designed to measure a level of independence in areas such as locomotion, sphincter control, transfers, self-care, communication, etc. Each variable within those categories is scored on a seven-point scale. The drawback to use of the FIM to show functional change in swallowing is that it is rated on a self-care scale called "eating." The eating scale focuses not just on the ability to eat/swallow, but on self-feeding skills like bringing the utensil to the mouth. Clinicians report it is not specific enough to measure change in swallowing. In addition, the eating scale does not have to be scored by an SLP.

To meet the demands on SLPs for data to demonstrate the value of services, ASHA has developed the *National Outcomes Measurement System* (NOMS) (ASHA, 1998). The NOMS measures change in a variety of areas through the use of seven-point rating scales called *Functional Communication Measures* (FCMs). These FCMs have been developed for areas including receptive and expressive communication, motor speech, voice, fluency, and of interest here, swallowing.

The swallowing FCM takes into account several factors which contribute to a change in functional ability to eat: kinds of solid foods patient can eat, kinds of liquids patient can swallow safely, amount of cueing needed/independent use of techniques, and how much of the patient's nutritional needs are met by mouth. For example, Level 1 indicates that the patient has no functional swallow and receives all nutrition and hydration by non-oral means. Level 3 indicates that an alternative method of feeding is still required, as the individual takes less than 50% of nutrition and hydration by mouth, and/or swallowing is safe with consistent use of moderate cues to use compensatory strategies, and/or patient requires maximum diet restrictions. At Level 7, the patient's ability to eat independently is not limited by swallow function and swallowing is considered safe and efficient for all consistencies. Compensatory strategies are effectively used when needed.

The registered user (an SLP) rates the patient's functional level on admit and at the end of therapy. These ratings, along with demographic information, diagnostic codes, treatment setting, and amount of treatment are submitted to ASHA's National Center for Treatment Effectiveness in Communication Disorders (NCTECD). The NCTECD compiles the data and prepares a national report card which can answer questions like:

- How many treatment units does it take for a patient with a CVA to move from a level 3 to a level 5?

- Do patients receive more or less treatment units in skilled nursing facilities compared to home health agencies, and is their amount of change affected by the amount of service?

- Do patients make more or less progress when seen in group treatment?

Such national data provides important information to the profession and to consumers and payers.

2. **Health Status of the Patient**
   Other analyses of the outcome of intervention look at whether the health status of the patient has changed. This includes looking at occurrences of pneumonia, weight loss, dehydration, or nutrition (Elmståhl et al., 1999). Elmståhl and colleagues studied 38 stroke patients and compared such ratings as plasma protein levels and body composition. They found that after treatment, 60% of cases showed improved levels of albumin and total iron-binding capacity. They concluded that swallowing treatment improves swallowing function and improved swallowing function is associated with improvements in nutritional parameters. Of course, attributing these changes to the treatment which took place is difficult because of many other related factors. Since outcomes research does not control variables, you cannot state that the outcome is the result of treatment.

Another group of researchers and clinicians working with Robbins (1998) are developing a scale to assess biological and physiological parameters. These measures would include a range of data from inexpensive and non-invasive to more costly and more invasive. The measures would include nutrition measures such as weight, body mass index, percent weight loss, hematocrit, albumin, etc. Hydration measures would include dry tongue, orthostatic blood pressure, BUN (blood urea nitrogen)/creatinine ratio, and serum osmolality.

3. **Patient/Caregiver Satisfaction**
While ability to eat and health status are important outcomes, they fail to consider whether the patient or caregiver is satisfied with that outcome. You may be thrilled that the patient has improved functional skills to the point that she can have her NG tube removed and eat soft foods with moderately thick liquids while using only a chin tuck. However, for the patient and caregiver, this may seem so far from normal that it is an unacceptable outcome.

Crary (1995) assessed the success of a direct intervention program for chronic neurogenic dysphagia secondary to brainstem stroke in three ways: immediate change in patient's ability to eat and drink more or eliminate tube feedings; changes in swallowing physiology; and long-term outcome. Success was determined via patient questionnaire. This questionnaire asked each patient to comment on their impressions of the success of the program.

The ASHA NOMS has a patient satisfaction component. At the end of the period of treatment, the patient is given a questionnaire to complete that asks for feedback with items like the following:

- My speech-language pathologist did a good job answering the questions I had about my problem.

- My SLP treated me with dignity and respect.

4. **Quality of Life**
Closely related to patient satisfaction are measures which assess the quality of the patient's life. Such measures will provide important information about the ultimate outcome of our intervention — is the patient's life enhanced by the intervention provided? Two quality of life measures are currently under development.

The Dysphagia Disability Index is under development by Silbergeit, Jacobson & Sumlin. It is a patient self-assessment of impairment, disability, and handicap due to dysphagia. It contains three subscales: physical, functional, and emotional, and has been standardized on patients with a variety of diagnoses. It promises to be quick and easy to administer, is standardized on pencil/paper or face-to-face administration, and the confidence interval will allow for tracking change. It is not suitable for patients with significant communication deficits and there is no caregiver version. The authors suggest that the scores on the subscales will provide useful information to help direct intervention and to educate the patient about deficit areas and prognosis.

McHorney and Rosenbek (1998), in an excellent article that reviews the measurement tools in use, provide information about the *Swallowing-Quality of Life* (SWAL-QOL). This is a comprehensive measure of quality of life and quality of care that is being developed by Robbins, Rosenbek, and McHorney at the Madison VA Medical Center. The measure was designed by conducting focus groups to obtain qualitative data that was used to delineate the major conceptual dimensions for the SWAL-QOL. It will include components such as symptoms, physical and eating sequelae (as a result from a disease or a consequence of a disease), emotional health, social functioning, and fear.

What Else Is Needed?

Outcomes measurement tools can yield important information about change in patient status over time. As described, these outcomes range from change in physiology to change in quality of life. Outcomes data can answer many questions as stated above. Outcomes data cannot, however, answer questions such as:

- Do patients get better as a result of the treatment provided?

- Do patients with impaired swallow improve more quickly as a result of treatment technique A or B?

For the answers to questions like these, efficacy data is needed.

Efficacy

Different authors define efficacy in different ways. Langmore (1995) uses efficacy to mean that "treatment is effective (yields the desired response) and efficient (more economical in terms of utilization of resources than the alternative)." Rosenbek (1995) provides a more rigorous definition. He states that efficacy is "improvement resulting from treatment applied in a rigidly controlled design when treatment and no-treatment conditions are compared. A comparison of two treatments of unproven efficacy is not an efficacy study." Rosenbek also considers efficacy to be different than efficiency. Using Rosenbek's definition, the first question listed above (Do patients get better as a result of the treatment provided?) would be an efficacy study if a treatment and no-treatment design were applied. In order for the second question (Do patients with impaired swallow improve more quickly as a result of treatment technique A or B?) to be an efficacy study, both treatment A and B would have to have undergone the rigorous treatment and no-treatment design and been shown to be efficacious.

For our purposes, we will use the less rigorous definition of efficacy. Examples will be provided about studies which have been completed to show

that treatment yields the desired response. Different researchers select different desired responses. Some studies analyze the results of treatment for patients within a specific population such as Parkinson's disease or head and neck cancer. Others show the effects of overall management of the dysphagia population or of specific treatment techniques. Still others select reduced cost of care or improved medical status as the desired outcome of dysphagia management. In fact, we will broaden our discussion of efficacy to include studies which demonstrate intended outcome of evaluation procedures as well as treatment.

What types of studies are found in the literature? Many of the studies are single subject design, which means the study describes the result of intervention for a particular patient. For example, Fonda, Schwarz, and Clinnick (1995) report in the form of a case study on a patient with Parkinson's disease whose dysphagia improved when the timing of his Levodopa was adjusted to one hour before meals. The power of a single subject design is minimal. It is impossible to know if the result will apply to other similar patients. To have more powerful data, the discipline needs more randomized studies of larger groups of patients. Rosenbek would argue that these studies need a no-treatment arm.

One example of a large scale randomized study is the work being done by the Communication Sciences and Disorders Research Group developed by ASHA to conduct randomized multi-center clinical trials (ASHA Leader, 1997). This work is funded by the largest-ever grant in communication sciences and disorders, a $5 million project to study the efficacy of treatments of disorders. The first randomized trial studied the efficacy of postural and diet interventions for swallowing disorders to determine if these interventions lower the risk of pneumonia.

As clinicians, it is important that we become sophisticated users of the research literature. We must not simply read the description of the study and the conclusions and then apply the technique to our patients. We must also analyze the methods used, population selected, dependent variables chosen, etc. In short, we must read every study the way we were taught in our research design course in graduate school. As critical consumers of research, we can decide when the information reported will be helpful to us and our patients.

It is not the intent of this chapter to scrutinize or critique the studies mentioned. Several excellent articles provide a review of efficacy literature and commentary on the state of our research (Langmore, 1995; Miller & Langmore, 1994; Rosenbek, 1995). The purpose of the following section is to make you aware of the kinds of studies available in the literature vs. those that are not available. There are instances when others demand proof that the method being used is the right method to use, or when others question whether your services really have an impact on the patient's health. Those instances, and others, demand that we have a good grasp of the current research findings.

Earlier it was mentioned that studies in the literature can be grouped according to the desired response or outcome that is being investigated. This chapter will briefly mention examples of studies which address:

- efficacy of overall management of patients with dysphagia

- efficacy of a particular treatment approach

- efficacy of bedside evaluations

- efficacy of clinical and instrumental exams

- reduced cost of care as the outcome of dysphagia management

- improvement in patient's medical status as outcome of dysphagia management

Examples of Studies in the Literature

1. **Efficacy of overall management of patients with dysphagia**

Some studies demonstrate that treatment of dysphagia results in patients being able to eat without pulmonary complications. Horner et al. (1991) found that treatment consisting exclusively of changes in posture and diet resulted in more than 80% of patients resuming a full oral diet with no incidence of pulmonary or nutritional complications.

In two separate articles, Neumann (1993, 1995) reported that swallowing therapy is associated with a successful outcome (defined in the different studies by exclusively oral feeding or progress in type, ease, and safety of feeding and by range of diet) with the groups of neurologic patients studied. These studies are examples of those which do not look specifically at a type of treatment, but at the efficacy (that is, the expected result was achieved) of a dysphagia treatment program.

2. **Efficacy of a particular therapy approach**

Chapter 7, which describes a variety of treatment techniques, lists efficacy studies associated with those techniques in Appendix D, pages 215-219. For purposes of example, let's consider the efficacy data available on thermal-tactile stimulation. In 1986, Lazzara, Lazarus, and Logemann demonstrated that "thermal sensitization" improved triggering of the swallowing reflex in 23 of the 25 neurologically-impaired patients on swallows of at least one food consistency. A study by Rosenbek et al. (1991) used a month-long trial of thermal application using a single-subject withdrawal (ABAB) design. This study failed to reveal strong evidence that two weeks of thermal application alternated with two weeks of no thermal application improved dysphagia following multiple strokes. In a later study, however, Rosenbek et al. (1996) found that thermal application reduced duration of stage transition (defined by Robbins as elapsed time between arrival of the head of the bolus at the posterior margin of the ramus and the and the beginning of maximum elevation of the hyoid bone) and total swallow duration. This is a beginning in the study of the efficacy of this one technique. We still don't know things such as:

- How frequently and with what intensity should the technique be used? (Rosenbek et al., 1998 found no single intensity emerges as the most therapeutic.)

- For which patients is the technique the most helpful?

- Does the technique result in elimination of aspiration?

- Does it matter if the mirror is cold or how firmly you push? (Results by Kaatzke-McDonald et al., 1996 would seem to indicate that a cold mirror is important.)

It will take time and the cooperative efforts of researchers and clinicians to answer these and other questions, not only about this technique, but about other techniques used as well.

3. **Efficacy of bedside evaluations**

In a study by Splaingard et al. (1988), 107 patients were involved in a blind study comparing videofluoroscopy with bedside clinical evaluations by speech-language pathologists in the diagnosis of aspiration. This study found that bedside evaluation identified only 42% of those who aspirated on the videofluoroscopy. Their conclusions were that the bedside evaluation alone underestimates the frequency of aspiration in patients with neurologic dysfunction.

In a more recent study, Logemann (1999) reported on the sensitivity and specificity of a 28-item screening test in identifying patients who aspirate, have an oral stage disorder, a pharyngeal delay, or a pharyngeal stage disorder. The results indicated there were a combination of variables which would classify patients correctly as having or not having aspiration 71% of the time. However, these authors, and most others, agree that being able to predict who will aspirate, while an important piece of information in patient management, does not provide the information needed to define the nature of the problem and plan appropriate treatment.

4. **Efficacy of clinical and instrumental exams**

Chapter 6 provides information on efficacy of both the videofluoroscopic and the fiber-endoscopic evaluations of swallowing. Those studies will not be repeated here. Most studies conclude that instrumental exams are effective in identifying aspiration, as well as in evaluating techniques and maneuvers which can be used to eliminate the aspiration. For example, Logemann et al. (1989) demonstrated via fluoroscopy that head rotation to the damaged side closes the vallecula and pyriform sinus on that side, sending food down the stronger side. Welch et al. (1993) used radiographic views to demonstrate that with the chin tucked, the dimensions of the pharynx changed. There was a posterior shift of the anterior pharyngeal structures, narrowing the laryngeal entrance. It also widened the angle of the epiglottis to the anterior tracheal wall.

5. **Reduced cost of care as the outcome of dysphagia management**

Smithard et al. (1996) studied 121 consecutive patients admitted with acute stroke. Among other findings, they noted that patients with an abnormal swallow on a bedside assessment had longer hospital stays. This study can be helpful when discussing the importance of a dysphagia management program with hospital administrators. Unfortunately, this study, like some others, credits the bedside assessment with the successful outcome of patients because it failed to recognize that treatment was planned based on the videofluoroscopic assessment.

6. **Improvement in patient's medical status as outcome of dysphagia management**

When documenting the effect that evaluation and management of dysphagia has on a patient's medical status, research has considered the survival of the patient, malnutrition, dehydration, pneumonia, and growth (for pediatric patients).

Mortality — Very few studies (Holas et al., 1994; Smithard et al., 1996; Croghan et al., 1994; Cowen et al., 1997) mention mortality related to dysphagia and dysphagia management programs. Smithard et al. found the presence of dysphagia was associated with an increased risk of death. Cowen et al. found that mortality was high in patients with severely abnormal swallowing studies who required non-oral feeding. It is very difficult to demonstrate that dysphagia management results in reduced mortality because dysphagia occurs with many other diseases which may cause the mortality.

Malnutrition and dehydration — Malnutrition and dehydration are both possible, and even probable, consequences of dysphagia. Malnutrition occurs in 47% of stroke patients when admitted to rehabilitation (Finestone, 1996), and it is estimated that 35-85% of institutionalized elderly (Nelson, 1993) are malnourished. Dysphagia increases the risk of malnutrition because patients often have reduced amount of oral intake, a restricted diet, and are tube fed. Dehydration probably occurs in most institutionalized elderly, and 33% may be clinically dehydrated (Lavizzo-Mourey, 1987). Despite the strong links between dysphagia and malnutrition and dehydration, there has been no cause and effect relationship established between these problems in patients with dysphagia who are or are not treated (Davalos et al., 1996; Keller 1993, 1995).

It is sometimes thought that dysphagia increases the risk of dehydration because we restrict patients from thin liquids, and therefore it is surmised that patients can't get enough fluids when taking only thickened liquids. Some programs try to counteract this fact by providing free water to their patients with dysphagia.

Garon et al. (1997) tested the hypothesis that patients become dehydrated on thickened liquids in a randomized control prospective study which examined two groups of stroke patients who had previously been identified as aspirating thin liquids. Control group subjects were given only thickened liquids and, over the course of the study, had a mean intake of 1210cc/day of thickened liquids. The study group subjects were allowed thickened liquids with additional thin water intake. They averaged combined fluid intake of 1318cc/day. No patient developed pneumonia, dehydration, or complications during the course of the study, or during a 30-day follow-up period. The patients, as expected, did not report satisfaction with thick liquids, and the study subjects reported high satisfaction with access to water. The authors expressed surprise that the study subjects did not drink less thickened liquid and more thin liquid.

In follow-up satisfaction surveys, the majority of the study patients reported that they drank water generally for oral dryness and to quench thirst. These authors recommend that water and ice chips presently be given only in instances of patient refusal to drink thickened liquids or when hydration issues cause medical concerns. They urge staff making decisions regarding water intake to follow a set protocol and examine outcomes. They also conclude that a larger scale research study is needed to assess safety of such a protocol. As yet, there is insufficient information in the literature to support widespread use of this approach, particularly with very ill, non-ambulatory patients.

Growth — In the pediatric population, a related issue is whether children are growing at the expected rate. Gisel and Alphonce (1995), Gisel (1994), and Gisel et al.(1996) studied children with cerebral palsy.

In the earlier study, the authors proposed a classification system for eating impairments that included growth, weight, height, and skin fold thickness. The authors concluded that oral sensorimotor therapy was effective in addressing oral-motor skills, but that the children needed caloric supplements for catch-up growth.

Pneumonia — The relationship between pneumonia and aspiration is muddy at best, and research has provided contradictory information. We know that not everyone who aspirates gets aspiration pneumonia. For example, Feinberg (1996) found that patients who aspirated liquids on fluoroscopy got no more pneumonia than patients who did not aspirate (unless they were tube fed). Corghan et al. (1994) reported no difference in number of patients who got pneumonia when comparing known aspirators to those who did not, yet Schmidt et al. (1994) reported patients were 7.6 times more likely to develop pneumonia if they aspirated on fluoroscopy.

We also do not know exactly who will develop pneumonia. It depends on how much is aspirated, what was aspirated, if the lungs were able to clear the material, and if the patient's pulmonary status was already compromised. We do, however, know the factors which increase the risk for developing pneumonia. Langmore (1998) found the best predictors for aspiration pneumonia to include:

- dependent for feeding

- multiple medical diagnoses

- current smoker

- tube fed

- dependent for oral care

- number of decayed teeth

- number of meds

What are some of the facts we know and can cite? Aspiration pneumonia has the highest mortality rate of any infection. Among the hospitalized elderly, development of pneumonia is associated with 43% mortality rate (Langmore, 1991). Pneumonia is the second most common infection in nursing homes, and up to 80% of nosocomial pneumonia may be aspiration pneumonia.

The only study, and it is not without its drawbacks, that actually compares a treatment to no-treatment group is one by Kasprisin et al. (1989) which compared two groups of treated patients with a group of untreated patients. Both treated groups had significantly less aspiration pneumonia than the untreated group. They state that even mildly dysphagic patients were at risk for the development of aspiration pneumonia, and that severely dysphagic patients responded to management of their swallowing problems.

What About Treatment Techniques/Protocols With No Published Efficacy Data?

In the area of dysphagia, perhaps more so than in other areas of speech-language pathology, clinicians seem willing to apply a technique or approach to their patients when no published proof exists. To a certain extent, that is a natural progression in a clinical field. If we waited until every technique had undergone careful treatment and no-treatment design studies, we would have few techniques at our disposal. However, we need to recognize the difference in published data compared to a presenter claiming "This has worked with 90% of my patients!" When the results of a study are submitted to a scientific journal, the article is subject to critical analysis and review by respected peers. If there are faults in the design of the study or in the interpretation of the results, these will be pointed out. Serious design flaws or misinterpretation of the data can keep the study from being published at all. This process used by scientific journals affords the readers some assurances that the study is scientifically sound.

Here are some questions you should ask yourself before beginning to use a technique you learned at a conference or heard about from a colleague if there is no published research to support it.

- *Does the technique make sense, given what you know about the physiology of the swallow?* For example, if a presenter told you that having the patient forcefully open and close the jaw would reduce pyriform sinus residue, you would quickly argue that jaw movement has nothing to do with laryngeal movement (which is largely responsible for reducing pyriform sinus residue).

- *Is there a possibility of harm to the patient?* Will the technique cause the patient any undo discomfort? For example, would a technique utilizing hot pepper sauce increase saliva flow and increase risk of aspirating bacteria laden secretions?

- *If there is no efficacy data published, why not?* Just having a presenter or colleague tell you that a technique works doesn't mean you should try it. Our Code of Ethics states that "individual statements to colleagues about professional services, research results, and products shall adhere to prevailing professional standards and shall contain no misrepresentations" (Principle IV. D, ASHA, 1994). If the researcher/clinician has been using the technique/protocol and is so confident of its efficacy that s/he is willing to teach others how to do it, then that individual has an obligation to submit the data for critical peer review.

- *If it seems to work for your patients, is that enough proof for you?* Remember the placebo effect. If you are excited about a

new technique and tell the patient how wonderful it is and how well it will work, that alone can have an effect on the patient. In addition to the placebo effect, just judging efficacy by how well it works for several patients does not help you determine what other variables you have failed to control that might be accounting for the change.

- *Are you taking time away from treatment with a more traditional technique that has been shown to be effective?* If you spend time in therapy having the patient hold a bag of ice, as you believe increasing sensitivity in the hand increases the speed of onset of the swallow, are you not taking time away from use of thermal-tactile stimulation, which has some support in the literature?

- *What do you tell a patient when you decide to use what must be considered an experimental approach?* You should disclose to the patient that the technique you are using does not yet have any published efficacy data to support it. The Code of Ethics again provides guidance to us in Principle I:

D. Individuals shall fully inform the persons they serve of the nature and possible effects of services rendered and products dispensed.

E. Individuals shall evaluate the effectiveness of services rendered and of products dispensed and shall provide services or dispense products only when benefit can reasonably be expected.

F. Individuals shall not guarantee the results of any treatment or procedure, directly or by implication; however, they may make a reasonable statement of prognosis.

How Do You Make Use of Data for Dysphagia Management?

It is readily apparent that the kinds of data described in this chapter have many uses in the management of patients with dysphagia. The following are just a few examples of problems you may encounter along with suggestions of the type of data you might need to address the problem.

1. **Development of clinical pathway**

   If the facility is developing a clinical pathway for stroke patients which will indicate when speech-language pathology will be called upon to see the patient regarding their dysphagia, you might want to have:

   - information about decreased length of stay for CVA patients when a dysphagia management program is in place

   - cost data comparing cost of tube feeding with cost of SLP services

2. **Refusal to allow referral for instrumental assessments**

   If the skilled nursing facility refuses to allow you to request instrumental assessments because they do not want to pay for the exam, what data might you want to have?

   - data about aspiration pneumonia rates and relationship between aspiration and the development of pneumonia

   - cost data regarding treating the pneumonia (when the patient returns from acute care after a hospital stay for the pneumonia)

   - data about cost of tube feeding compared to oral feeding plus therapy (noting that therapy cannot be planned without instrumental exam)

   - data about how many patients can resume oral feeding as result of instrumental exam

3. **Family needs information**

   The family of a patient with a new CVA wants to know if their father will be able to go home after rehabilitation and eat food without supervision. What information do you need to counsel the family? Outcomes data from a national data base, as well as specific information from your facility about similar patients, will allow you to give an informed answer about prognosis.

These are just a few examples of the way outcomes and efficacy data can be used in the management of patients with dysphagia. Not only must we be clinicians, we must become advocates as well. A successful advocate is one who has data to back her arguments. Every SLP who works with patients with dysphagia should:

- be in regular contact with her representatives in Congress to let them know of the negative effects that reimbursement changes have had on patient care

- use information from a variety of sources when counseling patients and families about the patient's disorder and prognosis

- use research data to supplement discussions with physicians concerning the value of dysphagia services

- use data to talk with administrators about the value and cost-benefit ratio of dysphagia services

- sign up to collect outcomes data for the national data base

- contact a researcher and volunteer to help with a research project on dysphagia, or better yet, suggest the topic for such a study and help identify the patients

These actions are examples of advocacy. For real change to take place, each of us must be an advocate in many ways.

Chapter 11

Sample Cases

The following nine cases will help you refine your skills in making recommendations and determining short- and long-term goals and treatment objectives based on findings from MBS studies. The cases are presented in summary form. Long-term goals and short-term goals are established for each patient. Cursory information from the MBS study is in the first column. The symptom is listed and the physiological cause of that symptom is indicated in italics. At the end of the findings, information about the effects of treatment strategies tried during the MBS are listed. The middle column contains recommendations based on the findings from the MBS study. If treatment for that finding is indicated, the corresponding short-term goals tried during the MBS are listed. The third column suggests possible treatment objectives for the problem(s) identified in the findings. The treatment objectives are based on the physiological cause of the symptom, and the codes indicate the short-term goal to which that objective is related.

For example, a significant finding for Case 1 shows that the patient could form a bolus with any food presented. The recommendation is that he can have any and all textures he feels he can handle. No specific treatment will be needed, so no short-term goal is listed. However, another finding showed that thin liquids trickled over the back of the tongue in a premature fashion, and the recommendation is for the patient to use chin-on-chest posture for thin liquids. Because this requires treatment, a short-term goal is listed. Treatment objectives were selected from those designed to address aspiration before the swallow due to reduced tongue control (AB/tc).

Treatment objectives can address more than one short-term goal. When you list them on your treatment plan, you can use the code that applies to the main reason you chose that objective or you can list both codes. For example, in Case 6, the patient has significant vallecular and pyriform sinus residue. The compensatory treatment objective that "Patient will remain seated upright at 90° without cues for 30 minutes after any PO intake" was chosen to reduce risk of food falling from valleculae and pyriforms into the airway. Therefore, it could be coded as AA/v/tb-3 (related to the short-term goal to reduce risk of aspiration after the swallow from the valleculae due to decreased tongue base strength) and AA/p/le-5 (related to the short-term goal to reduce risk of aspiration after the swallow from the pyriforms due to reduced laryngeal elevation). It could even be coded AA/V/ppw-3 (related to the short-term goal to reduce the risk of aspiration after the swallow from the valleculae due to reduced movement of the posterior pharyngeal wall) if you thought that was the main reason for the vallecular residue.

The last two cases (Case 8 and Case 9) are of patients considered inappropriate for therapy. Those case studies show how the recommendations are based on selected findings.

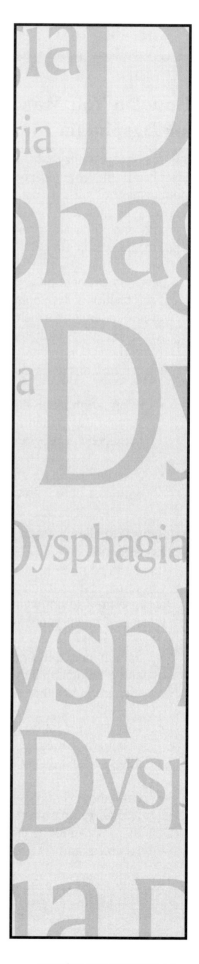

Case 1

History	acute cerebrovascular accident, primary brainstem hemorrhage secondary to hypertension
Long-Term Goal	Patient will be able to eat and drink without risk of aspiration pneumonia.
Short-Term Goal 11 (AB/tc)	Patient will improve back of tongue control to keep food from falling over the back of the tongue and into the airway.
Short-Term Goal 15 (AA/p/le)	Patient will increase laryngeal elevation to reduce residue in the pyriform sinus(es) and reduce risk of the residue falling into the airway after the swallow.
Short-Term Goal 16 (AA/p/hm)	Patient will increase anterior movement of the hypolaryngeal complex to reduce residue in the pyriform sinuses and reduce the risk of the residue falling into the airway after the swallow.
Short-Term Goal 18 (AA/lv/at)	Patient will improve arytenoid tipping/closure at entrance to airway to reduce penetration into the upper laryngeal vestibule to reduce the risk of the penetrated material being aspirated after the swallow.
Short-Term Goal 20 (AA/v/tb)	Patient will increase base of tongue movement to reduce vallecular residue (unilateral or bilateral) to reduce the risk of the residue being aspirated after the swallow.
Short-Term Goal 21 (AA/v/ppw)	Patient will increase movement of the posterior pharyngeal wall to reduce vallecular residue to reduce the risk of the residue being aspirated after the swallow.

Selected Findings: Symptoms and Physiology (Physiology shown in italics below)	Recommendations and Short-Term Goals Based on Findings	Treatment Objectives
Oral Preparatory Phase Patient is somewhat slow to masticate the cookie, but is able to form a good bolus.	any and all textures patient feels he can handle	
Oral Voluntary Phase If the patient isn't in a chin-down posture, thin liquids trickle over the back of the tongue in a premature fashion *due to decreased strength and control of back of tongue.*	chin-on-chest posture for all swallows (Short-Term Goal 11 - AB/tc) (Note: Sometimes it is easier for a patient to remember to use chin-down on all swallows than for selected textures only. This patient is aspirating only thin liquids, but later shows penetration of paste which could be eliminated with chin-down posture. Therefore, this patient should probably use chin-down for all consistencies.)	AB/tc-1 Patient will use chin-down posture for all consistencies without cues on 10 of 10 trials. (c) AB/tc-4 Patient will exert pressure with the back of tongue up against tongue depressor on 9 of 10 trials. (A helpful cue is to ask the patient to try to say a /k/.) (f) AB/tc-5 Patient will produce forceful /k/ at the end of words on 9 of 10 trials. (f)

Case **1**, *continued*

Selected Findings: Symptoms and Physiology (Physiology shown in italics below)	Recommendations and Short-Term Goals Based on Findings	Treatment Objectives
Pharyngeal Phase Bolus size 5cc with chin in neutral, aspirated small amount before the swallow without any reaction to this aspiration, confirming reduced back of tongue control.		
Significant vallecular residue after swallow indicating *reduced pressure from base of tongue and posterior pharyngeal wall*. Does not aspirate residue and clears some with multiple swallow, but amount of residue makes patient at risk to aspirate.	base of tongue exercises (Short-Term Goal 20 - AA/v/tb) and posterior pharyngeal wall exercises (Short-Term Goal 21 - AA/v/ppw) for better bolus propulsion through the hypopharynx to reduce vallecular residue	AA/v/tb-4 Patient will use multiple swallows with cues on 8 of 10 trials. (c) AA/v/tb-7 Patient will use effort swallow with/without cues on 8 of 10 trials. (c,f) AA/v/tb-9 Patient will demonstrate tongue base retraction on 8 of 10 trials. (f) AA/v/ppw-8 Patient will swallow saliva using tongue hold on 8 of 10 trials. (c)
Significant pyriform residue after the swallow due to *decreased laryngeal elevation and reduced anterior movement of hypolaryngeal complex*. At risk to aspirate.	laryngeal elevation exercises to eliminate pyriform sinus residue (Short-Term Goal 15 - AA/p/le). exercises to increase anterior movement of hypolaryngeal complex to reduce pyriform residue (Short-Term Goal 16 - AA/p/hm)	AA/p/le-6 Patient will use Mendelsohn maneuver for pudding consistencies with cues on 7 of 10 trials. (c,f) AA/p/le-8 Patient will produce /i/ in continuous fashion, including falsetto, on 10 of 10 trials. (f) AA/p/hm-7 Patient will perform head lift maneuver for 60 seconds on 2 of 2 trials. (f) AA/p/hm-8 Patient will perform 30 repetitive head lift maneuvers. (f)

Chapter 11
The Source for Dysphagia

264

Copyright © 2000 LinguiSystems, Inc.

Selected Findings: Symptoms and Physiology (Physiology shown in italics below)	Recommendations and Short-Term Goals Based on Findings	Treatment Objectives
Patient penetrated about 20% of the paste bolus during the swallow due to *limited closure at entrance to larynx.* He was able to cough on command and clear all material from his trachea. This penetration was eliminated with chin-down posture.	laryngeal entrance closure exercises to reduce penetration (Short-Term Goal 18 - AA/lv/at) (Note: You must decide whether a patient needs to use a technique some or all of the time as a compensation or in non-meal treatments as a facilitator. It was decided that since the patient could eliminate penetration with chin-down, it could be a simpler procedure to use at meals. The super-supraglottic will be used as a facilitator in treatment.)	AA/lv/at-4 Patient will use super-supraglottic swallow during treatment with cues on 9 of 10 trials. (f)
Effect of treatment strategies attempted: When the patient took uncontrolled amounts of thin liquid from a cup with chin-down posture, he eliminated most of the penetration and did eliminate all aspiration as a result of widening the valleculae and improving airway protection.	As a precaution, give 1 tsp. bolus size because patient continued to have some penetration with uncontrolled amounts.	AB/tc-2 Patient will control bolus size to teaspoon without cues on 10 of 10 trials. (c)
When using a straw, the patient aspirated small amounts before the swallow.	all liquids from cup; no straws	AB/tc-3 Patient will use a cup for all liquid intake without cues on 10 of 10 trials. (c)
Using a chin-down posture with paste significantly reduced the pooling in the valleculae and eliminated the aspiration and penetration. When using a good chin-down posture, a liquid wash helped to successfully clear most of the paste and there was no aspiration.	liquid wash okay with chin-down	AA/v/tb-5 Patient will use thin consistency liquid wash with chin-down to widen valleculae every several bites with cues on 9 of 10 trials. (c)

Case 2

History	Mild right CVA. History of prior right CVA. Wet vocal quality before, during, and after the initial bedside evaluation. Significant clinical signs of aspiration.
	Patient was reintubated secondary to increasing respiratory failure for seven days and had been extubated two days at time of this study.
	Breathy vocal quality, very wet quality after oatmeal, pureed fruit, and juice on bedside evaluation. She also coughed after oatmeal and pureed fruit. Patient has an NG tube in place.
Long-Term Goal	Patient will safely consume Level III diet with honey-thick liquids without complications such as aspiration pneumonia.
Short-Term Goal 7 (BP/tm)	Patient will increase tongue movement to improve the ability to move a bolus to the back of the mouth in a coordinated fashion to reduce the risk of it falling into the airway.
Short-Term Goal 13 (AD/lc)	Patient will increase closure of the true folds to keep food from falling into the airway during the swallow.
Short-Term Goal 20 (AA/v/tb)	Patient will increase base of tongue movement to reduce vallecular residue (unilateral or bilateral) to reduce the risk of the residue being aspirated after the swallow.

Selected Findings: Symptoms and Physiology (Physiology shown in italics below)	Recommendations and Short-Term Goals Based on Findings	Treatment Objectives
Oral Preparatory Phase Functional for the juice, honey-thick liquid, and paste; some difficulty with the cookie partly due to not wearing her dentures.		
Oral Voluntary Phase All consistencies trickle over the back of the tongue *due to mild weakness of back of tongue*.	sitting up at 90°; take small bites and sips	
There is only a small amount of trickle while most of the bolus remains in the oral cavity. Patient is not aspirating.	Note: Since this small amount of premature loss is not causing any functional problems, some recommendations are made as precaution only.	
Difficulty keeping the bolus in a cohesive fashion *due to reduced tongue movement*.	pureed — one regular vegetable to try chewing with dentures with SLP present (Short-Term Goal 7 - BP/tm)	BP/tm-6 Patient will move lemon swab placed between tongue and hard palate from front to back on 10 of 10 trials. (f)

Selected Findings: Symptoms and Physiology (Physiology shown in italics below)	Recommendations and Short-Term Goals Based on Findings	Treatment Objectives
		BP/tm-7 Patient will sweep tongue from alveolar ridge to junction of hard and soft palate on 9 of 10 trials. (f)
		BP/tm-11 Patient will eat only pureed and soft cohesive foods without cues on 10 of 10 trials. (d)
Pharyngeal Phase Shows aspiration of 10% of the bolus during the swallow with an immediate cough reaction with thin liquids.	laryngeal closure exercises (Short-Term Goal 13 - AD/lc). If voice is still breathy in a week to 10 days, ENT consult re: vocal fold closure*	AD/lc-6 Patient will use supra-glottic swallow for saliva consistencies with cues on 10 of 10 trials. (f)
		AD/lc-7 Patient will demonstrate Valsalva maneuver (breath hold) on 10 of 10 trials. (f)
Aspiration of 10% of the honey bolus during the swallow with no reaction when the aspiration occurred.		
Aspirates 10% of the paste bolus during the swallow with no reaction. *All due to reduced laryngeal closure.*		
Shows *reduced base of tongue pressure* which results in significant vallecular residue after the swallow which then trickles down to the pyriforms.	exercises to increase tongue base strength (Short-Term Goal 20 - AA/v/tb)	AA/v/tb-4 Patient will use multiple swallows without cues on 7 of 10 trials. (c)
		AA/v/tb-7 Patient will use effort swallow with cues on 9 of 10 trials. (f)
		AA/v/tb-9 Patient will demonstrate tongue base retraction on 10 of 10 trials. (f)

* Would presume at this point that decreased laryngeal closure is secondary to intubation. Primary physician usually prefers to wait two weeks after extubation before consulting ENT.

Selected Findings: Symptoms and Physiology (Physiology shown in italics below)	Recommendations and Short-Term Goals Based on Findings	Treatment Objectives
A-P View Revealed symmetrical pooling in the valleculae but slightly more pooling in the left pyriform. Asymmetrical movement of the vocal cords to midline with the left cord perhaps moving less than the right. **Effect of Treatment Strategies Attempted** After the A-P view revealed what appeared to be reduced movement of the left vocal fold to midline, patient was tried with head rotation to the left. It appeared the patient swallowed honey and paste in small amounts without aspiration, but aspiration of thin liquids continued with compensatory techniques.	thick liquids — moderate thick (honey); vegetables should be drained well since patient cannot safely take thin liquids; pills/tablets whole followed by thickened liquid or meds via tube; head turned to left encourage coughing Other: hold tube feedings prior to meals to increase appetite; MBS before advancing diet since patient often silently aspirates.	AD/lc-4 Patient will use head rotation to left for all swallows with cues on 10 of 10 trials. (c) AD/lc-8 Patient will take only liquids of honey consistency with cues on 10 of 10 trials. (d) AD/lc-9 Patient will avoid foods in liquid base with cues on 10 of 10 trials. (d)

268

Case 3

History	History of TIAs. Mild-moderate senile dementia, arteriosclerotic cardiovascular disease. Patient does not feed self. Coughing especially on liquids.
Long-Term Goal	Patient will safely consume Level V diet with thin liquids without complications such as aspiration pneumonia.
Short-Term Goal 13 (AD/lc)	Patient will compensate for decreased closure of true folds to keep food from falling into the airway during the swallow. (Note: Since treatment for this patient will involve compensating for the deficits and not trying to improve function, the wording of the short-term goal has been modified.)

Selected Findings: Symptoms and Physiology (Physiology shown in italics below)	Recommendations and Short-Term Goals Based on Findings	Treatment Objectives
Oral Preparatory Phase Within functional limits for all textures.	regular diet	
Oral Voluntary Phase Within functional limits.		
Pharyngeal Phase The initial presentations of thin liquids in 3cc and 5cc from a spoon were swallowed without difficulty. The reflex initiates adequately and there is no penetration or aspiration. However, patient took 10cc bolus from a cup during the swallow with an immediate cough reaction to the aspiration when it occurred. This appears to be due to *reduced ability to achieve laryngeal closure*. Patient was allowed to try 10cc from a straw and showed penetration on one trial and aspiration on the next. When the patient took controlled amounts from a straw, he showed aspiration on 1 of 3 trials. Syrup-thick liquids are swallowed without penetration or aspiration even in large amounts.	thin liquids in small sips from spoon to eliminate penetration (Short-Term Goal 13 - AD/lc) (Note: Patient does not feed himself. If he did, the Rolyan Millicup might be a good way to control size.)	AD/lc-1 Patient will control bolus size to one teaspoon with cues on 10 of 10 trials. (c) AD/lc-3 Patient will use spoon for liquid presentations with cues on 10 of 10 trials. (c)

Case 3, *continued*

Selected Findings: Symptoms and Physiology (Physiology shown in italics below)	Recommendations and Short-Term Goals Based on Findings	Treatment Objectives
A-P View Patient appears to exhibit bilateral movement of the vocal folds to midline, but adequacy of closure cannot be assessed.	ENT evaluation for more complete assessment of vocal fold closure probably not indicated because patient would not be able to follow therapeutic exercises. Laryngeal closure exercises are not recommended because patient can't readily follow directions.	
Effect of Treatment Strategies Attempted Syrup-thick - patient able to take uncontrolled amounts without aspiration or penetration. Chin-down posture with uncontrolled thin liquids does not eliminate aspiration.		
Patient is not very reliable at controlling the bolus size on his own. He can take uncontrolled amounts of syrup from a cup or straw without penetration or aspiration.	If patient isn't supervised for bolus size, consider keeping him on syrup-thick liquids.	AD/lc-8 Patient will take only liquids of syrup consistency without cues on 10 of 10 trials. (d)

Case 4

History	Difficulty tolerating her own secretions. Exhibited cough and continued wet vocal quality. Strangled on thin liquids presentations. Recent onset cerebrovascular accident, past history of multiple cerebrovascular accidents, but was eating regular diet.
Long-Term Goal 1	Patient will safely consume Diet Level II pudding-thick liquids without complications such as aspiration pneumonia. (Note: Too early to determine if Long-Term Goal 1 or possibly only 4, will be appropriate, but we are aiming for #1.)
Long-Term Goal 4	Patient will maintain nutrition/hydration via alternative means.
Short-Term Goal 5 (BF/tm)	Patient will increase tongue movement to improve the ability to put food and liquid into a cohesive bolus to reduce the risk of food falling into the airway.
Short-Term Goal 6 (BF/tc)	The tone in patient's cheek(s) will increase to improve the ability to put food and liquid into a cohesive bolus to reduce the risk of food residue falling into the airway.
Short-Term Goal 7 (BP/tm)	Patient will increase tongue movement to improve the ability to move a bolus to the back of the mouth in a coordinated fashion to reduce the risk of it falling into the airway.
Short-Term Goal 11 (AB/tc)	Patient will improve back of tongue control to keep food from falling over the back of the tongue and into the airway.
Short-Term Goal 12 (AB/dr)	Patient will decrease delay in initiation of pharyngeal swallow to reduce food falling into the airway during the delay before the swallow.
Short-Term Goal 15 (AA/p/le)	Patient will increase laryngeal elevation to reduce residue in the pyriform sinsus(es) and reduce risk of the residue falling into the airway after the swallow.

Selected Findings: Symptoms and Physiology (Physiology shown in italics below)	Recommendations and Short-Term Goals Based on Findings	Treatment Objectives
Difficulty tolerating her own secretions.	cue patient to clear wet vocal quality, frequent suctioning, aggressive oral care	BF/tm-9 Patient will click tongue against roof of mouth on 7 of 10 trials. (f)
Oral Preparatory Phase Decreased ability to adequately form a bolus within the oral cavity on all liquid presentations *due to limited tongue movement and decreased tone in cheeks*.	increase strength and accuracy of tongue movements to better form bolus (Short-Term Goal 5 - BF/tm)	BF/tm-11 Patient will push blade of tongue upward against tongue depressor on 7 of 10 trials. (f)
		BF/tm-12 Patient will push right and left lateral border of tongue against tongue depressor on 7 of 10 trials. (f)

Selected Findings: Symptoms and Physiology (Physiology shown in italics below)	Recommendations and Short-Term Goals Based on Findings	Treatment Objectives
	increase tone in cheeks for better bolus formation (Short-Term Goal 6 - BF/tc)	BF/tc-6 Patient will produce "oo" and then "ee" with exaggerated lip movement on 7 of 10 trials. (f) BF/tc-7 Patient will pucker lips, then move from side to side on 7 of 10 trials. (f)
Oral Voluntary Phase Some premature trickle over back of tongue while manipulating bolus secondary to *reduced strength of back of tongue.*	back of tongue exercises (Short-Term Goal 11 - AB/tc)	AB/tc-5 Patient will produce a forceful /k/ at the end of words on 8 of 10 trials. (f)
Piecemeal deglutition requiring two or three attempts to adequately clear the oral cavity. Patient *has reduced tongue strength.*	lingual exercises to improve bolus propulsion (Short-Term Goal 7 - BP/tm)	BP/tm-6 Patient will move lemon swab placed between tongue and hard palate from front to back on 10 of 10 trials. (f) BP/tm-7 Patient will sweep tongue from alveolar ridge to junction of hard and soft palate on 9 of 10 trials. (f) BP/tm-8 Patient will pop tongue against hard palate on 10 of 10 trials. (f)
Pharyngeal Phase Patient pushes bolus to valleculae and it falls to pyriforms with 3-5 second *delay* before patient swallows. Aspiration of a trace to approximately 25% of every bolus amount before the swallow from valleculae and pyriforms (as soon as patient begins the swallow)	increase speed of initiation of onset of swallow (Short-Term Goal 12 - AB/dr)	AB/dr-5 (a) Patient will decrease length of time from command to swallow to onset of swallow from 5 seconds to 1 second following thermal-tactile application on 7 of 10 trials. (c,f) AB/dr-5 (b) Patient will decrease length of time from command to swallow to onset of swallow from 5 seconds to 1 second following neurosensory stimulation on 7 of 10 trials. (c,f)

Selected Findings: Symptoms and Physiology (Physiology shown in italics below)	Recommendations and Short-Term Goals Based on Findings	Treatment Objectives
During second swallow, patient aspirated the residue from the pyriform sinuses and coughed in response to the aspiration; *residue is present because of reduced laryngeal elevation.*	increase laryngeal elevation to reduce amount of pyriform residue (Short-Term Goal 15 - AA/p/le)	AA/p/le-6 Patient will use Mendelsohn maneuver for saliva without cues on 7 of 10 trials. (f) AA/p/le-7 Patient will use super-supraglottic swallow for saliva without cues on 7 of 10 trials. (c,f) AA/p/le-8 Patient will produce /i/ in continuous fashion, including falsetto, on 8 of 10 trials. (f) AA/p/le-9 Patient will increase laryngeal elevation via SEMG biofeedback on 10 of 10 trials. (f)
Effect of Treatment Strategies Attempted Chin-down position did not increase airway protection, therefore aspiration of all materials continued. Head rotation to reduce pyriform sinus residue was not helpful. Patient had attempted to perform Mendelsohn at bedside during indirect dysphagic therapy and was unable to coordinate the sequences with dry swallows, so it was not attempted with PO swallows.	NPO; remove water pitcher repeat MBS prior to trying diet since patient is aspirating significant amounts	

Case 5

History	Massive CVA with anoxic brain damage. Patient is apraxic. Unable to follow commands. Bedside evaluation swallowed 90% of trials after oral stimulation. Fed by NG only since the CVA 2 months prior to this evaluation.
Long-Term Goal	Patient's quality of life will be enhanced through eating and drinking small amounts of food and liquid.
Short-Term Goal 2 (AL/lc)	Patient will improve lip closure to reduce anterior loss to keep food and liquid in the mouth while eating.
Short-Term Goal 5 (BF/tm)	Patient will increase tongue movement to improve the ability to put food and liquid into a cohesive bolus to reduce the risk of food falling into the airway.
Short-Term Goal 7 (BP/tm)	Patient will increase tongue movement to improve the ability to move a bolus to the back of the mouth in a coordinated fashion to reduce the risk of it falling into the airway.
Short-Term Goal 12 (AB/dr)	Patient will decrease delay in initiation of pharyngeal swallow to reduce food falling into the airway during the delay before the swallow.

Selected Findings: Symptoms and Physiology (Physiology shown in italics below)	Recommendations and Short-Term Goals Based on Findings	Treatment Objectives
Oral Preparatory Phase At times the patient was asked to hold the spoon in his hand to make the presentation since apraxia seems to be a major problem. He exhibits extremely poor lip closure with most material running out the right side of the mouth.	lip closure exercises (Short-Term Goal 2 - AL/lc) Note: Though patient has a difficult time performing oral movements secondary to apraxia, this is chosen as a goal to address major labial weakness.	AL/lc-2 Patient will achieve lip closure around object (Lifesaver on string, Popsicle, ice cube) for 6 seconds on 8 of 10 trials. (f) AL/lc-3 Patient will achieve lip closure against resistance provided by clinician placing fingers on upper and lower lips on 10 of 10 trials. (f) AL/lc-4 Patient will pucker lips (as if to blow a kiss) on 8 of 10 trials. (f) AL/lc-7 Patient will hold tongue depressor between closed lips (not teeth) for count of 10 on 7 of 10 trials. (f) AL/lc-8 Patient will grin (retracting corners of lips) as wide as possible without showing teeth on 8 of 10 trials. (f)

Selected Findings: Symptoms and Physiology (Physiology shown in italics below)	Recommendations and Short-Term Goals Based on Findings	Treatment Objectives
Oral Preparatory Phase, *cont.* Patient does not form a bolus with any of the materials presented, but lets them fall into the anterior and right lateral sulcus. He has some *tongue weakness*.	improve coordination of tongue movements (Short-Term Goal 5 - BF/tm)	BF/tm-8 Patient will push up with back of tongue against tongue depressor on 7 of 10 trials. (A helpful cue is to ask patient to try to make a /k/.) (f) BF/tm-9 Patient will click tongue against roof of mouth on 7 of 10 trials. (f) BF/tm-10 Patient will push tongue tip out against tongue depressor on 7 of 10 trials. (f) BF/tm-11 Patient will push blade of tongue upward against tongue depressor on 7 of 10 trials. (f)
Oral Voluntary Phase No coordinated anterior to posterior movement with the tongue to move the bolus back. The *tongue weakness* interferes, but *discoordination* is a major problem. The thin liquid bolus finally falls over the back of the tongue in an uncontrolled manner. With the other materials, the patient never propels any significant amount posteriorly.	improve tongue movement (Short-Term Goal 7 - BP/tm) Note: Short-Term Goal 8 to improve oral coordination involves only compensation and diet treatment objectives. Because this patient is being kept NPO, this goal will have to be deferred.	BP/tm-6 Patient will move lemon swab placed between tongue and hard palate from front to back on 6 of 10 trials. (f)

Case 5, *continued*

Selected Findings: Symptoms and Physiology (Physiology shown in italics below)	Recommendations and Short-Term Goals Based on Findings	Treatment Objectives
Pharyngeal Phase Thin liquids - Patient aspirated 50% of thin liquids before the swallow with an immediate cough reaction when the aspiration occurred. Pudding — able to propel only small amount over the back of the tongue. Penetrated a very small amount of food before the swallow. Patient probably aspirated at a later time from residue in upper laryngeal vestibule. **Effect of Treatment Strategies Attempted** An attempt was made to use a towel roll to place the patient in a chin-down posture and present more thin liquid. However, in this position, he lost all of the bolus anteriorly due to severe lip closure problems. **Summary** Patient has profound oral dysphagia, losing most of each bolus anteriorly and into sulci. When part of a bolus falls over the back of the tongue prematurely, the patient aspirates 50% of the bolus during the swallow. It is difficult to determine how much the pharyngeal component is actually involved.	Note: It is difficult to determine if patient actually has a delayed swallow or is simply unprepared for the swallow since the voluntary component is absent. Will treat as if it is a delay. (Short-Term Goal 12 - AB/dr) Patient should remain NPO. Proceed with PEG placement since NG tube has already been in over 8 weeks and prognosis for a rapid return to PO feeding is not good. Attempt oral stimulation and work on bolus formation and manipulation without presenting food to the patient. Repeat MBS before trying any PO.	AB/dr-5 (a) Patient will decrease length of time from command to swallow to onset of swallow from 5 seconds to 2 seconds following sour bolus (lemon swab) on 9 of 10 trials. (f) AB/dr-5 (b) Patient will decrease length of time from command to swallow to onset of swallow from 5 seconds to 2 seconds following thermal-tactile stimulation on 9 of 10 trials. (f)

Case 6

History	Essential tremor. Two recent hospitalizations for pneumonia. Previous MBS study four days prior revealed severe pharyngeal dysphagia characterized by aspiration of thin liquids during and after the swallow. Syrup-thick liquids were aspirated after the swallow. Severe risk for aspiration of paste after the swallow because of significant residue caused by reduced laryngeal elevation due to the patient's significantly decreased strength overall.
	It was recommended that the patient remain NPO and a PEG tube was to be placed, but physician reported patient seemed much stronger and requested we repeat this study before the tube was placed.
Long-Term Goal	Patient will be able to eat foods and liquids with more normal consistency.
Short-Term Goal 11 (AB/tc)	Patient will improve back of tongue control to keep food from falling over the back of the tongue and into the airway.
Short-Term Goal 14 (AD/mc)	Patient will improve rate of laryngeal elevation/timing of closure to keep food from falling into the airway during the swallow.
Short-Term Goal 15 (AA/p/le)	Patient will increase laryngeal elevation to reduce residue in the pyriform sinus(es) and reduce risk of the residue falling into the airway after the swallow.
Short-Term Goal 20 (AA/v/tb)	Patient will increase base of tongue movement to reduce bilateral vallecular residue to reduce the risk of the residue being aspirated after the swallow.
Short-Term Goal 21 (AA/v/ppw)	Patient will increase movement of the posterior pharyngeal wall to reduce vallecular residue to reduce the risk of the residue being aspirated after the swallow.

Selected Findings: Symptoms and Physiology (Physiology shown in italics below)	Recommendations and Short-Term Goals Based on Findings	Treatment Objectives
Oral Preparatory Phase Weakness and some decreased speed in forming a bolus, but patient is able to form a bolus with each material.	mechanical soft - ground	
Oral Voluntary Phase Some premature movement of thin liquid bolus over back of tongue *due to weakness*.	improve back of tongue control (Short-Term Goal 11)	AB/tc-4 Patient will exert pressure with back of tongue up against tongue depressor on 8 of 10 trials. (f) AB/tc-5 Patient will produce forceful /k/ at the end of words on 8 of 10 trials. (f)

Case 6, *continued*

Selected Findings: Symptoms and Physiology (Physiology shown in italics below)	Recommendations and Short-Term Goals Based on Findings	Treatment Objectives
Pharyngeal Phase Thin liquids — bolus falls over the back of the tongue *(due to weak back of tongue)* to valleculae and pyriforms, but then the reflex initiates in adequate time. Once the bolus size reaches 10cc, patient begins to aspirate before the swallow as the bolus falls over the back of the tongue and the *initiation of the swallow is mistimed.* Totally asymptomatic with this aspiration. Significant vallecular and pyriform sinus residue after the swallow *related to reduced base of tongue to posterior pharyngeal wall and reduced laryngeal elevation respectively.*	thin liquids in teaspoon amounts; no thin liquids at meals since patient probably can't handle thin liquids when pyriforms are full of other material; needs to improve timing of initiation of swallow (Short-Term Goal 14 - AD/mc)	AB/tc-2 Patient will control bolus size to thin liquids on teaspoon without cues on 10 of 10 trials. (c) AB/tc-7 Patient will avoid foods in liquid base without cues on 10 of 10 trials. (d) AD/mc-5 Patient will use super-supraglottic swallow for saliva with cues on 10 of 10 trials. (f)
Honey — minimal penetration but never any aspiration	moderate thick (honey) liquids with meals	
Vallecular residue and pyriform sinus residue due to *decreased laryngeal elevation and decreased base of tongue to pharyngeal wall pressure.*	laryngeal elevation exercises (Short-Term Goal 15 - AA/p/le)	AA/p/le-6 Patient will use Mendelsohn maneuver for paste consistencies with cues on 8 of 10 trials. (c,f) AA/p/le-8 Patient will produce /i/ in continuous fashion, including falsetto, on 8 of 10 trials. (f)
	increase base of tongue strength (Short-Term Goal 20 - AA/v/tb)	AA/v/tb-3 (or AA/p/le-5 or AA/v/ppw-3) Patient will remain seated upright at 90° without cues for 30 minutes after any PO intake. (c)

Selected Findings: Symptoms and Physiology (Physiology shown in italics below)	Recommendations and Short-Term Goals Based on Findings	Treatment Objectives
Paste — significant valleculae and pyriform sinus residue *due to decreased base of tongue to posterior pharyngeal wall pressure*		AA/v/tb-7 Patient will use effort swallow with cues on 10 of 10 trials. (c,f) AA/v/tb-9 Patient will demonstrate tongue base retraction on 8 of 10 trials. (f)
	increase posterior pharyngeal wall movement (Short-Term Goal 21 - AA/v/ppw)	AA/v/ppw-8 Patient will swallow saliva using tongue hold on 8 of 10 trials. (f)
Cookie — no new residue		
Effect of Treatment Strategies Attempted Second swallow spontaneously helped clear a lot of the material out of the pyriforms. Honey-thick liquid wash paired with the second or third swallow helped clear most of the residue. Chin-down posture with thin liquids did not eliminate the aspiration.	alternate honey liquid swallows every several bites; multiple swallows — needs cues to swallow 2-3 times	AA/p/le-1 Patient will alternate honey consistency liquid wash every several bites(s) with cues on 8 of 10 trials. (c) AA/p/le-2 Patient will use multiple swallows for each bite without cues on 10 of 10 trials. (c) AD/mc-7 Patient will only take liquids of honey consistency with cues on 8 of 10 trials. (d)

279

Case 7

History	Etiology unknown at time of evaluation. Migrating neck pain for the past two months and occipital headaches. Later determined to be a brain tumor.
Long-Term Goal 1	Patient will maintain nutrition/hydration via alternative means.
Long-Term Goal 2	Patient will be able to eat foods and liquids with more normal consistency.
Short-Term Goal 5 (BF/tm)	Patient will increase tongue movement to improve the ability to put food and liquid into a cohesive bolus to reduce the risk of food falling into the airway.
Short-Term Goal 7 (BP/tm)	Patient will increase tongue movement to improve the ability to move a bolus to the back of the mouth in a coordinated fashion to reduce the risk of it falling into the airway.
Short-Term Goal 12 (AB/dr)	Patient will decrease delay in initiation of pharyngeal swallow to reduce food falling into the airway during the delay before the swallow.

Selected Findings: Symptoms and Physiology (Physiology shown in italics below)	Recommendations and Short-Term Goals Based on Findings	Treatment Objectives
Oral Preparatory Phase Unable to manipulate a bolus; little to no tongue movement.	improve tongue movement for bolus formation and propulsion (Short-Term Goal 5 - BF/tm & Short-Term Goal 7 - BP/tm)	BF/tm-7 Patient will protrude tongue to try to touch the chin and nose with tongue tip on 6 of 10 trials. (f) BF/tm-8 Patient will push up with back of tongue against tongue depressor on 6 of 10 trials. (f) BF/tm-10 Patient will push tongue tip out against tongue depressor on 6 of 10 trials. (f)
Oral Voluntary Phase Patient tips head back to help propel the bolus posteriorly; able to propel it over the back of the tongue.		BP/tm-6 Patient will move lemon swab placed between tongue and hard palate from front to back on 6 of 10 trials. (f) BP/tm-8 Patient will pop tongue against hard palate on 5 of 10 trials. (f)

Selected Findings: Symptoms and Physiology (Physiology shown in italics below)	Recommendations and Short-Term Goals Based on Findings	Treatment Objectives
Pharyngeal Phase The initial bolus fell over the back of the tongue to valleculae and pyriform sinuses and remained there for greater than 30 seconds with *no noticeable elicitation of a swallow reflex*. There was no notable laryngeal closure or elevation despite the patient's tongue pumping and apparent repeated efforts to try to elicit a swallow reflex. Very small amounts of the bolus passed through the cricopharyngeus without any further superior or anterior movement of larynx.	Patient should remain NPO as he is at severe risk for aspiration. Because part of the problem appears to be severe delay and/ or lack of initiation of the swallowing reflex, techniques to elicit a swallow should be applied several times a day by Speech-Language Pathology and patient and family trained in technique. (Short-Term Goal 12 - AB/dr)	AB/dr-5 (a) Patient will decrease length of time from command to swallow to onset of swallow from 30 seconds to 10 seconds following thermal-tactile stimulation on 6 of 10 trials. (f) AB/dr-5 (b) Patient will decrease length of time from command to swallow to onset of swallow from 30 seconds to 10 seconds following neurosensory stimulation on 6 of 10 trials. (f) AB/dr-5 (c) Patient will decrease length of time from command to swallow to onset of swallow from 30 seconds to 10 seconds following suck-swallow on 6 of 10 trials. (f)

Case 8

| | History | Multi-infarct dementia. Recent respiratory arrest. Pureed diet with extra-thick liquids. Patient eats only 25% of her meal. Swallow reflex is delayed by 6 seconds and often up to 10+ seconds. Wet vocal quality. |

History   Multi-infarct dementia. Recent respiratory arrest. Pureed diet with extra-thick liquids. Patient eats only 25% of her meal. Swallow reflex is delayed by 6 seconds and often up to 10+ seconds. Wet vocal quality.

Long-Term Goal   Patient will maintain nutrition/hydration via alternative means.

Selected Findings: Symptoms and Physiology (Physiology shown in italics below)	Recommendations and Short-Term Goals Based on Findings	Treatment Objectives
Oral Preparatory Phase Significant anterior loss may not be due to poor oral prep skills but may be due instead to the fact that the patient is trying to avoid taking this material.		
Oral Pharyngeal Phase Each bolus falls over the back of the tongue in a premature fashion.		
Pharyngeal Phase Pharyngeal dysphagia with aspiration of thin liquid before, during, and after the swallow. The patient has *severely limited laryngeal elevation and closure* during the swallow. She aspirates thicker materials after the swallow from severe residue in the pyriforms. She is only *inconsistently able to elicit a swallow reflex* and then it is very weak at best.	This patient is not safe for any PO intake.	
Effect of Treatment Strategies Attempted She cannot elicit a second dry swallow on command. Postural changes did not eliminate the aspiration. Cognitive status precluded the consistent and reliable use of any other techniques.	There do not appear to be any textures or positions in which the patient can take these textures without severe aspiration. Patient might be best served by placement of a PEG tube. This would be preferred over an NG tube since the prognosis for any return to eating by mouth is extremely poor. Should patient and/or family decline a tube, they must understand that this patient will continue to aspirate and experience subsequent pulmonary complications such as aspiration pneumonia.	

Case 9

History	Parkinson's disease, multi-infarct dementia. Bedside evaluation revealed no oral movement, premature spill, and drooling. Severe choking episode. Currently on pureed and thickened liquids.

Selected Findings: Symptoms and Physiology (Physiology shown in italics below)	Recommendations and Short-Term Goals Based on Findings	Treatment Objectives
Oral Preparatory Phase Patient bunched his tongue and did not allow for presentation of thin liquids via spoon although several attempts were made. Presentation was then made via syringe* to try to bypass the oral phase, but patient still would not allow material to move over the back of his tongue. This material fell to the floor of the patient's mouth and remained there despite repeated verbal cues to swallow. **Pharyngeal Phase** This phase was not observed as the patient never initiated any posterior movement of the bolus.	Patient is a poor candidate for PO. It is not known whether he will aspirate because the pharyngeal stage could not be observed. It appears that the patient has totally forgotten how to manipulate and swallow a bolus. Family and physician need to discuss whether the patient should have G-tube placed or be maintained on fluids only per IV at this time. No treatment is indicated as the dysphagia is probably progressive in nature secondary to the severe dementia.	

* Some patients in Skilled Nursing Facilities are fed by syringe, although this is almost always contraindicated. However, since using syringes is the practice of some facilities, it's helpful to document what happens under fluoroscopy. Also, there is a rare patient with poor oral skills who has adequate pharyngeal phase and can swallow safely if material reaches pharyngeal phase.

Glossary

achalasia — failure of the smooth muscle fibers to relax at the top of the stomach resulting in food backing up

advance directive — a legal paper which allows a patient to state wishes about the use of life-support machines and medical treatment; also used to name someone else to make medical choices for the patient

albumin — a protein found in the blood; known as serum albumin

anticholinergics — blocking the passage of impulses through the parasympathetic nerves

antidepressants — effective against depressive illness

antihistamines — substances capable of counteracting the effects of histamine

antihypertensives — agents that prevent or relieve high blood pressure

arrhythmia — a variation from the normal heartbeat

atelectasis — incomplete expansion or collapse of pulmonary alveoli, or of a segment or lobe or lobes of the lung

beneficence — performing kind acts (principle of ethics)

bolus tube feeding — tube feeding given in a concentrated dose rather than spread out on a slower drip over time

BUN (blood urea nitrogen)/creatinine ratio — the ratio of urea nitrogen to creatinine found in the blood; the ratio provides a rough estimate of kidney function; an extremely high ratio of BUN to creatinine may indicate dehydration

cervical auscultation — in swallowing, generally describes listening with a stethoscope over the larynx for breath sounds during swallowing

cervical osteophyte — a bony growth on the anterior part of the cervical spine that protrudes into the esophagus

chronic obstructive pulmonary disease — a general term describing any obstructive breathing problem

cuffed trach tube — a tracheostomy tube with a cuff that can be inflated; the cuff rests below the vocal cords and serves as an anchor in the trachea

Current Procedural Terminology (CPT) — billing codes approved by the American Medical Association

deglutition — the oral, oral voluntary, and pharyngeal stages of swallowing

dehydration — a condition in which a patient is not getting enough fluids to keep cells hydrated

diuretics — medicines that stimulate the flow of urine

duodenum — the first part of the small intestine

dyspnea	shortness of breath
edema	swelling caused by an abnormal accumulation of fluid in the intercellular spaces
edentulous	without teeth
endoscope	a tubular instrument which usually has a light source that can be inserted into a body cavity to permit visualizing the interior
erythrocytes	mature red blood cells
esophageal reflux	as opposed to gastroesophageal reflux in which the contents of the stomach move up into the esophagus, esophageal reflux is generally used to mean that food remains in the esophagus and then moves back up toward the proximal esophagus
Fiberoptic Endoscopic Evaluation of Swallowing (FEES®)	a procedure in which an endoscope is passed transnasally into the pharynx for assessment of swallowing
gastroesophageal reflux	movement of the contents of the stomach up and out of the stomach into the esophagus
GER or GERD	gastroesophageal reflux or gastroesophageal reflux disease
GI	gastrointestinal; pertaining to the stomach and intestines
globus	feeling of fullness or sensation of a lump in the throat
gram negative bacilli	a type of bacteria found in the mouth
hematocrit	a lab value that reflects the amount of erythrocytes in a given volume of blood
infiltrate (pulmonary infiltrates)	indicates that some substance has passed into the lungs and is viewed on x-ray; does not necessarily mean that it is an aspirated substance
intubation	inserting a breathing tube through the larynx into the trachea to attach the patient to a ventilator
jejunum	the second part of the small intestine between the duodenum and the ilium
maleficence	harm or causing harm
malnutrition	the patient is not getting enough food to maintain adequate health or the patient's body may not be able to absorb and distribute the nutrition the patient is receiving
nasal cannula	small tubing that carries oxygen directly into the nose
neoplasm	tumor
neuroleptic drugs	drugs prescribed to treat psychotic behavior
nonmaleficence	do no harm to the patient (principle of ethics)
nosocomial pneumonia	pneumonia acquired in a health care facility

NPO	nothing by mouth
odynophagia	pain or a feeling of obstruction on swallowing
orthostatic blood pressure	blood pressure taken in an upright position
parenteral	any feeding route other than the digestive tract; can be used to describe intravenous, subcutaneous, intramuscular, or mucosal
parenteral nutrition	a patient's total caloric needs are being met by intravenous route (A deep line is surgically placed into the subclavian artery and nutrition in a clear solution is delivered directly into a chamber of the heart; sometimes called total parenteral nutrition [TPN] or parenteral hyperlimantation.)
paternalism	caring for people in a paternalistic way (i.e., making decisions for them)
patulous	distended
peristalsis	a wave-like progression of contraction and relaxation of muscle fibers in the esophagus
protein calorie malnutrition	the patient is malnourished in both calories and protein
rale	abnormal respiratory sound
reflux	see gastroesophageal reflux
rhonchi	coarse, dry rales in the bronchial tubes
sensitivity	accuracy identifying patients who have a particular characteristic
serum osmolality	a measure of particle concentration in the blood; a high osmolality may indicate dehydration
specificity	accuracy ruling out patients who do not have a particular characteristic
tardive dyskenesia	a form of hyperkinetic dysarthria that may develop after prolonged use of neuroleptic drugs
UGI (Upper GI)	a videofluoroscopic study of the lower (distal) esophagus, stomach, and the stomach emptying into the small intestine
upper esophageal sphincter	sphincter at the top of the esophagus formed by the cricopharyngeus
valleculae	depression created between base of tongue and epiglottis
Valsalva maneuver	trying to exhale forcefully while tightly closing the glottis; increases intrathoracic pressure
wheeze	whistling, respiratory sound

Resources

AliMed
297 High St.
Dedham, MA 02026-9135
800-225-2610
FAX: 800-437-2966
www.dysphagiatherapy.com
✓ variety of educational materials
   for SLPs and patients

Bernard Food Industries, Inc.
1125 Hartrey Ave.
Evanston, IL 60202
800-323-3663
FAX: 800-962-1546
www.bernardfoods.com
✓ variety of prepared food products

Bruce Medical Supply
411 Waverly Oaks Rd.
Dept. 10242
Waltham, MA 02154-9166
800-225-8446
FAX: 781-894-9519
✓ variety of food thickeners
✓ Menu Magic

Cliffdale Farms
181 Kelly Road
Quakertown, PA 18951
800-887-1553
FAX: 215-529-7409
www.cliffdale.com
✓ prepackaged foods with
   modified consistency

Diamond Crystal Brands, Inc.
(formerly Menu Magic Foods, Inc.)
43 W. 62nd St.
Indianapolis, IN 46268
800-732-5805
FAX: 317-216-2150
✓ NutraThik

Hormel Health Labs
(formerly American Institutional
Products, Inc.)
P.O. Box 800
Austin, MN 55912
800-866-7757
FAX: 507-437-9815
www.thickandeasy.com
✓ prepared food products

Imaginart
307 Arizona St.
Bisbee, AZ 85603
800-828-1376
FAX: 800-737-1376
www.imaginartonline.com
✓ laryngeal mirrors
✓ dysphagia supplies
✓ variety of educational materials

MenuDirect Corp.
865 Centennial Ave.
Piscataway, NJ 08854
888-MENU123 (636-8123)
FAX: 732-980-6770
www.menudirect.com
✓ variety of prepackaged
   consistency-modified foods

National Center for Treatment Effectiveness in Communication Disorders
ASHA
10801 Rockville Pike
Rockville, MD 20852
301-897-5700, ext. 9265
nctecd@asha.org
✓ ASHA NOMS

Northern Speech Services, Inc. & National Rehabilitation Services, Inc.
117 N. Elm St.
P.O. Box 1247
Gaylord, MI 49735
888-337-3866
FAX: 517-732-6164
www.nss-nrs.com
✓ variety of educational
   materials on dysphagia

Novartis Nutrition
Nutrition Dept.
445 State St.
Fremont, MI 49413-0001
800-777-8103
FAX: 888-828-2977
www.novartis.com
✓ variety of food thickeners

Posey Company
5635 Peck Rd.
Arcadia, CA 91006-0020
800-44-POSEY (447-6739)
FAX: 800-767-3933
www.posey.com
✓ manometer

Precision/Milani Foods Division
2150 N. 15th Ave.
Melrose Park, IL 60160
800-333-0003
FAX: 708-216-0709
www.precisionfoods.com
✓ Diafoods Thick-It
✓ modified food products

Smith & Nephew, Inc. — Rehabilitation Division
One Quality Dr.
P.O. Box 1005
Germantown, WI 53022-8205
800-558-8633
FAX: 800-545-7758
www.easy-living.com
✓ Rolyan Millicup

STERIS Corp. - Capital Equipment Group
(formerly Hausted, Inc.)
5960 Heisley Rd.
Mentor, OH 44060
800-428-7833
FAX: 440-639-4450
✓ modified chairs

The Triad Group
600 Perkins Dr.
Mukwonago, WI 53149
800-288-1288
FAX: 414-363-6933
www.hptriad.com
✓ lemon glycerine swabs

Vess Chairs, Inc.
9036 W. Schlinger Ave.
West Allis, WI 53214
414-476-2488
FAX: 414-476-3493
✓ Vess chairs

References ──────────────────────────────

Chapter 1

Baker, W. L. and S. L. Smith. "Pulmonary Aspiration and Tube Feedings: Nursing Implications." *Focus on Critical Care*, Vol. 11, No. 2, 1984, pp. 25-27.

Buchhol, D. W. "Cricopharyngeal Myotomy May Be Effective Treatment for Selected Patients with Neurogenic Otopharyngeal Dysphagia." *Dysphagia*, Vol. 10, 1995, pp. 255-258.

DePaso, W. J. "Aspiration Pneumonia." *Clinics in Chest Medicine*, Vol. 12, No. 2, 1991, pp. 269-284.

DeVita, M. and L. Spierer-Rundbach. "Swallowing Disorders in Patients with Prolonged Orotracheal Intubation or Tracheostomy Tubes." *Critical Care Medicine*, Vol. 18, No. 12, 1990, pp. 1328-1330.

Eisele, D. W., D. G. Koch, A. E. Tarazi, and B. Jones. "Aspiration from Delayed Radiation Fibrosis of the Neck." *Dysphagia*, Vol. 6, No. 2, 1991.

Ergun, G. A. and P. F. Miskovitz. "Aging in the Esophagus, Common Pathologic Conditions and Their Effect Upon Swallowing in the Geriatric Population." *Dysphagia*, Vol. 7, 1992, pp. 58-63.

Feinberg, M. "The Effects of Medications on Swallowing." *Dysphagia - A Continuum of Care.* Gaithersburg, MD: Aspen Publishers, Inc., 1997.

Fonda, D., J. Schwarz, and S. Clinnick. "Parkinson Medication One Hour Before Meals Improves Symptomatic Swallowing: A Case Study." *Dysphagia*, Vol. 10, 1995, pp. 165-166.

Galindo-Ciocon, D. "Tube Feeding: Complications Among the Elderly." *Journal of Gerontological Nursing*, 1993, pp. 17-21.

Hamilos, D. L. "Gastroesophageal Reflux and Sinusitis in Asthma." *Clinics in Chest Medicine*, Vol. 16, No. 4, 1995, pp. 683-697.

Henderson, C. "Safe and Effective Tube Feeding of Bedridden Elderly." *Geriatrics*, Vol. 46, No. 8, 1991, pp. 56-66.

Hendrix, T. "Art and Science of History Taking in the Patient with Difficulty with Swallowing." *Dysphagia*, Vol. 8, 1993, pp. 69-73.

Kayser-Jones, J. "The Use of Nasogastric Feeding Tubes in Nursing Homes: Patient, Family and Health Care Perspectives." *The Gerontologist*, Vol. 30, No. 4, 1990, pp. 469-479.

Kikendall, J. W., A. C. Friedman, and M. A. Oyewole. "Pill-induced Esophageal Strictures: Case Reports and Review of the Medical Literature." *Digestive Diseases and Sciences*, Vol. 28, No. 174, 1983.

Konstantinides, N. and E. Shronts. "Tube Feeding: Managing the Basics." *American Journal of Nursing*, 1983, pp. 1312-1320.

Koufman, J. A. "The Otolaryngologic Manifestations of Gastroesphageal Reflux Disease (GERD): A Clinical Investigation of 225 Patients Using Ambulatory 24-Hour pH Monitoring and an Experimental Investigation of the Role of Acid and Pepsin in the Development of Laryngeal Injury." *Laryngoscope*, Vol. 101, No. 4, Suppl. 53, 1991.

Langmore, S. "Managing the Complications of Aspiration in Dysphagic Adults." *Seminars in Speech and Language: Swallowing Disorders*, Vol. 12, No. 3, 1991, pp. 199-207.

Lazarus, C., J. Murphy, and L. Culpepper. "Aspiration Associated with Long-Term Gastric Versus Jejunal Feeding: A Critical Analysis of the Literature." *Archives of Physical Medicine and Rehabilitation*, Vol. 71, 1990, pp. 46-53.

Lazarus, C. L., J. A. Logemann, B. R. Pauloski, L. A. Colangelo, P. J. Kahrilas, B. B. Mittal, and M. Pierce. "Swallowing Disorders in Head and Neck Cancer Patients Treated with Radiotherapy and Adjuvant Chemotherapy." *Laryngoscope*, Vol. 106, 1996, pp. 1157-1166.

Little, A. G. "Nissen Fundoplication for Gastroesophageal Reflux Disease: How does Nissen Fundoplication Prevent Reflux?" *Diseases of the Esophagus*, 1996, pp. 247-250.

Martyn-Nemeth, P. and K. Fitzgerald. "Clinical Considerations, Tube Feeding in the Elderly." *Journal of Gerontological Nursing*, Vol. 18, No. 2, 1992, pp. 30-36.

Mitchell, C. and K. Parry-Billings. "Gastroesophageal Reflux Disease." *Nursing Standard*, Vol. 6, No. 24, 1992, pp. 25-28.

Mold, J. W., L. E. Reed, A. B. Davis, M. L. Allen, D. L. Decktor, and M. Robinson. "Prevalence of Gastroesophageal Reflux in Elderly Patients in a Primary Care Setting." *The American Journal of Gastroenterology*, Vol. 86, No. 8, 1991, pp. 965-970.

Nilsson, H. "Further Comments on Swallowing in Parkinson's Disease." *Dysphagia*, Vol. 12, 1997, pp. 98-99.

Park, R. H. R., M. C. Allison, J. Lang, E. Spence, A. J. Morris, B. J. Z. Danesh, R. I. Russell, and P. R. Mills. "Randomised Comparison of Percutaneous Endoscopic Gastrostomy and Nasogastric Tube Feeding in Patients with Persisting Neurological Dysphagia." *British Medical Journal*, Vol. 304, 1992, pp. 1406-1409.

Schultz, A., P. Niemtzow, S. R. Jacobs, and F. Naso. "Dysphagia Associated with Cricopharyngeal Dysfunction." *Archives of Physical Medicine and Rehabilitation*, Vol. 60, 1979, pp. 381-384.

Shaker, R., M. Milbrath, J. Ren, R. Toohill, W. J. Hogan, Q. Li, and C. L. Hofman. "Esophagopharyngeal Distribution of Refluxed Gastric Acid in Patients with Reflux Laryngitis." *Gastroenterology*, Vol. 109, 1995, pp. 1575-1582.

Spray, F., G. Zuidema, and J. Cameron. "Aspiration Pneumonia: Incidence of Aspiration with Endotracheal Tubes." *The American Journal of Surgery*, Vol. 131, 1986, pp. 701-703.

Sullivan, P. A. and A. M. Guilford. *Swallowing Intervention in Oncology*. San Diego: Singular Publishing Group, Inc., 1999.

Triadafilopoulos, G., A. Hallstone, H. Nelson-Abbot, and K. Bedinger. "Oropharyngeal and Esophageal Interrelationships in Patients with Nonobstructive Dysphagia." *Digestive Diseases and Sciences*, Vol. 37, No. 40, 1992, pp. 551-557.

Chapter 2

American Speech-Language-Hearing Association. "Code of Ethics." *Asha*, Vol. 36, Suppl. 13, 1994, pp. 1-2.

American Speech-Language-Hearing Association, Healthcare Financing Division, *1995 Fact Sheet Medicare Developments*.

American Speech-Language-Hearing Association, Healthcare Financing Division, *1995 Fact Sheet New Revised CPT Codes for 1996*.

References, *continued*

International Classification of Diseases, 9th Revision, Clinical Modifications (ICD-9-CM), Department of Health and Human Services Publication No. (PHS) 80-1260, Washington, D.C.

Kander, M. and S. White. *Medicare Handbook for Speech-Language Pathology and Audiology Services*. American Speech-Language-Pathology Association, Rockville, MD, 1994.

Klontz, H. A., J. P. McCarty, and S. C. White. *Private Health Plans Handbook for Speech-Language Pathology and Audiology Services*. Rockville, MD: ASHA.

Medicare Hospital Manual, Section 450, Baltimore: HCFA.

Medicare Intermediary Manual, Section 3910, Special Instructions for Medical Review of Dysphagia Claims, Baltimore: HCFA, 1990.

Medicare Outpatient Physical Therapy and Comprehensive Outpatient Rehabilitation Facility Manual, Section 504, Baltimore: HCFA.

Medicare Skilled Nursing Facility Manual, Section 543:4, Baltimore: HCFA.

Omnibus Budget Reconciliation Act, 1987: Rules and Regulations (February 2, 1989), Federal Register, Vol. 54:21.

Physician's Current Procedural Terminology, 4th Ed. (CPT), Chicago: American Medical Association.

Chapter 3

Agency for Health Care Policy and Research. "Research on Swallowing Problems in the Elderly Highlights Potential for Preventing Pneumonia in Stroke Patients." Press Release, Rockville, MD., March 30, 1999.

Davies, A. E., D. Kidd, S. P. Stone, and J. MacMahon. "Pharyngeal Sensation and Gag Reflex in Healthy Subjects." *The Lancet*, Vol. 345, No. 8948, 1995, pp. 487-488.

DeJong, R. *The Neurologic Examination*. New York: Hoeber Medical Division, Harper & Row, 1967.

DePippo, K. L., M. A. Holas, and M. J. Reding. "Validation of the 3-oz Water Swallow Test for Aspiration Following Stroke." *Archives of Neurology*, Vol. 49, 1992, pp. 1259-1261.

ECRI. "An Evidence Report on the Diagnosis and Treatment of Dysphagia/Swallowing Disorders in the Elderly." Rockville, MD: The Agency for Health Care Policy and Research, November 4, 1999.

Emick-Herring, B. and P. Wood. "A Team Approach to Neurologically-Based Swallowing Disorders." *Rehabilitation Nursing*, Vol. 15, No. 3, 1990, pp. 126-132.

Garon, B. R., M. Engle, and C. Ormiston. "Reliability of the 3-oz Water Swallow Test Utilizing Cough Reflex as Sole Indicator of Aspiration." *Journal of Neurological Rehabilitation*, Vol. 9, No. 3, 1995, pp. 139-143.

Gottlieb, D., M. Kipnis, E. Sister, Y. Vardi, and S. Brill. "Validation of the 50ml³ Drinking Test for Evaluation of Post-Stroke Dysphagia." *Disability and Rehabilitation*, Vol. 18, No. 10, 1996, pp. 529-532.

Hamlet, S., D. G. Penney, and J. Formolo. "Stethoscope Acoustics and Cervical Auscultation of Swallowing." *Dysphagia*, Vol. 9, 1994, pp. 63-68.

Hamlet, S. L., R. J. Nelson, and R. L. Patterson. "Interpreting the Sounds of Swallowing: Fluid Flow Through the Cricopharyngeus." *Annals of Otology, Rhinology, and Laryngology*, 1990, pp. 749-752.

Hamlet, S. L., R. L. Patterson, S. M. Flemming, and L. A. Jones. "Sounds of Swallowing Following Total Laryngectomy." *Dysphagia*, Vol. 7, 1992, pp. 160-165.

Hiiemae, K. M. and J. B. Palmer. "Food Transport and Bolus Formation During Complete Feeding Sequences on Foods of Different Initial Consistency." *Dysphagia*, Vol. 14, No. 1, 1999, pp. 31-42.

Hunter, P. C., J. Crameri, S. Austin, M. C. Woodward, and A. J. Hughes. "Response of Parkinsonian Swallowing Dysfunction to Dopaminergic Stimulation." *Journal of Neurology, Neurosurgery, and Psychiatry*, Vol. 63, No. 5, 1997, pp. 579-583.

Hutchins, B. and J. Giancarlo. "Developing a Comprehensive Dysphagia Program." *Seminars in Speech and Language: Swallowing Disorders*, Vol. 12, No. 3, 1991, pp. 209-215.

Kennedy, G. "The Role of The Speech-Language Therapist in the Assessment and Management of Dysphagia in Neurologically-Impaired Patients." *Post Graduate Medical Journal*, Vol. 68, 1992, pp. 545-548.

Leder, S. B. "Gag Reflex and Dysphagia." *Head & Neck*, Vol. 18, 1996, pp. 138-141.

Leder, S. B. "Videofluoroscopic Evaluation of Aspiration with Visual Examination of the Gag Reflex and Velar Movement." *Dysphagia*, Vol. 12, 1997, pp. 21-23.

Logemann, J. A. *Evaluation and Treatment of Swallowing Disorders*. Austin, TX: Pro-Ed, 1998.

Logemann, J. A., S. Veis, and L. Colangelo. "A Screening Procedure for Oropharyngeal Dysphagia." *Dysphagia*, Vol. 14, No. 1, 1999.

Martens, L., T. Cameron, and M. Simonsen. "Effects of a Multidisciplinary Management Program on Neurologically-Impaired Patients With Dysphagia." *Dysphagia*, Vol. 5, 1990, pp. 147-151.

Martin, B. J. W., J. A. Logemann, R. Shaker, and W. Dodds. "Coordination Between Respiration and Swallowing: Respiratory Phase Relationships and Temporal Integration." *Journal of Applied Physiology*, Vol. 26, No. 2, 1994, pp. 714-723.

Mody, M. and J. Nagia. "A Multidisciplinary Approach to the Development of Competency Standards And Appropriate Allocation for Patients with Dysphagia." *The American Journal of Occupational Therapy*, Vol. 44, No. 4, 1990, pp. 369-372.

Nathadwarawala, K. M., J. Nicklin, and C. M. Wiles. "A Timed Test of Swallowing Capacity for Neurological Patients." *Journal of Neurology, Neurosurgery, and Psychiatry*, Vol. 55, 1992, pp. 822-825.

Nowak, T. V. "Management of Upper Gastrointestinal Tract Dysfunction." *Seminars in Neurology*, Vol. 16, No. 3, 1996, pp. 281-288.

Poirier, N. C., I. Bonavina, R. Taillefer, A. Nosadini, A. Peracchia, and A. Duranceau. "Cricopharyngeal Myotomy for Neurogenic Oropharyngeal Dysphagia." *Journal of Thoracic and Cardiovascular Surgery*, Vol. 113, No. 2, 1997, pp. 233-240.

Selley, W. G., F. C. Flack, and W. A. Brooks. "Respiratory Patterns Associated with Swallowing, Part II. Neurologically Impaired Dysphagic Patients." *Age and Ageing*, Vol. 18, 1989, pp. 173-176.

Smith, C. H., J. A. Logemann, L. A. Colangelo, A. W. Rademaker, and B. R. Pauloski. "Incidence and Patient Characteristics Associated with Silent Aspiration in the Acute Care Setting." *Dysphagia*, Vol. 14, No. 1, 1999, pp. 1-7.

Smith, D., S. Hamlet, and L. Jones. "Acoustic Technique for Determining Timing of Velopharyngeal Closure in Swallowing." *Dysphagia*, Vol. 5, 1990, pp. 142-146.

Sorin, R., S. Somers, W. Austin, and S. Bester. "The Influence of Videofluoroscopy on the Management of the Dysphagic Patient." *Dysphagia*, Vol. 2, 1988, pp. 127-135.

Splaingard, M., B. Hutchins, L. Sulton, and G. Chaudhuri. "Aspiration in Rehabilitation Patients: Videofluoroscopy vs. Bedside Clinical Assessment." *Archives of Physical Medicine and Rehabilitation*, Vol. 69, 1988, pp. 637-640.

Takahashi, K., M. E. Groher, and K. Michi. "Stethoscope Acoustics and Cervical Auscultation of Swallowing." *Dysphagia*, Vol. 9, 1994, pp. 54-92.

Vice, F., J. Heinz, G. Guiriati, M. Hood, and J. Bosma. "Cervical Auscultation of Suckle Feeding in Newborn Infants." *Developmental Medicine and Child Neurology*, Vol. 32, 1990, pp. 760-768.

Vice, F. and J. F. Bosma. "Cervical Auscultation of Feeding in Adults." Videotape developed by University of Maryland School of Medicine, 1995.

Zenner, P. M., D. S. Losinski, and R. H. Mills. "Using Cervical Auscultation in the Clinical Dysphagia Examination in Long-Term Care." *Dysphagia*, Vol. 10, No. 1, 1995, pp. 27-31.

Chapter 4

Arsenault, J. and J. Atwood. "Development of a Competency-Based Training Model for Dysphagia Management in a Medical Setting." *Seminars in Speech and Language: Swallowing Disorders*, Vol. 12, No. 3, August 1991, pp. 236-244.

DePippo, K., M. Holas, and M. Reding. "Validation of the 3-oz. Water Swallow Test for Aspiration Following Stroke." *Archives of Neurology*, Vol. 49, 1992, pp. 1259-1261.

Donahue, P. A. "When It's Hard to Swallow — Feeding Techniques for Dysphagia Management." *Journal of Gerontological Nursing*, Vol. 16, No. 4, 1990, pp. 6-9.

Ekberg, O. "Posture of the Head and Pharyngeal Swallowing." *Acta Radiologica: Diagnosis* (Stockholm), Vol. 27, No. 6, 1986, pp. 691-696.

Emick-Herring, V. and P. Wood. "A Team Approach to Neurologically-Based Swallowing Disorders." *Rehabilitation Nursing*, Vol. 15, No. 3, 1990, pp. 126-132.

Garon, B. R., M. Engle, and C. Ormiston. "Reliability of the 3-oz. Water Swallow Test Utilizing Cough Reflex as Sole Indicator of Aspiration." *Journal of Neurological Rehabilitation*, Vol. 9, No. 3, 1995, pp. 139-143.

Gelfand, D. W. and D. J. Ott. "Barium Sulfate Suspensions: An Evaluation of Available Products." *American Journal of Roentgenology*, Vol. 138, 1982, p. 935.

Hutchins, B. *Managing Dysphagia: An Instrumentational Guide for the Client and Family*. San Antonio: Communication Skill Builders (a division of The Psychological Corporation), 1991.

Karnell, M. and S. Langmore. "Videoendoscopy in Speech and Swallowing for the Speech-Language Pathologist." In *Medical Speech-Language Pathology: A Practitioner's Guide*, New York: Thieme Medical Publishers, Inc., 1998, pp. 563-584.

Kidder, T. M., S. E. Langmore, and B. J. W. Martin. "Indications and Techniques of Endoscopy in Evaluation of Cervical Dysphagia: Comparison with Radiographic Techniques." *Dysphagia*, Vol. 9, No. 4, 1994, pp. 256-261.

Kolodny, V. and A. M. Malek. "Improving Feeding Skills." *Journal of Gerontological Nursing*, Vol. 17, No. 6, 1991, pp. 20-24.

Langmore, S. E. and T. M. McCulloch. "Examination of the Pharynx and Larynx and Endoscopic Examination of Pharyngeal Swallowing." In A. Perlman and K. Schultz (eds.). *Deglutition and Its Disorders*. San Diego: Singular Press, 1996, pp. 201-226.

Langmore, S., K. Schatz, and N. Olson. "Endoscopic and Videofluoroscopic Evaluations of Swallowing and Aspiration." *Annals of Otology, Rhinology, and Laryngology*, Vol. 100, 1991, pp. 678-681.

Langmore, S. E., K. Schatz, and N. Olsen. "Fiberoptic Endoscopic Examination of Swallowing Safety: A New Procedure." *Dysphagia*, Vol. 2, 1988, pp. 216-219.

Lazarus, C. L., J. A. Logemann, A. W. Rademaker, P. J. Kahrilas, T. Pajak, R. Lazar, and A. Halper. "Effects of Bolus Volume, Viscosity, and Repeated Swallows in Nonstroke Subjects and Stroke Patients." *Archives of Physical Medicine and Rehabilitation*, Vol. 74, No. 10, 1993, pp. 1066-1070.

Leder, S. B., C. T. Sasaki, and M. I. Burrell. "Fiberoptic Endoscopic Evaluation of Dysphagia to Identify Silent Aspiration." *Dysphagia*, Vol. 13, No. 1, 1998, pp. 19-21.

Linden, P. and A. Siebens. "Dysphagia: Predicting Laryngeal Penetration." *Archives of Physical Medicine and Rehabilitation*, Vol. 64, 1983, pp. 281-284

Linden, P., K. Kuhlemeier, and C. Patterson. "The Probability of Correctly Predicting Subglottic Penetrations and Clinical Observations." *Dysphagia*, Vol. 8, 1993, pp. 170-179.

Logemann, J. "Precautions for Feeding Dysphagic Patients." Videotape distributed by Northern Speech Services, Inc., 1989.

Logemann, J. *Evaluation and Treatment of Swallowing Disorders*. Austin, TX: Pro-Ed, 1998, pp. 54-62, 168-185.

Logemann, J. A., S. Veis, and L. Colangelo. "A Screening Procedure for Oropharyngeal Dysphagia." *Dysphagia*, Vol. 14, No. 1, 1999, pp. 44-51.

Logemann, J. A. and P. J. Kahrilas. "Relearning to Swallow After Stroke — Application of Maneuvers and Indirect Biofeedback: A Case Study." *Neurology*, Vol. 40, 1990, pp. 1136-1138.

Logemann, J. A., B. R. Pauloski, L. Colangelo, C. Lazarus, M. Fujiu, and P. J. Kahrilas. "Effects of a Sour Bolus on Oropharyngeal Swallowing Measures in Patients with Neurogenic Dysphagia." *Journal of Speech and Hearing Research*, Vol. 38, No. 3, 1995, pp. 556-563.

Martin-Harris, B., S. I. McMahon, and R. Haynes. "Aspiration and Dysphagia: Pathophysiology and Outcome." *Phonoscope*, Vol. 1, No. 2, 1998, pp. 123-132.

Neuman, S. "Swallowing Therapy with Neurologic Patients: Results of Direct and Indirect Therapy Methods in 66 Patients Suffering from Neurological Disorders." *Dysphagia*, Vol. 8, No. 2, 1993, pp. 150-153.

Ott, D. J. and D. W. Gelfand. "Gastrointestinal Contrast Agents: Indications, Uses, and Risks." *Journal of the American Medical Association*, Vol. 249, 1983, p. 2380.

Ott, D. J., R. G. Hodge, L. A. Pikna, M. Y. M. Chen, and D. W. Gelfand. "Modified Barium Swallow: Clinical and Radiographic Correlation and Relation to Feeding Recommendations." *Dysphagia*, Vol. 11, 1996, pp. 187-190.

Perlman, A. L. "Application of Instrumental Procedures to the Evaluation and Treatment of Dysphagia." *Dysphagia - A Continuum of Care*, Gaithersburg, MD: Aspen Publishers, Inc., 1997.

Ralsey, A., J. A. Logemann, P. J. Kahrilas, A. W. Rademaker, B. R. Pauloski, and W. J. Dodds. "Prevention of Barium Aspiration During Videofluoroscopic Swallowing Studies: Value of Change in Posture." *American Journal of Roentgenology*, Vol. 74, No. 12, 1993, pp. 1005-1009.

Robbins, J., R. L. Levine, A. Maser, J. C. Rosenbek, and G. B. Kempster. "Swallowing After Unilateral Stroke of the Cerebral Cortex." *Archives of Physical Medicine and Rehabilitation*, Vol. 74, No. 12, 1993, pp. 1295-1300.

Rubin-Terrado, M. and D. Linkenheld. "Don't Choke On This: A Swallowing Assessment." *Geriatric Nursing*, 1991, pp. 288-291.

Shanahan, T. K., J. A. Logemann, A. W. Rademaker, B. R. Pauloski, and P. J. Kahrilas. "Chin-down Posture Effect on Aspiration in Dysphagic Patients." *Archives of Physical Medicine and Rehabilitation*, Vol. 74, No. 7, 1993, pp. 736-739.

Smith, C. H., J. A. Logemann, L. A. Colangelo, A. W. Rademaker, and B. R. Pauloski. "Incidence and Patient Characteristics Associated with Silent Aspiration in the Acute Care Setting." *Dysphagia*, Vol. 14, No. 1, 1999, pp. 1-7.

Sorin, R., S. Somers, W. Austin, and S. Bester. "The Influence of Videofluoroscopy on the Management of the Dysphagic Patient." *Dysphagia*, Vol. 2, 1988, pp. 127-135.

Splaingard, M., B. Hutchins, L. Sulton, and G. Chaudhuri. "Aspiration in Rehabilitation Patients: Videofluoroscopy vs. Bedside Clinical Assessment." *Archives of Physical Medicine and Rehabilitation*, Vol. 69, 1988, pp. 637-640.

Chapter 5

American Speech-Language-Hearing Association (1994). Code of Ethics. *Asha*, 36 (March, Suppl. 13), pp 1-2.

Annas, G. J. "Do Feeding Tubes Have More Rights Than Patients?" *Hastings Center Report*, Vol. 16, 1986, pp. 26-28.

Banja, J. "Nutritional Discontinuation: Active or Passive Euthanasia?" *Journal of Neuroscience Nursing*, Vol. 22, No. 2, 1990, pp. 117-120.

Beauchamp, T. L. and J. F. Childress. "Principles of Biomedical Ethics." New York, Oxford University Press, 1994.

Brody, H. and M. Noel. "Dietitians' Role in Decisions to Withhold Nutrition and Hydration." *Journal of the American Dietetic Association*, Vol. 91, No. 5, 1991, pp. 580-585.

Campbell-Taylor, I. and R. H. Fisher. "The Clinical Case Against Tube Feedings in Palliative Care of the Elderly." *Journal of the American Geriatrics Society*, Vol. 35, 1987, pp. 1100-1104.

Davidson, B., R. Vander Lann, M. Hirschfeld, A. Norberg, E. Pitman, and L. Ying. "Ethical Reasoning Associated with the Feeding of Terminally Ill Elderly Cancer Patients: An International Perspective." *Cancer Nursing*, Vol. 13, No. 5, 1990, pp. 286-292.

Ely, J., P. Peters, F. Zweig, N. Elder, and F. Schneider. "The Physician's Decision to Use Tube Feedings: The Role of the Family, the Living Will, and the Cruzan Decision." *Journal of the American Geriatrics Society*, Vol. 40, 1992, pp. 471-475.

Groher, M. E. "Ethical Dilemmas in Providing Nutrition." *Dysphagia*, Vol. 5, 1990, pp. 102-109.

Klor, B. M. and F. J. Milianti. "Rehabilitation of Neurogenic Dysphagia with Percutaneous Endoscopic Gastrostomy." *Dysphagia*, Vol. 14, No. 3, 1999, pp. 162-164.

Meyers, R. and M. Grodin. "Decision Making Regarding the Initiation of Tube Feedings in the Severely Demented Elderly: A Review." *Journal of the American Geriatrics Society*, Vol. 39, No. 5, 1991, pp. 526-531.

Mitchell, S. L., D. K. Kiely, and L. A. Lipsitz. "Does Artificial Enteral Nutrition Prolong the Survival of Institutionalized Elders with Chewing and Swallowing Problems?" *Journal of Gerontology*, Vol. 53A, No. 3, 1998, pp. M207-M213.

O'Rourke, K. "The AMA Statement on Tube Feeding: An Ethical Analysis." *America*, Vol. 155, 1986, pp. 321-331.

Orr, R., J. Paris, and M. Seigler. "Caring for the Terminally Ill: Resolving Conflicting Objectives Between Patient, Physician, Family, and Institution." *Journal of Family Practice*, Vol. 33, No. 5, 1991, pp. 500-504.

Peck, A., C. Cohen, and M. Mulvihill. "Long-Term Enteral Feeding of Aged Demented Nursing Homes Patients." *Journal of the American Geriatrics Society*, Vol. 38, 1990, pp. 1195-1198.

"Position of the American Dietetic Association: Issues in Feeding the Terminally Ill Adult." *Journal of the American Dietetic Association*, Vol. 92, No. 8, 1992, pp. 996-1005.

Sandstead, H. "A Point of View: Nutrition and Care of Terminally Ill Patients." *American Journal of Clinical Nutrition*, Vol. 52, 1990, pp. 767-769.

Serradura-Russell, A. "Ethical Dilemmas in Dysphagia Management and the Right to a Natural Death." *Dysphagia*, Vol. 7, 1992, pp. 102-105.

Steinbrock, R. and B. Lo. "Artificial Feeding — Solid Ground, Not a Slippery Slope." *New England Journal of Medicine*, Vol. 318, 1988, pp. 286-290.

Vaux, K. "The Travail and Triumph of Sydney Greenspan." *Journal of Allied Health*, Winter 1991, pp. 1-3.

Watts, D., B. McCaulley, and B. Priefer. "Physician-Nurse Conflict: Lessons from a Clinical Experience." *Journal of the American Geriatrics Society*, Vol. 38, 1990, pp. 1151-1152.

Wilson, D. "Ethical Concerns in a Long-Term Tube Feeding Study." *IMAGE: Journal of Nursing Scholarships*, Vol. 24, No. 3, 1992, pp. 195-199.

Chapter 6

American Speech-Language-Hearing Association, "Instrumental Diagnostic Procedures for Swallowing." ASHA, Suppl. 7, 1992, pp. 25-33.

American Speech-Language-Hearing Association, "Roles of the Speech-Language Pathologist and Otolaryngologist in the Performance and Interpretation of Endoscopic Evaluations of Swallowing." In Press.

Arsenault, J. K. and J. Atwood. *Development of a Competency-Based Training Model for Dysphagia Management in a Medical Setting*. New York: Thieme Medical Publishing, Inc., 1991, pp. 236-246.

Aviv, J. E., J. H. Martin, R. L. Sacco, D. Zagar, B. Diamond, M. S. Keen, and A. Blitzer. "Supraglottic and Pharyngeal Sensory Abnormalities in Stroke Patients with Dysphagia." *Annals of Otology, Rhinology, and Laryngology*, Vol. 105, 1996, pp. 92-97.

Aviv, J. E., T. Kim, R. L. Sacco, S. Kaplan, K. Goodhart, B. Diamond, and L. G. Close. "FEESST: A New Bedside Endoscopic Test of the Motor and Sensory Components of Swallowing." *Annals of Otology, Rhinology, and Laryngology*, Vol. 107, 1998, pp. 378-387.

Aviv, J. E., T. Kim, J. E. Thomson, S. Sunshine, S. Kaplan, and L. G. Close. "Fiberoptic Endoscopic Evaluation of Swallowing with Sensory Testing (FEESST) in Healthy Controls." *Dysphagia*, Vol. 13, 1998, pp. 87-92.

Barofsky, I. and K. R. Fontaine. "Do Psychogenic Dysphagia Patients Have an Eating Disorder?" *Dysphagia*, Vol. 13, No. 1, 1998, pp. 24-28.

Beck, T. and B. Gaylar. "Image Quality and Radiation Levels in Videofluoroscopy for Swallowing Studies: A Review." *Dysphagia*, Vol. 5, 1990, pp. 118-128.

Briani, C., M. Marcon, M. Ermani, M. Costantini, R. Bottin, V. Iurilli, G. Zaninotto, D. Primon, G. Feltrin, and C. Angelini. "Radiological Evidence of Subclinical Dysphagia in Motor Neuron Disease." *Journal of Neurology*, Vol. 245, 1998, pp. 211-216.

Cook, I. "Investigative Techniques in the Assessment of Oral-Pharyngeal Dysphagia." *Digestive Diseases and Sciences*, Vol. 16, 1998, pp. 125-133.

Daniels, S. K., K. Brailey, D. H. Priestly, L. R. Herrington, L. A. Weisberg, and A. L. Foundas. "Aspiration in Patients With Acute Stroke." *Archives of Physical Medicine and Rehabilitation*, Vol. 79, No. 1, 1998, pp. 14-19.

Dodds, W., E. Steward, and J. Logemann. "Physiology and Radiology of the Normal Oral and Pharyngeal Phases of Swallowing." *American Journal of Roentgenology*, Vol. 154, 1990, pp. 965-974.

Ertekin, C., I. Aydogdu, N. Yüceyar, S. Tarlaci, N. Kiylioglu, M. Pehlivan, and G. Çelebi. "Electrodiagnostic Methods for Neurogenic Dysphagia." *Electroencephalography and Clinical Neurophysiology*, Vol. 109, 1998, pp. 331-340.

Feinberg, M. "Radiographic Techniques and Interpretation of Abnormal Swallowing in Adult and Elderly Patients." *Dysphagia*, Vol. 8, 1993, pp. 256-258.

Feinberg, M. and O. Ekberg. "Videofluoroscopy in Elderly Patients with Aspiration: Importance of Evaluating Both Oral and Pharyngeal Stages of Deglutition." *Journal of the American Geriatrics Society*, Vol. 156, 1991, pp. 293-296.

Feinberg, M. J., O. Ekberg, L. Segall, and J. Tully. "Deglutition in Elderly Patients with Dementia: Findings of Videofluorographic Evaluation and Impact on Staging and Management." *Radiology*, Vol. 183, 1992, pp. 811-814.

Functional Communication Measures. American Speech-Language-Hearing Association, Rockville, MD, 1998.

Garon, B. R., M. Engle, and C. Ormiston. "Silent Aspiration: Results of 1,000 Videofluoroscopic Swallow Evaluations." *Journal of Neurological Rehabilitation*, Vol. 10, 1996, pp. 121-126.

Gates, G. A. (ed.). *Dysphagia: The Methold of Haskins Kashima in Current Therapy in Otolaryngology —
Head and Neck Surgery.* Philadelphia: B. C. Decker, 1990.

Horner, J., J. E. Riski, J. Ovelmen-Levitt, and B. S. Nashold, Jr. "Swallowing in Torticollis Before and After
Rhizotomy." *Dysphagia*, Vol. 7, No. 3, 1992, pp. 117-125. (Duke Rating Scale)

Jones, B. and M. Donner. "Examination of the Patient with Dysphagia." *Radiology*, Vol. 167, No. 2, 1988,
pp. 319-326.

Karnell, M. and S. Langmore. "Videoendoscopy in Speech and Swallowing for the Speech-Language Pathologist."
In *Medical Speech-Language Pathology: A Practioner's Guide*. New York: Thieme Medical Publishers, Inc., 1998,
pp. 563-584.

Kidder, T. M., S. E. Langmore, and B. J. W. Martin. "Indications and Techniques of Endoscopy and Evaluation of
Cervical Dysphagia: Comparison with Radiographic Techniques." *Dysphagia*, Vol. 9, No. 4, 1994, pp. 256-261.

Kuhlemeier, K. V., P. Yates, and J. B. Palmer. "Intra- and Interrater Variation in the Evaluation of Videofluoroscopic
Swallowing Studies." *Dysphagia*, Vol. 13, No. 2, 1998, pp. 142-147.

Langmore, S. E. "Editorial: Laryngeal Sensation: A Touchy Subject." *Dysphagia*, Vol. 13, 1998, pp. 87-93.

Langmore, S. E. and T. M. McCulloch. "Examination of the Pharynx and Larynx and Endoscopic Examination
of Pharyngeal Swallowing." In A. Perlman and K. Schultz (eds.). *Deglutition and Its Disorders*. San Diego:
Singular Press, Inc., 1996, pp. 201-226.

Langmore, S., K. Schatz, and N. Olson. "Endoscopic and Videofluoroscopic Evaluations of Swallowing and
Aspiration." *Annals of Otology, Rhinology, and Laryngology*, Vol. 100, 1991, pp. 678-681.

Langmore, S. E. and M. Karnell. *Videoendoscopy in Speech and Swallowing for the Speech-Language Pathologist*.
New York: Thieme Medical Publishers, Inc., 1998, pp. 563-584.

Leder, S.B., C. T. Sasaki, and M. I. Burrell. "Fiberoptic Endoscopic Evaluation of Dysphagia to Identify Silent
Aspiration." *Dysphagia*, Vol. 13, No. 1, 1998, pp. 19-21.

Leder, S. B. "Serial Fiberoptic Endoscopic Swallowing Evaluations in the Management of Patients with Dysphagia."
Archives of Physical Medicine and Rehabilitation, Vol. 79, 1998, pp. 1264-1269.

Logemann, J. A. "Manual for the Videofluoroscopic Study of Swallowing." *Administrators in Radiology*, Vol. 3,
1993, pp. 20-23 & 43.

Logemann, J. "Non-invasive Approaches to Deglutive Aspiration." *Dysphagia*, Vol. 8, 1993, pp. 331-333.

Logemann, J. "Videofluoroscopic Swallowing Studies: Evaluation and Therapy Planning." Distributed by
Continuing Education Programs of America, 1988.

Logemann, J. *Evaluation and Treatment of Swallowing Disorders*. San Diego: College Hill Press, 1983.

Logemann, J. A. *Manual for the Videofluorographic Study for Swallowing*. (2nd ed.) Austin, TX: Pro-Ed, 1993.

Logemann, J. A., B. R. Pauloski, A. Rademaker, B. Cook, D. Graner, F. Milianti, Q. Beery, D. Stein, J. Bowman, C.
Lazarus, M. A. Heiser, and T. Baker. "Impact of the Diagnostic Procedure on Outcome Measures of Swallowing
Rehabilitation in Head and Neck Cancer Patients." *Dysphagia*, Vol. 7, No. 4, 1992, pp. 179-187.

Martin-Harris, B., S. I. McMahon, and R. Haynes. "Aspiration and Dysphagia: Pathophysiology and Outcome." *Phonoscope*, Vol. 1, No. 2, 1998, pp. 123-132.

Murray, J., S. Langmore, S. Ginsberg, and A. Dostie. "The Significance of Accumulated Oropharyngeal Secretions and Swallowing Frequency in Predicting Aspiration." *Dysphagia*, Vol. 11, 1996, pp. 99-103.

Nilsson, H., O. Ekberg, R. Olsson, and B. Hindfelt. "Dysphagia in Stroke: A Prospective Study of Quantitative Aspects of Swallowing in Dysphagic Patients." *Dysphagia*, Vol. 13, No. 1, 1998, pp. 32-38.

Odderson, I. R., J. C. Keaton, and B. S. McKenna. "Swallow Management in Patients on an Acute Stroke Pathway: Quality is Cost Effective." *Archives of Physical Medicine and Rehabilitation*, Vol. 76, No. 12, 1995, pp. 1130-1133.

Ott, D. J. "Editorial: Observer Variation in Evaluation of Videofluoroscopic Swallowing Studies: A Continuing Problem." *Dysphagia*, Vol. 13, No. 3, 1998, pp. 148-151.

Périé, S., L. Laccourreye, A. Flahault, V. Hazebroucq, S. Chaussade, and J. L. St. Guily. "Role of Videoendoscopy in Assessment of Pharyngeal Function in Oropharyngeal Dysphagia: Comparison with Videoendscopy and Manometry." *Laryngoscope*, Vol. 108, 1998, pp. 1712-1716.

Perlman, A., J. Grayhack, and B. Booth. "The Relationship of Vallecular Residue to Oral Involvement, Reduced Hyoid Elevation, and Epiglottic Functions." *Journal of Speech and Hearing Research*, Vol. 35, 1992, pp. 734-741.

Rosenbek, J., J. A. Robbins, E. Roecker, J. Coyle, and J. Wood. "A Penetration-Aspiration Scale." *Dysphagia*, Vol. 11, 1996, pp. 93-98.

Sonies, B. C. "Instrumental Procedures for Dysphagia Diagnosis." *Seminars in Speech and Language*, Vol. 12, No. 3, 1991, pp. 185-198.

Sonies, B. and B. Baum. "Evaluation of Swallowing Pathophysiology." *Otolaryngological Clinics of North America*, Vol. 21, No. 4, 1988, pp. 637-648.

Spiegel, J. R., J. C. Selber, and J. Creed. "A Functional Diagnosis of Dysphagia Using Videoendoscopy." *ENT-Ear, Nose & Throat Journal*, 1998, pp. 628-632.

Steefel, J. S. *Dysphagia Rehabilitation for Neurologically-Impaired Adults*. Springfield, IL: Charles C. Turner, 1981.

Yoshida, G., D. Maglinte, R. Hamaker, and S. Kelvin. "Evaluation of Swallowing Disorders: The Modified Barium Swallow." *Indiana Medicine*, Vol. 83, No. 12, 1990, pp. 892-895.

Chapter 7 (For specific references on the treatment techniques, see Appendix D, pages 215-219.)

Breslin, R. *Food: The Essence of Life: Creative Cooking for the Pureed Diet*. Branfort, CT: Connecticut Hospice Institute, 1988.

Casprisin, A., H. Clumeck, and M. Nino-Murcia. "The Efficacy of Rehabilitative Management of Dysphagia." *Dysphagia*, Vol. 4, 1989, pp. 48-52.

Curran, J. and M. Groher. "Development and Dissemination of an Aspiration Risk Reduction Diet." *Dysphagia*, Vol. 5, 1990, pp. 6-12.

Curran, J. "Nutritional Considerations." In M.E. Groher (ed.) *Dysphagia: Diagnosis and Management*. (2nd ed.) Boston: Butterworth-Heinemann, 1992.

Glickstein, J. *Reimburseable Geriatric Service Delivery*. Aspen: Aspen Publishing, 1993.

Groher, M. (ed.). *Dysphagia: Diagnosis and Management*. (2nd ed.) Boston: Butterworth-Heinemann, 1992.

Groher, M. (ed.). "Special Issue: Managing Dysphagia in a Chronic Care Setting Part I." *Dysphagia*, Vol. 5, No. 52, 1990, pp. 59-109.

Logemann, J. A. *Evaluation and Treatment of Swallowing Disorders*. San Diego: College Hill Press, 1983.

Lux, I. and K. Nash. *Continuous Quality Improvement in the Clinical Management of Dysphagia*. Gaylord, MI: Northern Speech Services, Inc., 1991.

Martin, A. "Dietary Management of Swallowing Disorders." *Dysphagia*, Vol. 6, 1991, pp. 129-134.

Mayes, C. "Pureed Diets: Come Alive with the Right Food Processor." *American Health Care Association Journal*, Vol. 11, 1985, pp. 24-28.

Mirro, J. and C. Patey. "Developing a Dysphagia Dietary Program." *Seminars in Speech and Language: Swallowing Disorders*, Vol. 12, No. 3, 1991, pp. 218-226.

Stanek, K., C. Hensley, and C. Van Ryser. "Factors Affecting Use of Food and Commercial Agents to Thicken Liquids for Individuals with Swallowing Disorders." *Journal of the American Dietetic Association*, Vol. 92, No. 4, 1992, pp. 488-490.

Chapter 9

American Speech-Language-Hearing Association. "Multiskilled Personnel." *Asha*, Vol. 39, Suppl. 17, 1997, pp. 13.

Bonanno, P. C. "Swallowing Dysfunction after Tracheostomy." *Annals of Surgery*, Vol. 174, 1971, pp. 29-33.

Bone, D. K., J. L. Davis, G. D. Zuidema, and J. L. Cameron. "Aspiration Pneumonia." *Annals of Thoracic Surgery*, Vol. 18, 1974, pp. 30-37.

Brandy, S. L., C. D. Hilldner, and B. F. Hutchins. "Simultaneous Videofluoroscopy Swallow Study and Modified Evans Blue Dye Procedure: An Evaluation of Blue Dye Visualization in Cases of Known Aspiration." *Dysphagia*, Vol. 14, No. 3, 1999, pp. 146-149.

Burgess, G. E., J. R. Cooper, and R. J. Marino. "Laryngeal Competence After Tracheal Extubation." *Anesthesiology*, Vol. 51, 1979, pp. 73-77.

Cameron, J., J. Reynolds, and G. Zuidema. "Aspiration in Patients with Tracheostomies." *Surgery, Gynecology, and Obstetrics*, Vol. 136, 1973, pp. 68-70.

Colice, G. L., T. A. Stukel, and B. Dain. "Laryngeal Complications of Prolonged Intubation." *Chest*, Vol. 96, No. 4, 1989, pp. 877-884.

Colice, G. L. "Resolution of Laryngeal Injury Following Translaryngeal Intubation." *American Review of Respiratory Disease*, Vol. 145, 1992, pp. 361-364.

Dettelbach, M. A., R. D. Gross, J. Mahlmann, and D. E. Eibling. "Effect of the Passy-Muir Valve on Aspiration in Patients with Tracheostomy." *Head & Neck*, Vol. 17, No. 4, 1995, pp. 297-302.

DeVita, M. A. and L. Spierer-Runback. "Swallowing Disorders in Patients with Prolonged Orotracheal Intubation or Tracheostomy Tubes." *Critical Care Medicine*, Vol. 18, No. 12, 1990, pp. 1328-1330.

Eibling, D. E. and R. Diez Gross. "Subglottic Air Pressure: A Key Component of Swallowing Efficiency." *Annals of Otology, Rhinology, and Laryngology*, Vol. 105, 1996, pp. 253-258.

Elpern, E. H., E. R. Jacobs, and R. C. Bone. "Clinical Studies in Respiratory Critical Care: Incidence of Aspiration in Tracheally Intubated Adults." *Heart & Lung*, Vol. 16, No. 5, 1987, pp. 527-531.

Elpern, E., M. Scott, L. Petro, and M. Ries. "Pulmonary Aspiration in Mechanically Ventilated Patients with Tracheostomies." *Chest*, Vol. 105, 1994, pp. 563-566.

Garon, K. C. and A. D. Meyers. "Editorial: Simultaneous Videofluoroscopy Swallow Study and Modified Evans Blue Dye Procedure: An Evaluation of Blue Dye Visualization in Cases of Known Aspiration." *Dysphagia*, Vol. 14, No. 3, 1999, pp. 150-151.

Higgins, D. M. and J. C. Maclean. "Dysphagia in the Patient with a Tracheostomy: Six Cases of Inappropriate Cuff Deflation or Removal." *Heart & Lung*, Vol. 26, No. 3, 1997, pp. 215-220.

Huxley, E. J., J. Virolax, W. R. Gray, and A. K. Pierce. "Pharyngeal Aspiration in Normal Adults and Patients with Depressed Consciousness." *American Journal of Medicine*, Vol. 64, 1978, pp. 654-658.

Ikari, T. and C. T. Sasaki. "Glottic Closure Reflex: Control Mechanisms." *Annals of Otology, Rhinology, and Laryngology*, Vol. 89, 1980, pp. 220-224.

de Larminat, V. P. Montravers., B. Dureuil, and J. M. Desmonts. "Alteration in Swallowing Reflex After Extubation in Intensive Care Unit Patients." *Critical Care Medicine*, Vol. 23, No. 3, 1995, pp. 486-490.

Leder, S. "Comment on Thompson-Henry and Braddock: The Modified Evan's (sic) Blue Dye Procedure Fails to Detect Aspiration in the Tracheotomized Patient: Five Case Reports." *Dysphagia*, Vol. 11, 1996, pp. 80-81.

Leder, S. B., J. M. Tarro, and M. I. Burrell. "Effect of Occlusion of a Tracheotomy Tube on Aspiration." *Dysphagia*, Vol. 11, No. 4, 1996, pp. 254-259.

Leder, S. B. "Effect of a One-Way Tracheotomy Speaking Valve on the Incidence of Aspiration in Previously Aspirating Patients with Tracheotomy." *Dysphagia*, Vol. 14, No. 2, 1999, pp. 73-78.

Leder, S. B., S. M. Cohn, and B. A. Moller. "Fiberoptic Endoscopic Documentation of the High Incidence of Aspiration following Extubation in Critically Ill Trauma Patients." *Dysphagia*, Vol. 13, No. 4, 1998, pp. 208-213.

Leder, S. B., D. A. Ross, M. I. Burrell, and C. T. Sasaki. "Tracheotomy Tube Occlusion Status and Aspiration in Early Post-surgical Head and Neck Cancer Patients." *Dysphagia*, Vol. 13, No. 3, 1998, pp. 167-172.

Logemann, J. Personal Communications. 1996.

Mason, M. F. *Speech Pathology for Tracheostomized and Ventilator Dependent Patients*. Newport Beach, VA: Voicing, 1993.

Murray, K. A. and L. A. Brzozowski. "Swallowing in Patients with Tracheotomies." *AACN Clinical Issues*, Vol. 9, No. 3, 1998, pp. 416-426.

Nash, M. "Swallowing Problems in the Tracheotomized Patient." *Otololaryngolic Clinics*, Vol. 21, 1988, pp. 701-709.

Physician's Desk Reference. Montvale, NJ: Medical Economics Company, 1996.

Rogers, B., M. Msall, and D. Shucard. "Hypoxemia During Oral Feedings in Adults with Dysphagia and Severe Neurological Disabilities." *Dysphagia*, Vol. 8, 1993, pp. 43-48.

Sellars, C., C. Dunnet, and R. Carter. "A Preliminary Comparison of Videofluoroscopy of Swallow and Pulse Oximetry in the Identification of Aspiration in Dysphagia Patients." *Dysphagia*, Vol. 13, No. 2, 1998, pp. 82-87.

Shaker, R., M. Milbrath, J. Ren, B. Campbell, R. Toohill, and W. Hogan. "Deglutitive Aspiration in Patients with Tracheostomy: Effect of Tracheostomy on the Duration of Vocal Cord Closure." *Gastroenterology*, Vol. 108, No. 5, 1995, pp. 1357-1360.

Spray, S., G. Zuidema, and J. Cameron. "Aspiration Pneumonia: Incidence of Aspiration with Endotracheal Tubes." *American Journal of Surgery*, Vol. 131, 1976, pp. 701-703.

Stauffer, J., D. Olson, and T. Petty. "Complications and Consequences of Endotracheal Intubation and Tracheostomy: A Prospective Study of 150 Critically-Ill Patients." *American Journal of Medicine*, Vol. 70, 1981, pp. 65-75.

Teramoto, S., Y. Fukuchi, and Y. Ouchi. "Oxygen Desaturation on Swallowing in Patients with Stroke. What Does It Mean?" *Age and Ageing*, Vol. 25, 1996, pp. 333-334.

Thompson-Henry, S. and B. Braddock. "The Modified Evan's (sic) Blue Dye Procedure Fails to Detect Aspiration in the Tracheotomized Patient: Five Case Reports." *Dysphagia*, Vol. 10, 1996, pp. 78-79.

Tippett, D.C. and A. A. Siebens. "Reconsidering the Value of the Modified Evan's (sic) Blue Dye Test: A Comment on Thompson-Henry and Braddock." *Dysphagia*, Vol. 11, 1996, pp. 78-79.

Tippett, D. C. and A. A. Siebens. "Using Ventilators for Speaking and Swallowing." *Dysphagia*, Vol. 6, No. 2, 1991, pp. 94-100.

Tolep, K., C. Leonard Getch, and G. J. Criner. "Swallowing Dysfunction in Patients Receiving Prolonged Mechanical Ventilation." *Chest*, Vol. 109, No. 1, 1996, pp. 167-172.

Whited, R. E. "A Prospective Study of Laryngotracheal Sequelae in Long-Term Intubation." *Laryngoscope*, Vol. 94, 1984, pp. 367-377.

Zaidi, N. H., H. A. Smith, S. C. King, C. Park, P. A. O'Neill, and M. J. Connolly. "Oxygen Desaturation on Swallowing as a Potential Marker of Aspiration in Acute Stroke." *Age and Ageing*, Vol. 24, 1995, pp. 267-270.

Chapter 10

American Speech-Language-Hearing Association. *National Outcomes Measuring Systems, Adult Speech-Language Pathology Component*, 1998.

Bartolome, G. and S. Neumann. "Swallowing Therapy in Patients with Neurological Disorders Causing Cricopharyngeal Dysphagia." *Dysphagia*, Vol. 8, 1993, pp. 146-149.

Bourel-Marchasson, I., F. Dumas, G. Pinganaud, J. P. Emeriau, and A. Decamps. "Audit of Percutaneous Endoscopic Gastrostomy in Long-Term Enternal Feeding in a Nursing Home." *International Journal for Quality in Health Care*, Vol. 9, No. 4, 1997, pp. 297-302.

Chouninard, J., E. Lavigne, and C. Villeneuve. "Weight Loss, Dysphagia, and Outcome in Advanced Dementia." *Dysphagia*, Vol. 13, No. 3, 1998, pp. 151-155.

Cowen, M. E., S. L. Simpson, and T. E. Vettese. "Survival Estimates for Patients with Abnormal Swallowing Studies." *Journal of General Internal Medicine*, Vol. 12, No. 2, 1997, pp. 88-94.

Crary, M. A. "A Direct Intervention Program for Chronic Neurogenic Dysphagia Secondary to Brainstem Stroke." *Dysphagia*, Vol. 10, No. 1, 1995, pp. 6-18.

Croghan, J. E., E. M. Burke, S. Caplan, and S. Denman. "Pilot Study of 12-month Outcomes of Nursing Home Patients with Aspiration on Videofluoroscopy." *Dysphagia*, Vol. 9, No. 3, 1994, pp. 141-146.

Davalos, A., W. Ricart, F. Gonzalez-Huix, S. Soler, J. Marrugat, A. Molins, R. Suner, and D. Genis. "Effect of Malnutrition After Acute Stroke on Clinical Outcome." *Stroke*, Vol. 27, No. 6, 1996, pp. 1028-1032.

Dejonckere, P. H. and G. J. Hordijk. "Prognostic Factors for Swallowing After Treatment of Head and Neck Cancer." *Clinical Otolaryngology*, Vol. 23, 1998, pp. 218-223.

Elmståhl, S., M. Bülow, O. Ekberg, M. Petersson, and H. Tegner. "Treatment of Dysphagia Improves Nutritional Conditions in Stroke Patients." *Dysphagia*, Vol. 14, No. 2, 1999, pp. 61-66.

Finestone, H. M., L. S. Greene-Finestone, E. S. Wilson, and R. W. Teasell. "Prolonged Length of Stay and Reduced Functional Improvement Rate in Malnourished Stroke Rehabilitation Patients." *Archives of Physical Medicine and Rehabilitation*, Vol. 77, 1996, pp. 340-345.

Finucane, T. E. and J. P. Bynum. "Use of Tube Feeding to Prevent Aspiration Pneumonia." *The Lancet*, Vol. 348, 1996, pp. 1421-1424.

Fonda, D., J. Schwarz, and S. Clinnick. "Parkinson Medication One Hour Before Meals Improves Symptomatic Swallowing: A Case Study." *Dysphagia*, Vol. 10, 1995, pp. 165-166.

Frattali, C. M. *Measuring Outcomes in Speech-Language Pathology*. New York: Theime Medical Publishers, Inc., 1998.

Garon, B. R., M. Engle, and C. Ormiston. "A Randomized Control Study to Determine the Effects of Unlimited Oral Intake of Water in Patients with Identified Aspiration." *Journal of Neurological Rehabilitation*, Vol. 11, 1997, pp. 139-148.

Gisel, E. G., T. Applegate-Ferrante, J. Benson, and J. F. Bosma. "Oral-Motor Skills Following Sensorimotor Therapy in Two Groups of Moderately Dysphagic Children with Cerebral Palsy: Aspiration vs. Nonaspiration." *Dysphagia*, Vol. 11, No. 1, 1966, pp. 59-71.

Gisel, E. G. "Oral-Motor Skills Following Sensorimotor Intervention in the Moderately Eating-Impaired Child with Cerebral Palsy." *Dysphagia*, Vol. 9, 1994, pp. 180-192.

Gisel, E. G. and E. Alphonce. "Classification of Eating Impairments Based on Eating Efficiency in Children with Cerebral Palsy." *Dysphagia*, Vol. 10, No. 4, 1995, pp. 268-274.

Groher, M. E. "Ethical Dilemmas in Providing Nutrition." *Dysphagia*, Vol. 5, 1998, pp. 102-109.

Groher, M. E. and T. N. McKaig. "Dysphagia and Dietary Levels in Skilled Nursing Facilities." *Journal of American Geriatrics Society*, Vol. 43, 1995, pp. 528-532.

Gross, C. R., R. D. Lindquist, A. C. Woolley, R. Granieri, K. Allard, and B. Webster. "Clinical Indicators of Dehydration Severity in Elderly Patients." *Journal of Emergency Medicine*, Vol. 10, 1992, pp. 267-274.

Gustafsson, B., L. M. Tibbling, and T. Theorell. "Do Physicians Care About Patients with Dysphagia? A Study on Confirming Communication." *Family Practice*, Vol. 9, No. 2, 1992, pp. 203-209.

Hillel, A. E., R. M. Miller, K. Yorkston, E. McDonald, F. H. Norris, and N. Konikow. "Amyotrophic Lateral Sclerosis Severity Scale." *Neuroepidemiology*, Vol. 8, 1989, pp. 142-150.

Holas, M. A., K. L. DePippo, and M. J. Reding. "Aspiration and Relative Risk of Medical Complications Following Stroke." *Archives of Neurology*, Vol. 51, 1994, pp. 1051-1053.

Horner, J., F. G. Buoyer, M. J. Alberts, and M. J. Helms. "Dysphagia Following Brainstem Stroke: Clinical Correlates and Outcome." *Archives of Neurology*, Vol. 48, 1991, pp. 1170-1173.

Horner, J., E. W. Massey, J. E. Riski, M. A. Lathrop, and K. N. Chase. "Aspiration Following Stroke: Clinical Correlates and Outcome." *Neurology*, Vol. 38, 1988, p. 1359.

Kaatze-McDonald, M. N., E. Post, and P. J. Davis. "The Effects of Cold, Touch, and Chemical Stimulation of the Anterior Faucial Pillar on Human Swallowing." *Dysphagia*, Vol. 11, 1996, pp. 198-206.

Kasprisin, A. T., H. Clumeck, and M. Nino-Murcia. "Letters to the Editor — Response to Kasprisin et al.: The Efficacy of Rehabilitative Management of Dysphagia." *Dysphagia*, Vol. 6, 1990, pp. 166-168.

Kasprisin, A. T., H. Clumeck, and M. Nino-Murcia. "The Efficacy of Rehabilitative Management of Dysphagia." *Dysphagia*, Vol. 4, 1989, pp. 48-52.

Kaw, M. and G. Sekas. "Long-term Follow-up of Consequences of Percutaneous Endoscopic Gastrostomy (PEG) Tubes in Nursing Home Patients." *Digestive Diseases and Sciences*, Vol. 39, 1994, pp. 738-743.

Keller, H. H. "Malnutrition in Institutionalized Elderly: How and Why?" *Journal of the American Geriatrics Society*, Vol. 41, No. 11, 1993, pp. 1212-1218.

Keller, H. H. "Weight Gain Impacts Morbidity and Morality in Institutionalized Older Persons." *Journal of the American Geriatrics Society*, Vol. 43, No. 2, 1995, pp. 165-169.

Langmore, S. E. "Efficacy of Behavioral Treatment for Oropharyngeal Dysphagia." *Dysphagia*, Vol. 10, 1995, pp. 259-262.

Langmore, S. E. "Managing the Complications of Aspiration in Dysphagic Adults." *Seminars in Speech and Language*, Vol. 12, No. 3, 1991, pp. 199-207.

Langmore, S. E., M. S. Terpenning, A. Schork, Y. Chen, J. T. Murray, D. Lopatin, and W. J. Loesche. "Predictors of Aspiration Pneumonia: How Important is Dysphagia?" *Dysphagia*, Vol. 13, No. 2, 1998, pp. 69-81.

Lavizzo-Mourey, R. J. "Dehydration in the Elderly: A Short Review." *Journal of the National Medical Association*, Vol. 79, No. 10, 1987, pp. 1933-1938.

Lazarus, C. L. "Editorial: Comments on the Effects of Cold, Touch, and Chemical Stimulation of the Anterior Faucial Pillar on Human Swallowing." *Dysphagia*, Vol. 11, 1996, pp. 207-208.

Lazzara, G. L., C. Lazarus, and J. A. Logemann. "Impact of Thermal Stimulation on the Triggering of the Swallowing Reflex." *Dysphagia*, Vol. 1, 1986, pp. 73-77.

List, M. A., C. Ritter-Sterr, and S. B. Lanksy. "A Performance Status Scale for Head and Neck Cancer Patients." *Cancer*, Vol. 66, 1990, pp. 564-569.

Logemann, J. A. "Criteria for Studies of Treatment for Oral-Pharyngeal Dysphagia." *Dysphagia*, Vol. 1, 1987, pp. 193-199.

Logemann, J. A., P. Kahrilas, M. Kobara, and N. Vakil. "The Benefit of Head Rotation on Pharyngoesophageal Dysphagia." *Archives of Physical Medicine and Rehabilitation*, Vol. 70, 1989, pp. 767-771.

Logemann, J. A., B. R. Pauloski, A. W. Rademaker, F. M. S. McConnell, M. A. Heiser, S. Cardinale, D. Shedd, J. Lewin, S. R. Baker, D. Graner, B. Cook, F. Milianti, S. Collins, and T. Baker. "Speech and Swallowing Function After Anterior Tongue and Floor of Mouth Resection With Distal Flap Reconstruction." *Journal of Speech and Hearing Research*, Vol. 36, 1993, pp. 267-276.

Logemann, J. A., B. R. Pauloski, A. W. Rademaker, F. M. S. McConnell, M. A. Heiser, S. Cardinale, D. Shedd, D. Stein, Q. Beery, J. Johnson, and T. Baker. "Speech and Swallow Function After Tonsil/Base of Tongue Resection With Primary Closure." *Journal of Speech and Hearing Research*, Vol. 36, 1993, pp. 918-926.

Logemann, J. A., S. Veis, and L. Colangelo. "A Screening Procedure for Oropharyngeal Dysphagia." *Dysphagia*, Vol. 14, 1999, pp. 44-51.

Martin, B. J. W., M. M. Corlew, H. Wood, D. Olson, L. A. Golopol, M. Wingo, and N. Kirmani. "The Association of Swallowing Dysfunction and Aspiration Pneumonia." *Dysphagia*, Vol. 9, 1994, pp. 1-6.

McHorney, C. A. and J. C. Rosenbek. "Functional Outcome Assessment of Adults with Oropharyngeal Dysphagia." *Seminars in Speech and Language*, Vol. 19, No. 3, 1998, pp. 235-247.

Miller, R. M. and S. E. Langmore. "Treatment Efficacy for Adults with Oropharyngeal Dysphagia." *Archives of Physical Medicine and Rehabilitation*, Vol. 75, 1995, pp. 1256-1262.

Moore, M. "Clinical Trials Research Group Begins Open Protocols." *ASHA Leader*, Vol. 2, No. 14, 1997.

Murray, J., S. E. Langmore, S. Ginsberg, and A. Dostie. "The Significance of Accumulated Oropharyngeal Secretions and Swallowing Frequency in Predicting Aspiration." *Dysphagia*, Vol. 11, No. 2, 1996, pp. 99-103.

Nelson, K. J., A. M. Coulston, K. P. Sucher, and R. Y. Tseng. "Prevalence of Malnutrition in the Elderly Admitted to Long-term Care Facilities." *Journal of the American Dietetic Association*, Vol. 93, No. 4, 1993, pp. 459-461.

Neumann, S. "Swallowing Therapy with Neurologic Patients: Results of Direct and Indirect Therapy Methods in 66 Patients Suffering from Neurological Disorders." *Dysphagia*, Vol. 8, 1993, pp. 150-153.

Odderson, I. R., J. C. Keaton, and B. S. McKenna. "Swallow Management in Patients on an Acute Stroke Pathway: Quality is Cost Effective." *Archives of Physical Medicine and Rehabilitation*, Vol. 76, 1995, pp. 1130-1133.

O'Neil, K. H., M. Purdy, J. Falk, and L. Gallo. "The Dysphagia Outcome and Severity Scale." *Dysphagia*, Vol. 14, No. 3, 1999, pp. 139-145.

Peck, A., C. E. Cohen, and M. N. Mulvihill. "Long-Term Enteral Feeding of Aged Demented Nursing Home Patients." *Journal of American Geriatrics Society*, Vol. 38, 1990, pp. 1195-1198.

Rademaker, A. W., J. A. Logemann, B. R. Pauloski, J. B. Bowman, C. L. Lazarus, G. A. Sisson, F. J. Milianti, D. Graner, B. S. Cook, S. L. Collins, D. W. Stein, Q. C. Beery, J. T. Johnson, and T. M. Baker. "Recovery of Postoperative Swallowing in Patients Undergoing Partial Laryngectomy." *Head & Neck*, 1993, pp. 325-334.

Robbins, J., J. W. Hamilton, and G. B. Kempster. "Oropharyngeal Swallowing in Normal Adults of Different Ages." *Gastroenterology*, Vol. 103, 1992, p. 829.

Rosenbek, J. C. "Efficacy in Dysphagia." *Dysphagia*, Vol. 10, 1995, pp. 263-267.

Rosenbek, J. C., J. Robbins, B. Fishback, and R. L. Levine. "Effects of Thermal Application on Dysphagia After Stroke." *Journal of Speech and Hearing Research*, Vol. 34, 1991, pp. 1257-1268.

Rosenbek, J .C., J. Robbins, W. Willford, G. Kirk, A. Schitz, T. W. Sowell, S. E. Deutsch, F. J. Milanti, J. Ashford, G. D. Gramigna, A. Fogarty, K. Dong, M. T. Rau, T. E. Prescott, A. M. Lloyd, M. T. Sterkel, and J. E. Hansen. "Comparing Treatment Intensities of Tactile-Thermal Application." *Dysphagia*, Vol. 13, 1998, pp. 1-9.

Rosenbek, J. C., E. B. Roecker, J. L. Wood, and J. Robbins. "Thermal Application Reduces the Duration of Stage Transition in Dysphagia After Stroke." *Dysphagia*, Vol. 11, pp. 225-233.

Salassa, J. R. "A Functional Outcome Swallowing Scale (FOSS) for Staging Dysphagia." Paper presented at the 39th Meeting of the American Society for Head and Neck Surgery, Scottsdale, AZ, 1997.

Schmidt, J., M. Holas, K. Halvorson, and M. Reding. "Videofluoroscopy Evidence of Aspiration Predicts Pneumonia and Death But Not Dehydration Following Stroke." *Dysphagia*, Vol. 9, 1994, pp. 7-11.

Silbergeit, A., B. Jacobson, and T. Sumlin. *Dysphagia Disability Index*. In development.

Smithard, D. G., P. A. O'Neill, C. Park, J. Morris, R. Wyatt, R. England, and D. F. Martin. "Complications and Outcome After Acute Stroke." *Stroke*, Vol. 27, No. 7, 1996, pp. 1200-1204.

Splaingard, M. L., B. Hutchins, L. D. Sulton, and G. Chaudhuri. "Aspiration in Rehabilitation Patients: Videofluoroscopy vs. Bedside Clinical Assessment." *Archives of Physical Medicine and Rehabilitation*, Vol. 69, 1988, pp. 637-641.

Strand, E. A., R. M. Miller, K. M. Yorkston, and A. D. Hillel. "Management of Oral-Pharyngeal Dysphagia Symptoms in Amyotrophic Lateral Sclerosis." *Dysphagia*, Vol. 11, No. 2, 1996, pp. 129-139.

Swigert, N. "Functional Outcomes and Dysphagia Management." In B. Cornett (ed.). *Clinical Practice Management in Speech-Language Pathology*. Gaithersburg, MD: Aspen Publishers, 1999.

Teichgraeber, J., J. Bowman, and H. Goepfert. "New Test Series for the Functional Evaluation of Oral Cavity Cancer." *Head and Neck Surgery*, Vol. 8, No. 1, 1985, pp. 9-20.

Unossom, M., A. C. Ek, P. Bjurulf, H. vonSchenck, and J. Larsson. "Feeding Dependence and Nutritional Status After Acute Stroke." *Stroke*, Vol. 25, 1994, pp. 366-371.

Welch, M. A., J. A. Logemann, A. W. Rademaker, and P. J. Kahrilas. "Changes in Pharyngeal Dimensions Effected by Chin Tuck." *Archives of Physical Medicine and Rehabilitation*, Vol. 74, 1993, pp. 178-181.

Winstein, C. J. "Neurogenic Dysphagia: Frequency, Progression, and Outcome in Adults Following Head Injury." *Physical Therapy*, Vol. 63, 1983, pp. 1992-1997.

Yorkston, K. M., E. Strand, R. Miller, A. Hillel, and K. Smith. "Speech Deterioration in Amyotrophic Lateral Sclerosis: Implications for the Timing of Intervention." *Journal of Medical Speech-Language Pathology*, Vol. 1, No. 1, 1993, pp. 35-46.

26-05-987